INDUSTRIAL FIRST AID

A REFERENCE AND TRAINING MANUAL

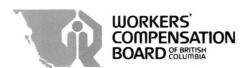

WORKERS' COMPENSATION BOARD OF BRITISH COLUMBIA

Canadian Cataloguing in Publication Data
Main entry under title:
Industrial first aid

   Includes index.
   Edited by Ronald L. Hazelton . . . et al. Cf. pref.
material.
   ISBN 0-7718-9153-9

   1. First aid in illness and injury – Handbooks,
manuals, etc. 2. Medical emergencies – Handbooks,
manuals, etc. 3. Medicine, Industrial – Handbooks,
manuals, etc. I. Hazelton, Ronald L. II. Workers'
Compensation Board of British Columbia.

RC88.9.I5I52 1992   616.02'52   C92-092053-5

**DECEMBER
1994**

Printed on recycled paper

Preface

The role of the Workers' Compensation Board in industrial first aid is to ensure that the standards of training in British Columbia are maintained at a high level and that Industrial First Aid Attendants are appropriately certified.

This manual is an essential part of the program offered by industrial first aid training agencies in the province. We know that the course can be demanding; however, we believe that workers have a right to expect the highest professional level of care from Attendants who may be called upon to assist them. First Aid Attendants in British Columbia have an outstanding reputation for the high level of service they provide to our work force.

Since the original manual was produced in 1969, procedures have been standardized and improved significantly for emergency pre-hospital care. This manual reflects the most current medical thinking in the field of first aid, to ensure a consistent approach among pre-hospital care workers and a smooth transition of care through each stage of the emergency setting.

We have drawn on numerous sources and have received input from many individuals and organizations. The result is a comprehensive training and reference resource that offers the student — and graduate — the information necessary to understand the principles of emergency care and how to provide the best possible assistance to the injured worker.

Editorial Advisory Committee

Acknowledgements

The Workers' Compensation Board expresses appreciation for the valuable contribution of the Editorial Advisory Committee Authors during the preparation of this publication. The committee members are grateful for the assistance of Nicole Hansford, Secretary and Glenda Troup, Word Processing Operator. Special mention is given to our Editor, Brenda Whittingham, Manager, Editorial Services, WCB Community Relations.

Other people and organizations who have generously contributed time and information to this book include:

Association of B.C. Optometrists

B.C. Ambulance Service

B.C. Drug and Alcohol Commission, Try Program

B.C. Ministry of Health, B.C. Centre for Disease Control

B.C. and Yukon Heart Foundation

Michael Bright, M.D., F.R.C.S., Ophthalmologist

Elaine R. Drysdale, M.D., F.R.C.P.(C); Psychiatrist, Vancouver General Hospital Psychiatry Consultant Liaison Service; Staff Psychiatrist, Burnaby Mental Health Unit and Shaughnessy Hospital

Emergency Health Services Academy, Justice Institute of British Columbia

Fleck Bros.

Fletcher Challenge Canada Ltd., Pitt Lake Division

Sue Greer, R.N.

Brian M. Hunt, M.D., F.R.C.S.(C), F.A.C.S.; Neurosurgeon, Lions Gate Hospital; Recent Past Director of Acute Trauma Life Support Programs for B.C.

Michael Lepawsky, B.A., M.D., C.C.F.P.(C); Medical Director, Vancouver General Hospital Hyperbaric Unit; Senior Consultant in Hyperbaric Medicine, Vancouver General Hospital; Hyperbaric Medical Consultant, Workers' Compensation Board of B.C.

Safety Supply Canada

Charles Snelling, M.D., F.R.C.S.(C); Division of Plastic Surgery, Vancouver General Hospital

Brenda St. Pierre, R.N.

S.O.S. Emergency Response Technologies

G.A. Willis, B.C. Drug and Information Centre

U.S. Department of Health and Human Services, Public Health Service Centre for Disease Control

Table of Contents

PART VI   HEAD AND NERVOUS SYSTEM

PART VII   FACIAL TRAUMA

Part I
Introduction to Industrial First Aid

THE PURPOSE OF THE INDUSTRIAL FIRST AID ATTENDANT IN INDUSTRY

Attendants perform a unique service in industry. They are in the position to alleviate suffering and on occasion save lives through their skills at an accident scene. Effective injury management can often shorten the healing time of the injury, allowing the worker to resume normal activities sooner.

Although many injuries are reported to the Workers' Compensation Board of British Columbia (WCB) each year, those do not include injuries that only needed first aid treatment. The ratio of first aid treatments to reportable injuries is about thirty to one. This indicates that over six million first aid treatments are given each year by Industrial First Aid Attendants.

QUALITIES OF THE INDUSTRIAL FIRST AID ATTENDANT

Attendants must perform their duties to the best of their ability. It is equally important that they recognize their own limitations.

A pleasant personality and a calm, cool attitude under stress are important for good patient care. A gentle but authoritative approach is desirable. That will allay anxiety in the patient and will expedite assessment and treatment.

AUTHORITY OF THE INDUSTRIAL FIRST AID ATTENDANT

The Attendant must be in complete charge of all first aid treatment of injured workers. Decisions of First Aid Attendants relating to first aid and the need for medical attention shall not be overruled by supervisory personnel. However, the decision to send the worker home lies with the attending physician or with the employer.

When the Attendant believes that a worker should be transported to a hospital, then — unless the worker objects — the person must be transported to the nearest hospital or physician. If the Attendant thinks it necessary to accompany the injured worker during transportation (e.g. the patient requires a stretcher for transport), he or she should do so. The patient is the responsibility of the Attendant until becoming the responsibility of pre-hospital emergency medical personnel or hospital staff.

The WCB First Aid Regulations strengthen the position of the Industrial First Aid Attendant in times of emergency by giving formal authority. Usually, the Attendant need not invoke this authority if a firm but courteous manner is used where patient welfare is concerned.

WORKERS' COMPENSATION ACT

The *Workers' Compensation Act* of British Columbia (Section 70[1]) states *Employers in any industry in which it is deemed proper may be required to install and maintain such first aid equipment and service as the Board may by order or regulation direct. Where an employer fails, neglects, or refuses to install or maintain the first aid equipment and service, the Board may:*

a) *Install the first aid equipment and service and charge the cost thereof to the employer; and the Board may enforce payment thereof, and for that purpose has the same powers and is entitled to the same remedies for enforcing payment as it possesses or is entitled to in respect of assessments.*

b) *Impose a special rate of assessment.*

c) *Order the employer to close down forthwith the whole or any part of the employment or place of employment and the industry carried on therein.*

INDUSTRIAL FIRST AID REGULATIONS

Under the First Aid Regulations passed by the Board pursuant to the Act, employers must provide and maintain first aid equipment and services suitable to the hazards of the work project, its remoteness and number of employees on the job. The regulations also make the employer responsible for providing suitable care and transportation of injured workers from the scene of the accident to the nearest hospital, physician, or qualified practitioner for initial treatment. Suitably equipped vehicles to serve as ambulances must be maintained where deemed necessary by the Board. Other regulations deal with location and layout of suitable first aid rooms. These are only highlights, and the Attendant must become familiar with all the First Aid Regulations.

LEGAL ASPECTS OF FIRST AID

Under the *Workers' Compensation Act,* a worker who is accidentally injured by another worker is barred from suing that other worker for those injuries where both were in the course and scope of employment at the time of the injury. This means that a First Aid Attendant who renders

first aid services to a worker as part of his or her employment duties will be protected from liability for inadvertent
injury caused by some negligent act or omission.

A First Aid Attendant who, in British Columbia, provides first aid services to an injured fellow worker or
renders emergency aid to a non-worker will seldom, if
ever, have to be concerned about legal liability for ordinary negligent acts or omissions that result in additional
injury or even death.

A First Aid Attendant does not have the protection of
the *Good Samaritan Act* when rendering first aid services
to a fellow worker as part of his or her employment
duties. That protection is excluded by Section 2(a) of the
Act. In those circumstances, however, Section 10(1) of
the *Workers' Compensation Act* provides equivalent protection from liability.

In the case of emergency aid to non-workers, the *Good
Samaritan Act* of British Columbia provides protection to
persons who in good faith render aid. This short and
clearly worded Act reads as follows:

GOOD SAMARITAN ACT

CHAPTER 155

**NO LIABILITY FOR EMERGENCY AID UNLESS
GROSS NEGLIGENCE**

1. A person who renders emergency medical services
   or aid to an ill, injured or unconscious person at the
   immediate scene of an accident or emergency that has
   caused the illness, injury or unconsciousness is not
   liable for damages for injury to or death of that person
   caused by his act or omission in rendering the medical
   services or aid unless he is grossly negligent.

EXCEPTIONS

2. Section 1 does not apply where the person rendering
   the medical services or aid
   (a) is employed expressly for that purpose; or
   (b) does so with a view to gain.

For gross negligence to apply, a person would have to
be reckless or wantonly indifferent to the results likely to
follow from his actions.

Part II
Basic Anatomy

The human body is a complex structure uniquely suited to survival in our environment. In order to provide first aid, the Attendant must have a basic understanding of human anatomy and function.

CELLS, TISSUES AND ORGANS

The basic unit of life is the **cell**. A bacterium is an organism composed of only one cell. The human body is made up of billions of cells.

In the course of growth and development, cells become specialized and are organized into **tissues.** Tissues are groups of cells with similar functions. For example, mus-

cle cells are grouped together to form the various muscles of the body. Connective tissue is made up of various cells that give structural support to the different parts of the body.

Organs are composed of different tissues that are structurally organized to perform a single function. The heart, for example, is composed primarily of specialized muscle tissue and connective tissue.

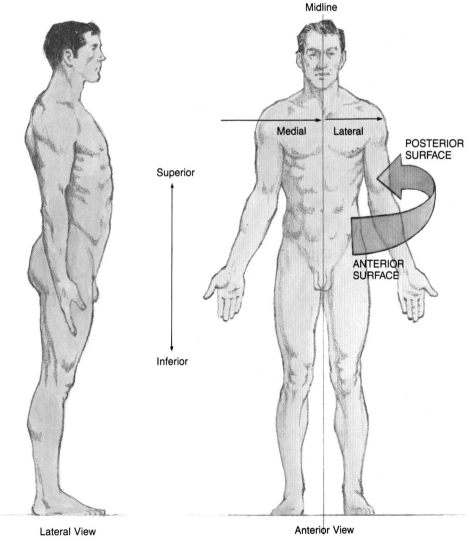

Figure II-1 Anatomical Position

SYSTEMS

The organs and tissues of the body are also organized into specific systems that perform all the major functions of the body. These are the major systems of the body:

- **The Respiratory System** is responsible for the intake of oxygen, an essential nutrient, and the elimination of carbon dioxide, a waste product.
- **The Circulatory System (Cardiovascular System)** is the transportation system of the body. It delivers oxygen, glucose and other essential nutrients to the tissues and carries away waste products.
- **The Nervous System** is the control centre and network that coordinates all the systems of the body. It allows us to interpret and respond to our environment.
- **The Digestive System** is made up of the stomach, intestines and other internal organs required to process the food that we ingest.
- **The Urinary System** is made up of the kidneys, ureters and bladder. It is responsible for filtering the blood and excreting most of the body's waste products.
- **The Genital System** is made up of the reproductive organs.
- **The Musculoskeletal System** is composed of the bones that provide the body's framework and all the body's muscles, tendons and ligaments.

ANATOMICAL LANGUAGE

Anatomy is the study of the structure and composition of the human body. The surface of the body has many specific visible features or landmarks that serve as guides to the underlying tissues and organs. SURFACE ANATOMY is the identification and recognition of those landmarks.

Visual inspection of the human body is of utmost importance for the provision of first aid. Much information regarding the extent of injury or illness is obtained through visual inspection. Therefore, the IFA Attendant must have adequate knowledge of surface anatomy in order to identify and communicate the patient's physical findings.

Physical findings are usually described in terms of their location relative to specific points or landmarks. In order to communicate properly with ambulance attendants, nurses and physicians, Attendants must learn the "language" of surface anatomy. For example, a laceration may be located two inches above the elbow on the inner aspect of the arm. As the Attendant will learn, this is best described as being "proximal" to the elbow and located on its "medial" aspect.

The anatomical position is the reference position for the human body (see Figure II-1). The terms used to describe surface anatomy are all based on the anatomical position. As shown, the anatomical position is the erect human body facing the examiner. Left and right refer to the patient's left and right, not the Attendant's left and right.

An imaginary vertical line drawn from the top of the head through the nose and the navel (belly button) is called the midline. It divides the body into two halves, right and left. All points further from the midline are referred to as lateral structures; those closer to the midline are called medial structures. For example, the shoulder lies on the lateral aspect of the trunk. The inner and outer corners of the eye are referred to as the medial and lateral corners of the eye.

The terms lateral, medial, superior and inferior are also used to describe various points in relation to specific landmarks. Lateral means away from the midline. Medial means towards the midline. Superior means above or towards the head. Inferior means below or towards the feet. For example, the head is superior to the chest but the abdomen is inferior to the chest. Figure II-2 shows a wound located on the face. It is described as lateral to the nose but medial to the earlobe. It is inferior to the eye but superior to the mouth.

The anterior surface refers to the front part of the body, i.e. the part that faces the examiner. For example, the face is on the anterior surface. The posterior surface refers to that aspect of the body that faces away from the examiner. The back is located on the posterior surface.

Because of the structure of the limbs, specific anatomical terms have been devised to describe their surface anatomy. Referring to Figure II-1, the Attendant should note that in the anatomical position the arms are maintained with the palms facing forward. Therefore, the palm of the hand is anterior. The back of the hand is posterior. Similarly, the legs are positioned with the toes pointing forward. Therefore, the knee cap (patella) is on the anterior suface. The Achillles tendon connected to the heel is posterior.

When describing landmarks on the limbs, proximal means towards the trunk and distal means away from the trunk. For example, the radial pulse at the wrist is distal to the elbow but proximal to the thumb. Similarly, the ankle is distal to the knee but proximal to the foot. The key anatomical terms are listed in Table II-a.

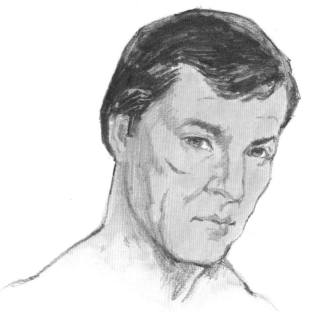

Figure II-2 Wound Location

TABLE II-a

Trunk — the torso of the body including the chest, abdomen and pelvis. The head and neck, arms and legs are all attached to the trunk.

Supine — the patient is lying down on his or her back.

Prone — the patient is lying down on the stomach.

Erect — the patient is standing upright.

Anterior — in front. The front of the body is the anterior surface.

Posterior — in back, behind. The back of the body is the posterior surface.

Midline — the imaginary line through the nose and the navel dividing the body into left and right halves.

Superior — above or closer to the head. Not used for points on a limb.

Inferior — below or closer to the feet. Not used for points on a limb.

Medial — closer to the midline.

Lateral — the side of the body, away from the midline.

Proximal — towards the trunk. Only used with respect to specific points on a limb.

Distal — away from the trunk. Only used with respect to specific points on a limb.

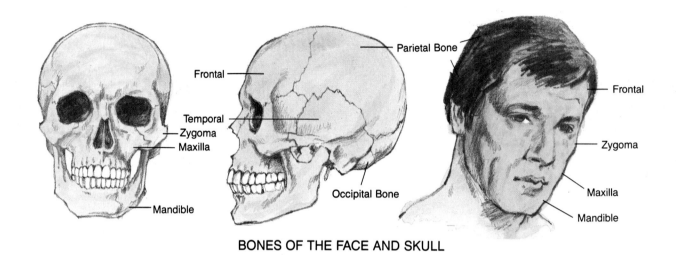

BONES OF THE FACE AND SKULL

ANATOMY

Head and Neck

The bones of the skull resemble a series of bony plates that are fused together to form the cranial cavity. The brain is encased within the cranial cavity.

The primary facial bones are the mandible (lower jaw), the maxilla (upper jaw), the zygoma (cheek bone), the bones of the orbit and the nasal bones. The lower jaw (mandible) is connected to the skull at a point just anterior to the ear. The action of opening and closing the mouth can be felt at this joint. The lower teeth are set into the mandible. The upper jaw is called the maxilla and is relatively fixed. The upper teeth are set into the maxilla. The hard palate, located in the roof of the mouth, is part of the maxilla.

The nose is only partially formed of bone — at the bridge of the nose. The remainder is made up of cartilage.

The eyes are set into the bony orbits which protect them. The zygoma (cheek bone) forms part of the network of orbital bones.

The neck contains many vital structures, including the airway, trachea, esophagus and carotid arteries. Figures II-3 and II-4 show lateral and anterior views of the neck. The Attendant should feel the thyroid cartilage, commonly known as the Adam's Apple. The thyroid cartilage forms part of the structural framework for the larynx or voice box. Inferior to the thyroid cartilage, the Attendant is able to palpate the rings of the trachea. Lateral to the trachea but medial to the sternomastoid muscles, the Attendant should palpate the pulse of the carotid artery. Posteriorly, the Attendant should palpate the bones of the cervical vertebrae. The most prominent vertebra is the seventh cervical vertebra.

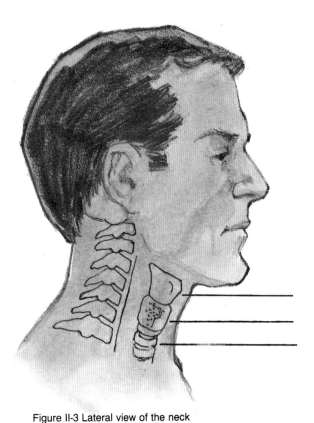

Thyroid Cartilage

Cricoid Cartilage

Tracheal Rings

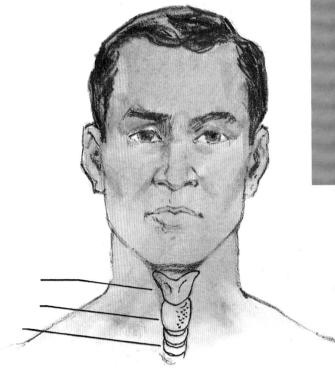

Figure II-3 Lateral view of the neck

Figure II-4 Anterior view of the neck

Thorax

The thorax (chest) contains the heart, lungs, esophagus and the great vessels, all within the thoracic cavity. The thoracic cavity is formed posteriorly by the 12 thoracic vertebrae. Twelve pairs of ribs wrap around from the thoracic vertebrae. The first seven connect anteriorly to the sternum (breast bone). Superiorly lie the clavicles (collar bones), which connect the shoulder to the sternum. Posteriorly are the scapulae (shoulder blades). Inferiorly, the thoracic cavity is separated from the abdominal cavity by the diaphragm (see Figure II-6). The superior end of the sternum forms a notch which may be palpated (the suprasternal notch). Inferiorly, the sternum ends with a narrow projection called the xiphoid process. The xiphoid process is an important landmark for the application of closed chest massage (CPR) and abdominal thrusts (Heimlich manoeuvre).

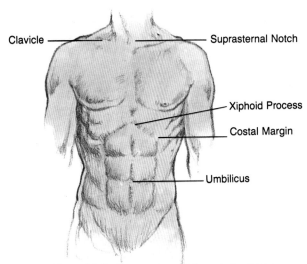

Clavicle

Suprasternal Notch

Xiphoid Process

Costal Margin

Umbilicus

Figure II-5 Surface anatomy of the anterior thorax

The inferior border of the ribs may be palpated anteriorly as the costal margin. The free ends of the 11th and 12th ribs may be palpated in the soft tissue on the lateral aspect of the trunk. The vital structures within the thoracic cavity are outlined in Figure II-6.

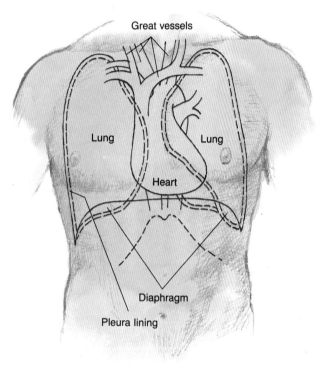

Figure II-6 Anatomy of the thorax

The Abdomen

The abdomen contains the organs of the digestive system, the spleen and the urinary-reproductive systems, as well as the aorta and its major branches. The abdomen is bounded superiorly by the diaphragm and inferiorly by the pelvis. Posteriorly, the lumbar vertebrae give structural support, but the back, flanks and anterior abdominal wall are all composed of muscle and connective tissue. The abdominal cavity is contained within the abdomen and contains most of the digestive organs, the liver, the spleen and the female reproductive organs. The pancreas, kidneys, bladder, parts of the large intestine and the major blood vessels are all located posteriorly to the abdominal cavity, embedded in the soft tissue of the back, flank and pelvis respectively.

The anterior surface of the abdominal cavity is divided into four quarters or quadrants by the midline and a horizontal line through the navel. Location of injuries or complaints of abdominal pain are identified by their relationship to these quadrants. The superior borders of the quadrants are the costal margins on both sides. The inferior borders are the inguinal ligaments that connect the anterior, superior iliac spines and the symphysis pubis.

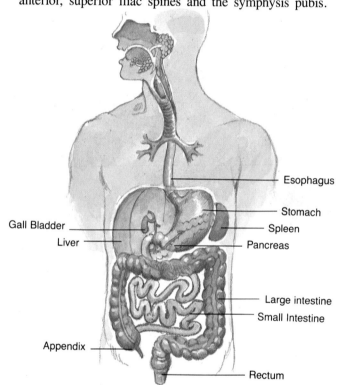

Figure II-7 Abdominal organs

Figure II-7 illustrates the anatomical relationship of the abdominal organs to the anterior abdominal wall. Pain or injury to a specific quadrant of the abdomen usually arises from or involves the organs located in that particular quadrant. Therefore, liver injury must be suspected with right upper quadrant trauma. Similarly, fractures of the left lower ribs may be associated with rupture of the spleen because of its location. The appendix is a small tubular structure attached to the cecum which is the first part of the large intestine or colon. Inflammation of the appendix is called appendicitis and because of its location usually presents with pain in the right lower quadrant.

The femoral arteries are palpable on both sides lateral to the symphysis pubis and inferior to the inguinal ligament.

Posteriorly, the surface of the back is not divided into quadrants. The area adjacent to the vertebral column on both sides is called the paraspinal region. Superiorly, the 12th rib forms the upper boundary. Inferiorly, the sacrum and iliac crests are palpable. The kidneys are located in the angles between the 12th rib and the vertebral column (see Figure II-8).

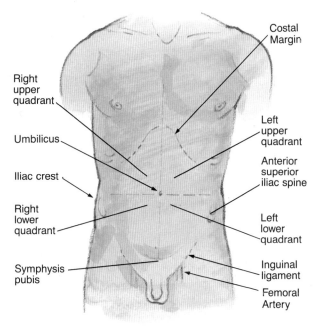

Surface anatomy of the abdomen

The Upper Extremity

The upper extremity includes the shoulders, the upper arm, the elbow, the forearm, the wrist and the hand. The shoulder is a complex structure. The shoulder girdle is composed of the bony structures that make up the shoulder. It consists of the clavicle (collar bone) located anteriorly, the scapula (shoulder blade) located posteriorly and the proximal end of the humerus (the bone of the upper arm). The clavicle is connected to a bony process of the scapula called the acromion at the acromioclavicular joint (A-C joint). This is palpable as a bony prominence on the superior aspect of the shoulder.

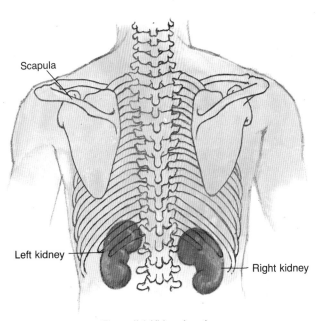

Figure II-8 Kidney location

The supporting bone of the upper arm, as previously mentioned, is the humerus. The proximal end of the humerus forms the shoulder joint with the scapula. The distal end joins with the radius and ulna (the supporting bones of the forearm) to form the elbow. The bony processes of the distal humerus are palpable on the medial and lateral aspects of the elbow. The posterior aspect of the elbow is the olecranon process, which forms the proximal end of the ulna. The ulna may be palpated along its entire course just beneath the skin on the posterior aspect of the forearm. A brachial pulse may be palpated on the anteromedial aspect of the elbow. Changes in the brachial pulse

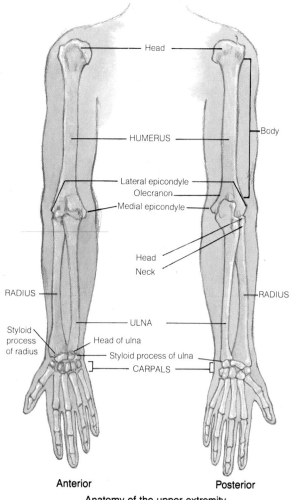

Anterior   Posterior
Anatomy of the upper extremity

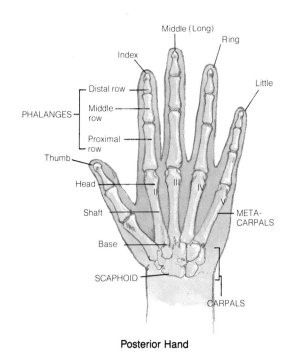

Posterior Hand

from inflation and deflation of the blood pressure cuff are recorded as the patient's blood pressure.

The two bones of the forearm, the radius and the ulna end at the wrist. The two bones of the forearm permit rotation of the hand. The wrist is a complicated joint by virtue of the complex movements that it performs. It has eight small bones arranged in two rows of four that connect the radius and ulna to the thumb and the metacarpal bones of the hand. The radial pulse is palpable on the anterior surface of the wrist on its lateral aspect.

The hand is made up of the palm, the thumb and four fingers. There are five bones called metacarpals, which form the structural framework of the palm. The distal ends of the metacarpals are the knuckles. Each finger consists of three small bones called phalanges, whose joints are readily identifiable on the fingers. The thumb has only two phalanges and joins the wrist via one of the metacarpal bones.

The Lower Extremity

The lower extremity consists of the hip, thigh, knee, calf, ankle and foot. The hip joint is formed by the articulation of the femur with the pelvis. A bony projection of the femur (greater trochanter) is palpable on the lateral aspect of the hip.

The main supporting structure of the thigh is the femur — the longest bone in the body. The femur articulates with the tibia to form the knee. The proximal end of the fibula extends to the knee but does not form part of the joint. The patella (knee cap) is located on the anterior aspect of the knee. With the knee extended and the thigh muscles relaxed, the patella is very mobile.

The two bones of the lower leg are the tibia (the shin bone) and the fibula, located lateral and parallel to the tibia. The distal end of the fibula is palpable at the ankle on its lateral aspect. The medial prominence of the ankle joint is the distal end of the tibia. The tibia and fibula articulate with the talus to form the ankle joint.

Situated posterior to or behind the medial prominence of the ankle is the pulse of the posterior tibial artery.

The foot is a complex structure made up of several tarsal bones, metatarsal bones and the toes. One of the tarsal bones is the heel bone or calcaneus. The big toe, like the thumb, is made up of only two phalanges, while all the other toes have three phalanges. Because of the direction of the foot in the anatomical position, there really is no true anterior or posterior aspect. The top of the foot is referred to as the dorsal aspect of the foot while the sole is referred to as the plantar aspect. On the dorsal surface of the foot anterior to the ankle, the dorsalis pedis pulse may be palpable.

SUMMARY

The Attendant must learn the language of surface anatomy. This section highlights the most important landmarks of the body. The location of the major arterial pulse points has also been emphasized.

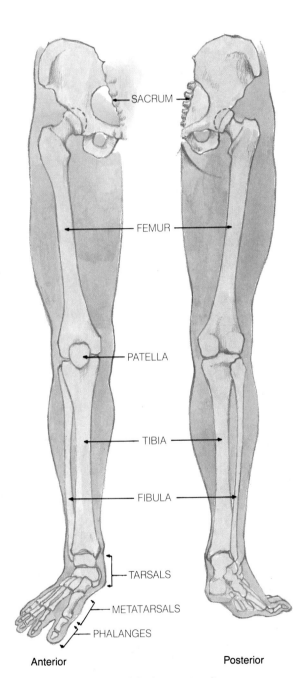

SACRUM

FEMUR

PATELLA

TIBIA

FIBULA

TARSALS

METATARSALS

PHALANGES

Anterior   Posterior

Anatomy of the lower extremity

Part III
Initial Evaluation of the Trauma Patient

TRAUMA CARE IN PERSPECTIVE

The major cause of death and disability in the young-adult age group (21 to 44) is trauma. Major strides in trauma care have evolved primarily from military experience, such as the Korean and Vietnam Wars. The Vietnam War has shown that, by using specially trained medics in the field, rapid transport by helicopter and specially designated hospitals, morbidity and mortality can be significantly reduced. The United States military demonstrated that rapid access to trauma care saves lives and reduces morbidity.

This concept has been extended to the civilian sector. We have witnessed the introduction of specialized trauma centres, life-flight helicopters and paramedic-staffed ground ambulances in efforts to improve the care of the injured patient.

Medical studies have firmly established the importance of rapid access to definitive care. The seriously injured patient has to be in the operating room within 60 minutes of injury in order to survive. This is called the "golden hour".

THE IFA ATTENDANT PERFORMS A UNIQUE AND CRITICAL SERVICE IN INDUSTRY. THE IFA ATTENDANT IS THE INITIAL ACTIVATOR OF THE ENTIRE SYSTEM DESIGNED TO OPTIMIZE TRAUMA CARE FOR WORKERS.

As part of his or her duties, the IFA Attendant therefore shoulders the responsibility of providing adequate care to the injured patient and at the same time ensuring that there are no unnecessary delays in getting the seriously injured patient to the hospital. Remember the "golden hour". Any time wasted may severely compromise the patient's survival down the road.

How then does the IFA Attendant handle this dilemma — to perform a thorough yet rapid assessment? The solution lies in the use of a PRIORITY ACTION APPROACH to patient assessment. The guidelines also provide a set of RAPID TRANSPORT CRITERIA to determine which patient has to be transported to the hospital without delay and which patient can be assessed and treated further in the field.

PRIORITY ACTION APPROACH

By fully understanding the concept of the "golden hour", the IFA Attendant will develop the skill of assessing and treating every trauma patient in a rapid, logical and orderly manner.

The following truths must always be remembered by IFA Attendants:
1. Major trauma patients cannot be "stabilized" in the field. Although splinting, bandaging, etc. are generally helpful for most patients, only critical interventions (i.e. airway maintenance, breathing, cervical spine immobilization and hemorrhage control) are necessary in major trauma patients. All other treatments only consume valuable minutes of the "golden hour".
2. Many trauma victims die because they do not make it to the operating room in time.
3. Trauma care demands efficient use of time so that the patient is transported to hospital as quickly as possible.

As the first person on the scene to initiate care, the Attendant's judgment and speed can often determine the trauma victim's fate. The patient's chance of survival can be maximized when Attendants have done their homework before accidents occur. The operative motto is "Be Prepared". First aid cannot be given if the patient cannot be found. It is important to get to know all the ins and outs of the plant or job site. It may be difficult to extricate a patient on the stretcher from certain locations. Precious time is wasted if the Attendant discovers this only during a true emergency. Attendants must learn how to quickly access the ambulance or helicopter service from their location. Emergency phone numbers must be adjacent to all phones for quick reference.

Immediate availability of equipment may be a serious problem. All essential equipment must be brought to the scene by the Attendant or a co-worker, to save precious time used running back and forth. The Attendant must think ahead to anticipate the patient's needs. The following equipment is usually necessary to complete the primary survey:
1. Oxygen and airway equipment, suctioning device if available
2. First aid kit with pressure bandages, scissors, etc.

3. Long spine board with a cervical spine immobilization device.

Furthermore, the equipment must be checked regularly. Precious time is lost if the oxygen cylinder is found to be empty or the suctioning device is inoperable when needed.

Finally, as much information as possible should be obtained when the first call is received: Where is the accident? What happened? How many victims? Are there any scene dangers? Will special equipment be required?

BE PREPARED!

THINK AHEAD!

INITIAL ASSESSMENT OF THE INJURED WORKER

The initial assessment of the injured worker follows the Priority Action Approach — a step-by-step flow chart for you to follow. The Priority Action Approach is divided into the following four stages:
1. Scene Assessment
2. Primary Survey
3. Transport Decision/Critical Interventions
4. Secondary Survey

SCENE ASSESSMENT

While approaching the patient:
1. Assess the scene for hazards.
2. Determine the mechanism of injury.
3. Note the number of victims.

REMEMBER TO CHECK THE SCENE FOR HAZARDS. DO NOT BECOME A VICTIM YOURSELF! Are there wires down? Toxic gases? Risk of explosion? Fire? Immediately determine whether or not special equipment is required (e.g. self-contained breathing apparatus.)

Also decide if the patient needs to be extricated immediately because of these hazards (e.g. leaking propane). DO NOT PROCEED WITH PATIENT ASSESSMENT IF IT EXPOSES YOU AND/OR THE PATIENT TO FURTHER RISK. Load the patient onto a lifting device, move to a safe environment, and then proceed with the assessment.

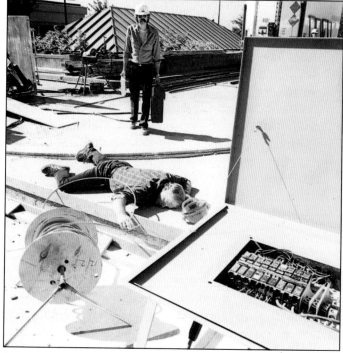
Assess the scene on approach.

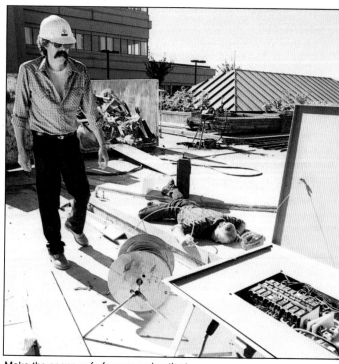
Make the scene safe for you and patient.

Many life-threatening injuries are not initially apparent. Learning how to suspect serious injuries and preparing to treat them as they develop is a special skill requiring study and experience. Understanding the mechanism of injury allows the IFA Attendant to predict serious injury. In general, injuries result from the transfer of sufficient energy to all or part of the body. For example, if a person falls onto soft ground, which absorbs some of the energy, the likelihood of injury is less than if a person had fallen onto a hard surface such as rock or concrete. By understanding the basic principles involved, the IFA Attendant should try to answer the following questions at every scene assessment:

1. What happened?
2. How much force or energy was applied?
3. To which part of the body and in what direction was the force applied?

As an example, a fall from a height of 2 metres (6 feet) would not cause as significant an injury as a fall from 10 metres (30 feet). The velocity gained by falling the extra distance from the greater height allows a considerably larger amount of energy to transfer to the body. Every organ of the body has a particular energy limit above which injury will occur. For example, an increasing force (or energy) can be applied to a bone until it finally breaks. A number of research studies have shown that certain types of accidents have a higher risk of serious internal injury. Because these injuries may not be readily apparent, the Attendant should consider the mechanism of the injury during the assessment. Patients with the potential for serious injury must be rapidly transported to hospital with only critical interventions performed. **"Remember the golden hour."** Table III-a below outlines these mechanisms of injury. TREATMENT OF THESE PATIENTS MUST BE LIMITED TO CRITICAL INTERVENTIONS ONLY.

TABLE III-a

Mechanisms of Injuries Requiring Rapid Transport to Hospital

1. Free-fall from a height greater than 6.5 metres (20 feet)
2. Severe deceleration in a motor vehicle accident (e.g. logging truck):
   - High-speed accident and/or major vehicular damage
   - Broken windshield, bent steering wheel, or other significant damage to passenger compartment
   - Victim thrown from vehicle
   - One or more vehicle occupants killed
   - Victim involved in roll-over type accident (e.g. forklift)
3. Pedestrian, bicyclist or motorcyclist struck at greater than 30 km per hour (20 miles per hour)
4. Severe crush injuries

The final step in the scene assessment is to determine the number of victims. Are all victims accounted for? Ask witnesses. Ask the other conscious patients. If there is more than one victim, get help immediately. Do not try to be a hero and do it all. Remember the "golden hour" applies to each individual patient. You cannot attend to more than one critical patient at a time. Recognize that, in the setting of multiple victims, patients may have to be transported to hospital without full assessments completed. You should be more concerned about getting all the patients transported to medical care, rather than worrying about doing a full assessment on one patient and leaving the others. Essentially, your energies should be directed to prioritizing patients for transport. The multi-victim scenario will be dealt with separately in more detail in Part XVI, Section B, page 363.

Summary

The scene assessment accomplishes the following goals:
1. Determines the presence of additional hazards to the Attendant as well as for the patient
2. Establishes the mechanism of injury

3.   Determines the number of victims

The information gained from the scene assessment allows some immediate transport decisions to be made and sets the basis for patient assessment.

PRIMARY SURVEY

The next stage of the Priority Action Approach is the primary survey. This is a rapid exam designed to determine the presence of any immediate life-threatening injuries. THE EXAM ITSELF SHOULD NOT TAKE MORE THAN TWO MINUTES. The primary survey should proceed in a rapid step-by-step manner, completing each one before proceeding to the next. The only intervention would be the treatment of life-threatening conditions such as: airway obstruction, cardiac arrest, open chest wound or major arterial bleeding. The primary survey is based on the assessment of the ABCs:

A   = Airway with C-spine control
B   = Breathing
C   = Circulation

The primary survey begins immediately after the scene assessment. Even if the victim is trapped and extrication is in process, patient care must be initiated, beginning with the primary survey.

A = AIRWAY

Approach the victim from the front, if possible. Briefly identify yourself: "I am an IFA Attendant. I am here to help you. What happened?" The patient's response or lack of response will give immediate information as to the level of consciousness and the status of the airway. If the patient is able to speak clearly, then the airway is clear and you should immediately proceed to the next step. If the patient cannot speak, you must evaluate the airway further.

Unless the patient is actively vomiting or there are obvious signs of major bleeding from the mouth or nose, the primary survey and all subsequent assessment is done best in the supine position rather than ¾ prone. If the patient is found prone, it is best to manually stabilize the neck and roll the patient to the lateral position to assess the airway. If the airway is clear, the patient may be rolled supine onto a long spine board or lifting device (if one is readily available and prepared for use), and the primary survey is completed. However, if the Attendant is alone and the conscious patient

is found prone or ¾ prone with a clear airway, the primary survey may be completed in the position found until help is available to roll the patient supine. The correct techniques for positioning injured patients are thoroughly described in Part IV, Section B, page 42.

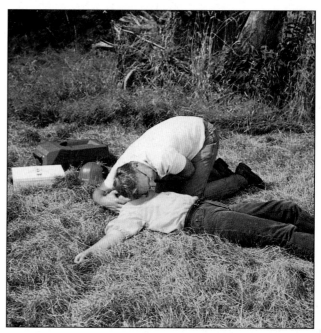

Assessing airway with C-spine control using a jaw thrust

The Attendant looks, listens and feels for the movement of air in and out of the mouth or nose. If necessary, the mouth is opened and the airway is cleared. If an obstructed or partially obstructed airway is suspected, it must be cleared before proceeding to the next step of the primary survey. ALL TRAUMA PATIENTS WITH A DECREASED LEVEL OF CONSCIOUSNESS SHOULD ALSO BE ASSUMED TO HAVE A CERVICAL SPINE INJURY AND TREATED ACCORDINGLY. Bystanders may be used to maintain the neck after you have moved it to the anatomical position. If the Attendant is alone, rocks, wood, even small mounds of earth can be used to maintain the neck in the anatomical position while the primary survey is done. REMEMBER, NEVER EXTEND THE NECK TO OPEN THE AIRWAY OF A TRAUMA PATIENT. The modified jaw thrust, as illustrated in the section on airway management, should be used in an attempt to open the airway. An oral airway may have to be inserted. Patients may have to be ventilated with supplemental oxygen using a pocket mask and/or a bag-valve mask device. Airway management is reviewed in greater detail in Part IV, Section B, page 39. REMEMBER THAT ALL PATIENTS WITH AIRWAY PROBLEMS ARE IN THE RAPID TRANSPORT CATEGORY.

For patients with airway problems, the Attendant must complete the primary survey rapidly, perform critical interventions and transport the patient to hospital. In these cases, the secondary survey and all further treatment must be performed en route. A critically ill trauma patient cannot be stabilized in the field and requires definitive care that can be provided only in the hospital.

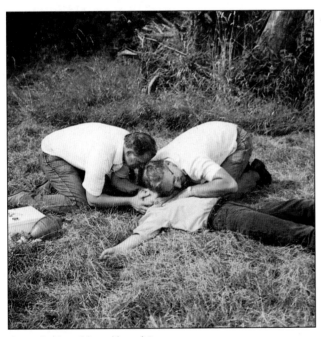

Assessing breathing with assistance

B = BREATHING

The status of the patient's breathing or respiration is the focus of the next step of the primary survey. The respiratory rate can be determined by counting the patient's breaths over a period of 15 seconds and multiplying by 4 to give the number of breaths per minute.

Counting the chest wall movements is probably the best method. The patient's chest wall may have to be exposed in order to adequately assess the breathing and look for obvious chest injuries. Alternatively, the Attendant can look, listen or feel for movement of air as the patient exhales and count the number of breaths.

The quality of the patient's respirations should be noted. Are the respirations shallow or laboured? Shallow breathing is characterized by minimal movements of the chest wall. Laboured breathing is characterized by shortness of breath in patients who are working hard at breathing. If the patient is breathing too slowly (10 or fewer per minute), he/she will require assisted ventilation with supplementary oxygen, using a pocket mask or bag-valve mask. If the patient is breathing too quickly (greater than 30 per minute), supplemental oxygen by mask will be required (10 litres per minute [Lpm]). If the respirations are also shallow or laboured, assisted ventilation with a bag-valve mask or pocket mask may be required. If bystanders are available, they may be used to provide pocket mask ventilations while the Attendant completes the primary survey.

Remember to manually stabilize the neck if a cervical spine injury is suspected, especially if assisted ventilation is required. A simple technique is to stabilize the patient's head between the knees while kneeling. This method frees up both hands to ventilate the patient. (See Figure III-1.) Alternatively, using a pocket mask to ventilate the patient allows the neck to be stabilized by the Attendant's hands and forearms. (See Figure III-2.)

Patients with a respiratory rate less than 10 or greater than 30 also fall into the Rapid Transport Category. Oxygen must be provided with assisted ventilation as required. If the patient is struggling because of respiratory distress, assisted ventilation with a bag-valve mask device must be attempted. If the patient resists the attempt, stop assisted ventilation but keep the mask with the high flow of oxygen near the patient's face. The remainder of the primary survey is then completed and the patient is transported. The secondary survey and all further treatment must be performed en route.

FINALLY, AS A GENERAL RULE, SUPPLEMENTAL OXYGEN BY FACE MASK MUST BE PROVIDED AT 10 LITRES PER MINUTE TO ALL PATIENTS IN THE RAPID TRANSPORT CATEGORY.

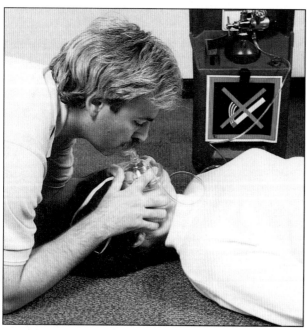

Figure III-1 Securing the head with the knees

Figure III-2 Using the pocket mask

C = CIRCULATION

Circulation is assessed best by feeling the patient's pulse, either at the wrist (the radial pulse), neck (carotid pulse) or groin (femoral pulse). The Attendant should use the fingers — not the thumb — to feel for the pulse to avoid confusing one's own pulse with that of the patient.

Generally, the pulse is assessed by noting its rate, strength and regularity. However, for purposes of the primary survey, only the presence or absence of the radial pulse is crucial.

With a healthy adult worker, loss of the radial pulse correlates approximately with a blood pressure of 90 mm Hg systolic. That is why the actual measurement of blood pressure is not an important skill for the IFA Attendant to learn. If the Attendant can feel the radial pulse then the blood pressure is at least 90 mm Hg. If the radial pulse is not palpable then the patient's blood pressure is less than 90. INABILITY TO FEEL THE RADIAL PULSE IMMEDIATELY PUTS THE PATIENT IN THE RAPID TRANSPORT CATEGORY. Accurately measuring the blood pressure only represents loss of precious minutes within the "golden hour".

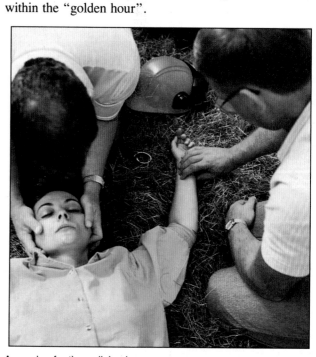

Assessing for the radial pulse

If the radial pulse is absent and confirmed, the patient is in shock and requires rapid transport to hospital. The patient requires supplemental oxygen by mask at 10 litres per minute, cervical spine immobilization if indicated, and preparation for rapid transport. Only modified immobilization techniques for limb fractures should be done at the scene for these critical patients.

In rare cases, loss of the radial pulse is related to direct vessel injury of the upper extremity. For example, a displaced fracture of the elbow may injure the artery. This can result in loss of the radial pulse on the injured side, and is not necessarily an indication of shock. Therefore, it is important that the IFA Attendant, when presented with an unpalpable radial pulse, examine the opposite wrist for a pulse and look for other symptoms associated with the presence of shock.

Within the context of the primary survey, it is only important to detect critical emergencies. Life-threatening external hemorrhage (i.e. major bleeding) needs to be controlled at this time with pressure dressings, bandages or, rarely, tourniquets. Assessment of the circulation is therefore limited to feeling the radial, carotid or femoral pulse, and performing a rapid body survey for massive external hemorrhage and obvious fractures. These sites of injury will have to be exposed to be examined properly (e.g. cutting heavy outer clothing or rain gear). THIS RAPID BODY SURVEY MUST NOT TAKE LONGER THAN 30 SECONDS. The Attendant must initiate any critical intervention that is required.

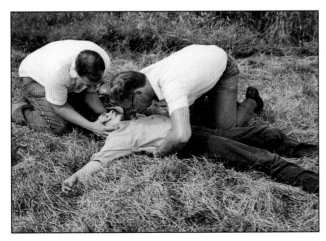

Performing a rapid body survey

RAPID TRANSPORT CRITERIA

Earlier in this section, reference has been made to the Rapid Transport Criteria. By now, the IFA Attendant should appreciate the importance of ensuring that critically injured patients are transported rapidly to hospital for definitive care. The question then becomes: How do I, as the IFA Attendant, determine which patient requires rapid transport and which patient can be transported at a more leisurely pace? By using the mechanism of injury, anatomy of injury and your primary survey, you have all the necessary tools. Specialists in trauma care have devised a short list of conditions that, once recognized, place the patient in the Rapid Transport Category. The following criteria must be memorized and carried with you in your kit for handy reference. Because head injury is the most important cause of morbidity and mortality in trauma patients, severe head injury and its definition is listed under the heading "Anatomy of Injury" below. The details of the neurological examination are covered in greater detail later in this section as well as in Part VI, Sections C and D, pages 133 and 143.

Rapid Transport Criteria for Injured Workers

The criteria can be established by:
A. Mechanism of injury
B. Anatomy of injury
C. Findings in the primary survey

A. Mechanism of Injury

1. Free fall greater than 6.5 metres (20 feet)
2. Severe deceleration in a motor vehicle accident (e.g. logging truck):
    * High-speed accident and/or major vehicular damage
    * Broken windshield, bent steering wheel, or other significant damage to passenger compartment
    * Victim thrown from vehicle
    * One or more vehicle occupants killed
    * Victim involved in roll-over type accident (e.g. forklift)
3. Pedestrian, motorcyclist or bicyclist struck at greater than 30 kph (20 mph)
4. Severe crush injuries

PRIORITY ACTION APPROACH FLOW CHART

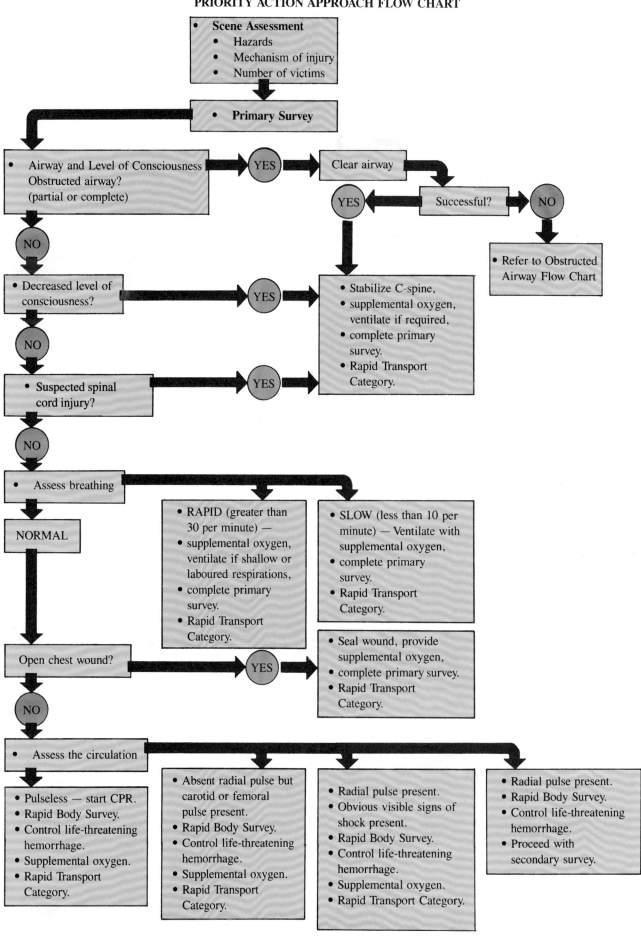

B. Anatomy of Injury

1. Severe head injury defined as:
   - Glasgow Coma Score less than or equal to 13 (details of GCS on page 26)
   - decreasing GCS by 2 or more
   - pupillary inequality greater than 1 mm and sluggish response to light
   - extremity weakness or paralysis, regardless of the GCS
   - depressed skull fracture
2. Penetrating injury to the head, neck, chest, abdomen or groin
3. Two or more proximal long-bone fractures, i.e. femur, humerus
4. Flail chest
5. Extensive facial burns, inhalation injury or burns greater than 10% body surface area, especially if associated with any other trauma
6. Amputation of extremity other than toe or fingertip
7. Spinal cord injury, paraplegia or quadriplegia

C. Findings in the Primary Survey

1. Partial or complete airway obstruction
2. Decreased Level of Consciousness (LOC) (does not respond to verbal command.)
3. Respiratory rate (less than 10 or greater than 30 per minute) or severe dyspnea
4. Absent radial pulses
5. Obvious circulatory shock

If the patient meets any of the above criteria, rapid transport is indicated. The treatment should be limited to the critical interventions only (see below). The secondary survey and further treatment should be done only en route. More importantly, the list of Rapid Transport Criteria is not intended to be "all or nothing". If there is any doubt whether or not the patient meets the Rapid Transport Criteria or special concerns are raised, the Attendant should rapidly transport the patient to hospital. IT IS IMPERATIVE TO REASSESS THE PATIENT FREQUENTLY BECAUSE PATIENTS WHO APPEAR TO BE STABLE INITIALLY MAY DETERIORATE. IN THOSE CASES, THE PATIENT MUST BE UPGRADED INTO THE RAPID TRANSPORT CATEGORY.

CRITICAL INTERVENTIONS

Given the time constraints of the "golden hour", it is imperative that patients in the Rapid Transport Category receive only essential treatment. These are referred to as the CRITICAL INTERVENTIONS. All other treatment, although important, should be performed en route to hospital. Do not delay transport of a seriously injured trauma patient. The following table summarizes the critical interventions.

TABLE III-b

Critical Interventions for the Seriously Injured Worker

1. Airway — clear an obstructed or partially obstructed airway
2. Breathing — supplemental oxygen by mask for all seriously injured (Rapid Transport Category) patients
   — ventilation with supplemental oxygen using bag-valve mask or pocket mask
   — seal an open sucking chest wound
3. Circulation — CPR if in cardiac arrest (pulseless, apnea)
   — control life-threatening hemorrhage with direct pressure, pressure points and/or tourniquet
4. Cervical spine immobilization with an appropriate hard collar on a well-padded spine board
5. Limited immobilization for major or open fractures or dislocations

PATIENT IMMOBILIZATION AND PACKAGING FOR RAPID TRANSPORT

From the time the Attendant has determined that the patient's condition warrants rapid transport to hospital, it is imperative that aside from attending to life-threatening situations involving AIRWAY, BREATHING and CIRCULATION, all efforts should be directed to "packaging" the patient for *safe* transport as rapidly as possible.

This means that if, during the primary survey, the Attendant reaches the decision that the patient falls into the Rapid Transport Category, the Attendant should only:
- complete the primary survey;
- carry out critical interventions relating to compromised airway, breathing and circulation;
- conduct a rapid body survey.

THE PRIMARY SURVEY, CRITICAL INTERVENTIONS AND PATIENT SECURING SHOULD NOT TAKE LONGER THAN 15 MINUTES!

The Attendant should then immediately proceed to "package" the patient and direct others to arrange for the appropriate transportation. The vital signs and secondary survey should be conducted AFTER the patient is packaged and en route to hospital or while the patient is waiting for the transport vehicle.

These recommended techniques are used for patient packaging for rapid transport. This way the patient is thoroughly immobilized and secured to a padded long spine board or stretcher. As the long spine board is the universal transport device available throughout industry, it is used in the following examples.

The term "patient packaging" is used so that the Attendant will think of the patient as a fragile, priceless article that must be shipped some distance and may be exposed to inadvertent rough handling and/or moved through all manner of positions. For example, in transit, the patient may be exposed to the shaking and thumping of a rough logging road or to air turbulence in an air evacuation. Alternatively, the patient may have to be turned rapidly as a unit into the lateral position to protect the airway if vomiting occurs, or the spine board may have to be put on its side to get it into an aircraft. For the multiple trauma patient with suspected C-spine injury, it is imperative that the patient be firmly secured with appropriate padding to the spine board, so that the patient does not move and associated injuries are protected and not aggravated.

THE TECHNIQUES USED FOR PATIENT IMMOBILIZATION AND PACKAGING FOR RAPID TRANSPORT SUPERSEDE AND REPLACE ALL OTHER IMMOBILIZATION AND SPLINTING TECHNIQUES TAUGHT IN THIS COURSE *ONCE* THE PATIENT FALLS INTO THE RAPID TRANSPORT CATEGORY.

Summary of Advantages of Rapid Transport Patient Packaging

- Patient is rapidly prepared for transport.
- The airway can be more easily managed while protecting the cervical spine.
- The method affords some chest wall stabilization for associated chest injuries.
- There is effective immobilization of other injuries, reducing their aggravation (e.g. spine injuries, pelvic fractures or lower limb fractures).
- The patient is protected from further injury en route.
- Have effective control of the delirious patient.

Equipment Required

1. A hard cervical collar of appropriate size.
2. Long spine board.
3. At least seven 2 metres x 5 cm (6′ x 2″) heavy Velcro® straps or, alternatively, safety-belt-type straps with quick-release buckles. These are the preferred straps. However triangular bandages and/or 5 cm (2″) tape may be used.
   - one to secure the head;
   - two to cross the upper chest. Each strap passes under the axilla on one side and over the opposite shoulder;
   - two to crisscross the pelvis;
   - one to secure the knees;
   - one to secure the ankles.
4. Six regular blankets or comparable padding:
   - one to fold and place on the spine board for padding;
   - one folded to fit between the legs;
   - two folded longways to run from the axilla to below the ankles on each side;
   - one folded as a horseshoe or cut in half and rolled to secure the head and neck; (NOTE: Acceptable alternative padding and support for the head and neck include 4.5 kg sandbags or large foam blocks.)
   - one to cover the patient if necessary, depending on the weather.
5. A triangular bandage to secure the feet and ankles with a figure-of-eight tie.

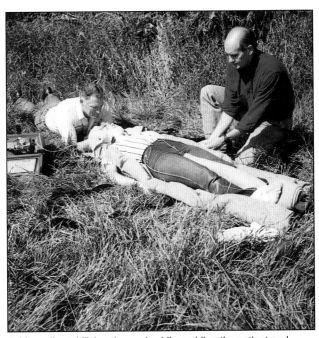

1. Manually stabilizing the neck while padding the patient and spine board

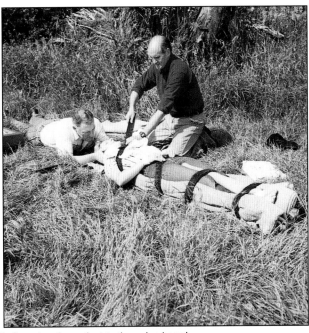

2. Securing the patient to the spine board

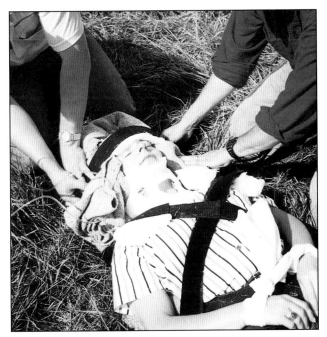

3. Securing the head to the spine board last

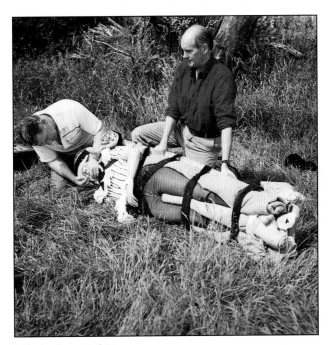

4. Packaging complete

Figure III-3

Procedure for Packaging of Patients in the Supine Position

The patient should be moved into the supine position according to the protocols outlined in the section on spinal injuries and their management (Part VI, Section D, page 149).

THE HEAD AND NECK SHOULD BE SECURED LAST! THE HEAD AND NECK SHOULD BE MAINTAINED IN THE ANATOMICAL POSITION MANUALLY OR WITH SANDBAGS WHILE THE REST OF THE PACKAGING IS APPLIED.

Industrial First Aid Attendants should follow the steps outlined pictorially (see Figure III-3). However, the sequence of strap application may have to be varied depending on the circumstances. THE ONLY FIRM RULE IS TO APPLY THE STRAPPING TO THE HEAD LAST.

While packaging is being carried out, it is imperative that the patient's condition, especially relating to the airway, breathing and circulation, be regularly reassessed. If necessary, the Attendant may have to delegate the packaging procedures to others while attending critical interventions (e.g. airway management, assisted ventilation, control of major hemorrhage, etc.). In this instance, the Attendant would supervise others from the head and then check all the strapping and padding once the critical interventions have been concluded.

All strapping should line up with the other side and should cross over the midline anteriorly to allow rapid access to the patient for further assessment. It should be firmly secured so that the patient will not move on the spine board during transportation. If Velcro® straps are used, it is recommended that the straps overlap one another at least 25-30 cm (10″-12″) in order to ensure a solid contact. It is important that the Velcro® straps be applied fuzzy side towards the patient. When they are pulled through the slots in the spine board, they should be twisted 180°, cinched-up firmly and applied to themselves, fuzzy side to hooked side.

The situation may arise where the Attendant must delegate some critical interventions (i.e. assisted ventilations) to assistants. In such cases, it is imperative that the Attendant recheck the effectiveness of the treatment rendered by the other helper(s) frequently and not become so distracted with packaging or other activities that the patient's condition deteriorates without the Attendant's knowledge and the appropriate intervention.

Although it is important to try to reduce patient discomfort and the aggravation of injuries, it may sometimes be necessary to roll the patient onto an injured part (e.g. fractured pelvis). The need may arise because of airway and C-spine concerns, which take precedence over other injuries. The Attendant must focus on treatment procedures that maintain the airway, breathing and circulation, and expedite the patient's rapid transport.

Such a situation might arise (for instance) if the Attendant is concerned for a patient's airway. The patient may have to be rolled onto a fractured pelvis, or possibly a fractured femur on that side, in order to manage the airway efficiently. Though this is perhaps less than ideal from the point of view of the fracture, the airway problem, being potentially life-threatening, takes precedence!

Procedure for Packaging of Patients in the Lateral Position

The patient should be moved into the lateral position according to the protocols in the section on spinal injuries and their management (see Part VI, Section D, page 147).

The major indications for transporting the patient with suspected cervical injury in the lateral position are:

- facial injuries with active bleeding in the nasal or oral airway;
- active vomiting;
- patients with a decreased level of consciousness who cannot be continuously monitored by the Attendant;
- stretcher limitations, i.e. inability to rotate the spine board or stretcher should the patient vomit;
- helicopter evacuations; if the stretcher is suspended below the helicopter during rescue operations, the patient cannot be monitored effectively so the lateral position is required.

THE HEAD AND NECK SHOULD BE SECURED LAST! The head and neck should be maintained in a neutral position manually, with sandbags, or with padding, while the rest of the packaging is applied.

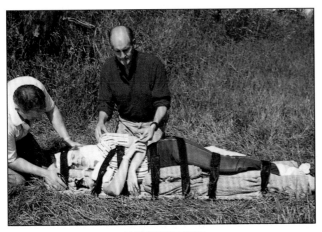

ANTERIOR VIEW
Securing the patient in the lateral position for rapid transport

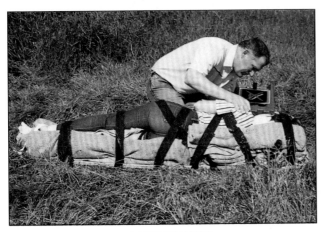

POSTERIOR VIEW
Note the padding to maintain the lateral position.

The Attendant should follow the same steps as outlined pictorially for the supine patient. However, the sequence of strap application may have to be varied depending on the circumstances. THE ONLY FIRM RULE IS TO APPLY THE STRAPPING TO THE HEAD LAST.

IT IS IMPORTANT TO CAREFULLY PAD THE SPINE BOARD AND ALL PARTS OF THE PATIENT THAT CONTACT THE BOARD IF TRANSPORTING THE PATIENT IN THE LATERAL POSITION.

More attention must be paid to filling in hollows and spaces, both anteriorly and posteriorly, not only for the comfort of the patient but also to ensure the patient will not move around during transport.

Please review again all the instructions for packaging the supine patient as they are, for the most part, equally applicable to packaging the patient in the lateral position.

SECONDARY SURVEY

The purpose of the secondary survey is to perform a rapid and complete head-to-toe assessment. A patient that is not in the rapid transport category should have this done at the scene. THE SECONDARY SURVEY SHOULD NOT TAKE MORE THAN TEN MINUTES.

With patients in the rapid transport category, the secondary survey should be initiated at the scene while awaiting a transport vehicle and completed en route.

The basics of the secondary survey are:

1. Vital signs
2. Chief complaint and history of current injury or illness
3. Medications
4. Allergies
5. Head-to-toe examination

Vital Signs

Once the primary survey has been completed, the Attendant should take the vital signs which are:

- respiratory rate
- pulse and capillary refill
- level of consciousness (LOC)
- pupils
- temperature

The respiratory rate and pulse have already been explained in the primary survey. They should be reassessed now, as part of the vital signs.

Respiratory rate

Assessing the respiratory rate has already been discussed.

Pulse and Capillary Refill

Assessment of the patient's pulse (circulatory status) is the next step in the taking of vital signs. If the patient has lost a considerable amount of blood (either internally or externally), the body responds by attempting to improve the output of the heart (i.e. it pumps faster, causing the heart rate and therefore the pulse to speed up). As blood loss increases in severity, the body responds by preserving the blood flow to the critical organs (brain, lungs, heart and kidneys) and diverting blood from non-critical areas (e.g. the skin and extremities).That is why the patient becomes pale from blood loss. The body constricts the blood vessels supplying the skin, reducing the blood flow and making the patient look pale. Similarly, the blood vessels supplying the extremities constrict, thereby reducing blood flow. As a result, the extremities (feet and hands) are cool to the touch. As part of the body's response to shock, sweating usually develops. As a result, the skin, in addition to being pale and cool, is also moist or wet with perspiration. The IFA Attendant should now recognize that these are the earliest signs of hemorrhagic or hypovolemic shock, which is covered in greater detail in Part V, Section B, page 100.

As blood loss continues, the radial pulse becomes weak and "thready". The carotid and femoral pulses may feel relatively stronger. This reflects the shifting of blood flow away from the peripheral extremities to the more important central organs.

As discussed in the primary survey, it is more important to assess the patient's pulses — particularly the radial, femoral and carotid pulses — than measure blood pressure. In the secondary survey, the Attendant should note the strength, the rate and the regularity of the pulse.

While assessing the pulse, the Attendant should note whether the extremities are cool to touch. The Attendant should also note the patient's colour, particularly looking for the presence of pallor or cyanosis. As shock deepens, the capillary refill test will become delayed. This test is performed by depressing the victim's fingernail and releasing quickly. The normal response is for the colour to return within two seconds. If it takes longer than two seconds, the test is delayed and provides strong evidence of shock. However, if the capillary refill is normal, shock may still be developing and the patient should be reassessed frequently. The capillary refill test cannot be interpreted in the hypothermic patient because the skin is already vasoconstricted due to the cold. Given the triad of findings — pallor, cool extremities and rapid pulse — the Attendant should recognize those as the signs of shock. In the setting of a traumatic injury, this must *always* be attributed to blood loss, either internal or external. The Attendant must then organize rapid transport of this patient to hospital.

Cyanosis is a bluish discolouration of the skin related to low levels of oxygen in the blood (hypoxia) and increased levels of carbon dioxide. It is usually most noticeable in the lips, fingertips and nail beds. The Attendant should compare the colour of his or her own fingertips to those of the patient. The presence of cyanosis usually indicates a cardio-respiratory emergency. If the airway is clear or has been stabilized, these patients require assisted ventilation with supplemental oxygen. Arrangements for rapid transport to hospital must be made.

To calculate pulse rate, count beats in a 15-second interval and multiply by 4 to determine the number of beats per minute. The pulse is usually regular. Skipped beats or an irregular pulse must be noted. To detect irregularities of the pulse, it may be necessary to monitor the pulse for a full 60 seconds. Irregularities of the pulse are most significant in the setting of a cardiac or respiratory emergency and less so with trauma patients. With trauma patients, remember the "golden hour". Do not lose precious minutes checking for irregularities of the pulse unless it is done en route to hospital.

Level of Consciousness

The next step in the vital signs is an assessment of the patient's level of consciousness. This is especially important for patients with head injury. Unfortunately, it has been difficult to assess level of consciousness because of the subjective nature of the words used to describe consciousness. For example, drowsiness means different things to different people. Therefore, the use of descriptive terms is to be avoided. The level of consciousness is assessed best by using the Glasgow Coma Score (GCS). This was initially developed as a score to predict outcome for patients with head injury. The advantage of the score is that its measurements are objective, easily reproducible and simple to use.

Glasgow Coma Score — GCS

The GCS measures three different functions of the nervous system as shown below.
a)   Eye-opening response
b)   Motor response
c)   Verbal response

The eye-opening response is measured by observing whether or not the patient opens the eyes to a stimulus. If the patient opens the eyes spontaneously, score a "4". If the eyes open to verbal command — ask the patient to open the eyes, shout if necessary — score a "3". If the patient opens the eyes only to a painful stimulus, score a "2". To provide a painful stimulus, press on the fingernails, using a hard object like a pen or pencil. Alternatively, the trapezius muscles located between the neck and the shoulder may be squeezed to provide a painful stimulus.

The motor response is similarly assessed using verbal and/or painful stimuli. The *best* response is noted by the Attendant. If the patient is paralyzed on one side, the motor response of the unaffected or better side would be used. The highest score in this category is "6" and indicates that the patient is responding appropriately by moving a limb as instructed. If the patient does not respond to verbal stimuli but localizes to painful stimuli, score "5". If there is withdrawal only to a painful stimulus, score a "4". It may be difficult to distinguish between a "4" and a "5". The following examples will help illustrate the differences. If patients are able to tell you to "stop squeezing my finger" (if that is the painful stimulus applied) they are localizing the pain because they can identify its source. Similarly, if they reach over with the opposite hand and tries to push the Attendant away, they are also localizing the pain. Simple withdrawal is a reflex action and if the patient does not appear to localize or identify the source of the pain then score a "4". The simple withdrawal reflex that you have when you touch a burning pot is an example of a simple withdrawal response.

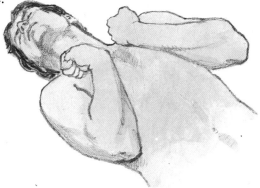

Figure III-4 Decorticate posturing

As the level of consciousness decreases, the nervous system responds to painful stimuli with a primitive postural reflex. The first type of reflex is called the decorticate (flexion) response or decorticate posturing. It is usually manifested by simultaneous flexion of the upper extremities and extension of the lower extremities. See Figure III-4. The other reflex is called decerebrate (extensor) posturing and is manifested by extension and internal rotation of one or both upper extremities and extension of one or both lower extremities. See Figure III-5. In the motor response category of the GCS, a decorticate response scores a "3" and a decerebrate response scores a "2". If there is no motor response at all to any stimulus, the score is "1".

The final category of the Glasgow Coma Score (GCS) assesses the patient's verbal response or speech. If the patient's speech is reasonably clear and coherent, the score is "5". If the patient's speech is confused but at least understandable, the score is "4". If the patient responds with simple inappropriate words or only curses, the patient scores a "3". If the patient's speech is unintelligible or incomprehensible (e.g. moaning), the score is a "2". Finally, if the patient is unresponsive and cannot speak at all, score a "1".

The GCS is summarized in Table III-c. The lowest possible score is "3" and the best score is "15". The unconscious patient typically does not open the eyes (eye opening response is "1"), withdraws only to painful stimuli (motor response = "4") and moans at times (verbal response = "2"). The GCS, in this example, is therefore "1 + 4 + 2 = 7". When reporting the score, the Attendant always follows the same order: eye opening, motor response and verbal response, followed by the total score. By telephone, the Attendant will report that the patient's level of consciousness is a "1-4-2", total "7", on the GCS. The Glasgow Coma Score's interpretation will be reviewed in Part VI, Section C on page 132, Head Injuries. Patients with a GCS of "13" or less are in the Rapid Transport Category. Similarly, if the patient's level of consciousness is decreasing, as measured by a falling GCS of "2" or more, the patient must be upgraded into the Rapid Transport Category.

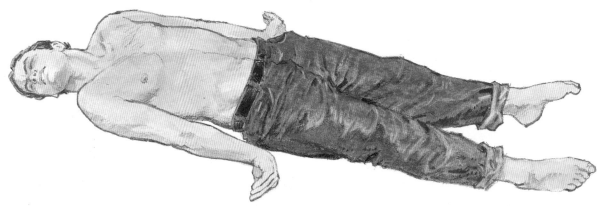

Figure III-5 Decerebrate posturing

TABLE III-c

GLASGOW COMA SCORE

EYE OPENING

Spontaneous	4
To Voice	3
To Pain	2
None	1

MOTOR RESPONSE

Obeys Commands	6
Localizes to Pain	5
Withdrawal to Pain	4
Decorticate Response (Flexion)	3
Decerebrate Response (Extensor)	2
No Response	1

VERBAL RESPONSE

Normal	5
Confused but Coherent	4
Simple Inappropriate Words	3
Incomprehensible Speech	2
No Speech	1

TOTAL

Highest Possible Score is 15
Lowest Possible Score is 3

Pupils

The Attendant must examine the pupils, especially if a head injury is suspected. The pupil is the dark central disk in the middle of the eye. The pupils are normally round and are equal to each other in diameter. In bright light, they each constrict (the diameter gets smaller). In darkness, they dilate (diameter gets larger). Shining a bright light (e.g. a flashlight) into one eye normally causes *both* pupils to constrict equally. Once the light is removed, the pupils *both* dilate back to their previous size. The Attendant should examine both eyes and determine if the pupils are constricted, normal or dilated and whether or not they are equal to each other. The Attendant should then shine a light into one eye and note the pupillary response. Remember, the pupils should both constrict quite briskly. If no light is available, the Attendant can close the patient's eyelids and then open them quickly. The pupillary response to uncovering the eyes should be noted. Once again, the normal response is a constriction.

A dilated, poorly reactive pupil caused by head injury is usually associated with a significant decrease in the patient's level of consciousness. If one pupil is dilated and poorly responsive to light, the Attendant must suspect a serious head injury and treat the patient accordingly (see Part VI, Section C, page 134, on Head Injuries). The Attendant must transport such patients to hospital rapidly.

A significant percentage of normal individuals have one pupil that is slightly larger than the other. The key difference between these individuals and those with serious head injury is that the slightly larger pupil of the normal

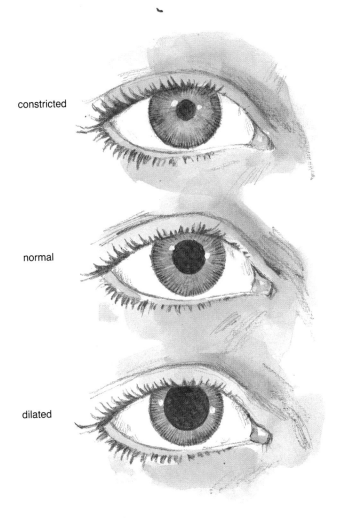

constricted

normal

dilated

Pupil reaction

a narrow temperature range. Extreme changes in body temperature are life-threatening. Too low a temperature (hypothermia) and too high (heat stroke) are equally life-threatening conditions. Body temperature is not usually measured in the field. Critically ill patients require rapid transport to hospital and there is not usually time to measure it. Minor injuries do not usually require the measurement of temperature for treatment purposes.

When hypothermia is a consideration (e.g. from exposure or near drowning), the only reliable temperature recording is a rectal recording. It is usually inconvenient, difficult or embarrassing to measure rectal temperature on your patient. Furthermore, ordinary thermometers cannot be used to measure hypothermia because the scale on ordinary thermometers does not go low enough. Special thermometers are required.

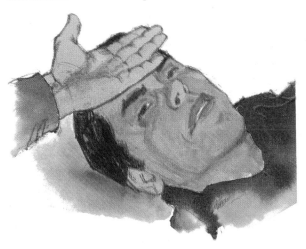

Assessing body temperature

individual constricts briskly to light while the dilated pupil in the head injury patient responds sluggishly or not at all. Furthermore, head injury patients with a dilated and poorly reactive pupil will usually have an altered level of consciousness.

The Attendant must not be fooled by patients with previous eye injuries or conditions (eye surgery, prescription eye drops or even a glass eye) that might result in unusual pupillary appearance. This underscores once again the value of obtaining the past medical history either from the patient or co-workers.

Temperature

Changes in body temperature are important because the complex metabolism of the body cells is dependent on

Nevertheless, recording the temperature is important when evaluating someone for a possible wound infection and anyone with a medical illness (as opposed to traumatic injury). The Attendant should feel the patient's skin temperature (forehead or abdominal wall) with the back of the hand just as mother used to do. Significant fever is usually readily noticeable.

Once the vital signs have been completed, the Attendant proceeds with the remainder of the secondary survey.

Chief Complaint and History of Current Injury or Illness

Obtain a history of the illness or injury, e.g. what happened? Determine the chief complaint by asking the patient what is bothering him/her the most. In general, allow patients to answer in their own words. Try to avoid "rapid-fire interrogation".

Sometimes the patient cannot remember or doesn't know what happened. In those instances, witnesses may be the only source of information.

Obtaining and recording the history of the injury is extremely important.

Most patients with injuries usually complain of pain of the affected region. Using the following mnemonic will help you gather all the necessary information related to a complaint of "pain", caused by injury or otherwise. Remember the mnemonic **PQRST.**

P = Position. Where is the pain located? Can the patient point to the pain?

Q = Quality of the Pain. What does it feel like? Sharp? Throbbing? Aching? Pressure-like?

R = Radiation. Is the pain localized to one region or does it spread (or radiate) to another area?

S = Severity. Have you ever had pain like this before? On a scale of 1 to 10, with 1 being minimal pain and 10 being excruciating pain, how would you rate the pain? What relieves the pain? What makes it worse? Changing position? Breathing?

T = Timing. How long ago did the pain start? Does it come and go or is it constant? Is it getting worse, better or staying the same?

Here is an example of how to use the mnemonic.

Example: Patient hurt back while lifting a heavy object:

P — "Low back pain."

Q — "Severe stabbing pain."

R — "Radiates down my left leg and up my back."

S — "Severe — 8/10." "It feels better if I don't move."

T — "Started when I lifted that heavy object half an hour ago and it's getting worse."

The next important part of the history is to determine the presence of associated problems. For example, if the patient complains of chest pain, ask if the pain is associated with shortness of breath. In general, associated problems are directly related to the region of injury. In the previous example of the patient complaining of back injury, it would be important to ask if there is any associated weakness or numbness of the lower extremities. In general, think of the injury (the back) and then ask about problems associated with the spinal cord or spinal nerves. This would manifest itself as weakness and/or numbness of the lower extremities.

Many injuries are associated with nausea, vomiting, general weakness, dizziness or sweating, and it is often helpful to specifically enquire about these symptoms.

Past Medical History

The next step in the history-taking process is to enquire about other medical illnesses (e.g. diabetes, heart disease, respiratory illness, seizures) and to ask about past illnesses related to the major complaint. Using the same example of the patient with back injury, it would be helpful to find out if the patient has had similar problems in the past; in this example, the patient has had previous surgery for a slipped disc in the lower back. The IFA Attendant should also enquire about previous hospitalizations.

Review of Systems

The next stage of the history-taking process is called the review of systems. Many patients will not volunteer all their problems during the initial questioning. Often, they focus only on the most painful region, "forgetting" the others. The careful Attendant will ask if the patient has any injuries to the head, face, neck, chest, abdomen or extremities, if they have not already been covered. In view of the importance of the ABCs (i.e. airway, breathing, circulation), the Attendant should always ask about any shortness of breath. Because of the frequency of neck and back injuries, ask specifically about those areas. Also, ascertain the presence of weakness or numbness in the extremities in all patients with head, cervical or back injuries.

Medications and Allergies

The last stage of the history is to record the patient's current medications and allergies. If possible, the Attendant should document the name, dose and frequency of use of current medication.

Head-To-Toe Examination

HEAD

The general approach to physical examination is inspection and palpation, i.e. look and feel, starting with the head and proceeding with the various regions; neck, chest, abdomen, extremities and back.

The Attendant observes the patient's head and face for open wounds, lacerations, swellings or deformities. The nose and oral cavity should be inspected for lacerations, blood or broken/displaced teeth. The patient's eyes also require careful assessment. If the patient is awake and alert enough, enquire about quality of vision; ask about contact lenses. The pupils have already been examined under vital signs above but may be reassessed here.

Open wounds and deep lacerations should not be probed, as the Attendant may cause excessive bleeding or cause further injury to delicate structures such as nerves or blood vessels. Bleeding from open wounds is controlled best by direct pressure. The facial bones and scalp should be palpated for areas of deformity or tenderness. Patients with suspected facial fractures are at particular risk for developing airway obstruction from soft tissue swelling or bleeding. All patients with severe facial injury should be assumed to have a cervical spine injury as well and be immobilized accordingly.

The Attendant should examine the ear canals for evidence of bleeding. The area just behind the ear should also be examined for bruising. These may be some of the signs of fracture of the base of the skull indicating head injury (see Part VI, Section C, page 129).

NECK

The neck is also inspected for evidence of injury, looking for swelling, deformity or open wounds. Patients with injuries to the anterior aspect of the neck may develop airway obstruction. Listen for evidence of hoarseness or stridor (high-pitched noise on inspiration and/or expiration). Because of the presence of major arteries and veins in the neck, penetrating injuries are potentially life-threatening. Therefore, penetrating injuries of the neck are in the Rapid Transport Category. Open wounds should not be probed and bleeding must be controlled by direct pressure. Direct pressure applied to wounds of the neck usually will not cause airway obstruction. Care must be taken not to apply pressure simultaneously to both sides of the anterior neck. (See Part V, Section C, page 110, on Bleeding and its Management.) Swelling of the neck from blunt or penetrating injury is also particularly dangerous because it may extend internally and precipitate airway obstruction.

All patients with a decreased level of consciousness must be assumed to have a cervical spine injury and be properly immobilized. The conscious patient should be asked about the presence of neck pain. If the answer is positive, the cervical spine should be fully immobilized. If the patient is conscious and denies neck pain, the cervical spine may be gently palpated for tenderness without moving the victim. If tenderness is elicited, the patient's cervical spine should also be immobilized. If the mechanism of injury is associated with a high risk of cervical spine injury, the cervical spine should be immobilized. (See Part VI, Section D, page 154, on Spinal Injuries.)

CHEST AND ABDOMEN

The chest and abdomen are then examined for evidence of injury. The Attendant must look for bruising or open wounds and palpate the chest and abdomen for tenderness. Chest wall or abdominal wall injuries must alert the Attendant to the presence of serious internal injuries. The motion of the chest wall should be observed during deep inspiration and expiration for evidence of pain, flail chest or pneumothorax. (See Part IV, Section C, page 59, on Traumatic Respiratory Emergencies.) Normally, when an individual breathes in, the chest wall rises and then falls on expiration. In the presence of multiple rib fractures, a segment of the chest wall may become disconnected from the rest of the bony thorax. On inspiration, this segment will not rise but will paradoxically fall inward. On expiration, as the chest wall falls in, this segment will expand outward. The condition is known as a flail chest and is usually associated with severe pulmonary injury and dysfunction. Therefore, as previously mentioned, patients with a flail chest fall into the Rapid Transport Category. Similarly, penetrating injuries of the chest and abdomen, because of their tendency to cause serious internal injuries, are also in the Rapid Transport Category.

The Attendant should note whether or not the abdomen is tender to palpation or if it is distended. These signs may indicate internal bleeding. The bony pelvis should be palpated for evidence of instability or tenderness.

BACK

The back must also be examined for evidence of injury. An initial examination can be performed by gently palpating the back for obvious bleeding, tenderness or deformity. A more complete examination, including visual inspection, can be done most efficiently while log-rolling the patient onto the spine board or other lifting device. Otherwise, the patient must be specifically log-rolled at the end of the secondary survey to examine the back. If a spinal injury has already been diagnosed, this step should not be done. (See page 145—Spinal Injuries and their Management.)

THE EXTREMITIES

The extremities are examined for evidence of trauma. Both upper and lower extremities must be checked for evidence of lacerations, swelling or gross deformity. Fractures are usually detected by the presence of pain, swelling and deformity of the affected limb. The limb should be palpated for signs of deformity or pain. In a patient with a decreased level of consciousness, the Attendant may have to rely on evidence of swelling and/or deformity. However, when a fracture or deep laceration is suspected, it is crucial that the Attendant examine the pulses distal to the injury site to determine whether or not a vascular injury is present. For injuries of the upper extremities, the radial pulse on the affected side must be checked. For injuries of the lower extremities, the Attendant must check the dorsalis pedis pulse (on the top of the foot — see Figure III-6) and the posterior tibialis pulse (on the inside of the foot, behind the ankle — see Figure III-7). Alternatively, capillary refill of the fingers or toes on the affected limb can be checked. Capillary refill is the return of colour to the nail bed or skin after squeezing the tip of the finger or toe. Measuring skin temperature of the corresponding hand or foot may also be helpful. Distal sensory and motor function must also be assessed in all patients with fractures or deep lacerations.

Because of the energy (or force) required to fracture two or more proximal long bones of the body (i.e. femur or humerus), these patients usually have other associated internal injuries which may not be detected by the Attendant. That is why these patients are in the Rapid Transport Category.

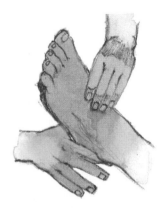

Figure III-6 Assessing the dorsalis pedis pulse

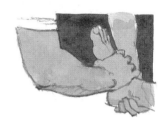

Figure III-7 Assessing the posterior tibialis pulse

NEUROLOGICAL EXAMINATION

A NEUROLOGICAL EXAMINATION MUST BE PERFORMED, ESPECIALLY IF A HEAD OR SPINAL CORD INJURY IS SUSPECTED. Assessment of the level of consciousness and pupillary response has already been discussed. The Attendant should assess both motor and sensory function.

Motor function is assessed by testing the various muscle groups of the body. For simplicity's sake and to conserve precious minutes, the Attendant should focus on motor function of the face, the upper extremities and the lower extremities. Motor function of the face can be assessed by having the patient smile or noting the facial features in response to a painful stimulus. A facial droop is a sign of paralysis of the facial muscles and represents an inability to lift the corner of the mouth when smiling or grimacing (i.e. drooping). Motor function of the upper extremities is tested by examining hand grips (ask the patient to squeeze the Attendant's fingers with one hand) or by arm raising (have the patient raise both arms upwards and perpendicular to the body). The best method is left to the judgment of the Attendant, taking into consideration any upper extremity injury. The Attendant should specifically look for any weakness not related to direct extremity injury. Special note should also be made of any difference (asymmetry) between the left and right arms. In the patient with a decreased level of consciousness, the Attendant should observe the response to a painful stimulus applied to each extremity (e.g. pressure on the nail bed). Again, the Attendant should note any asymmetry in the response.

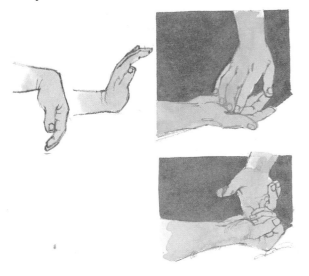

Assessing motor and sensory function in the upper limbs

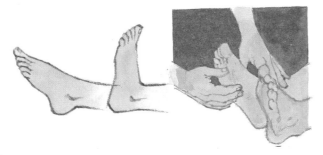

Assessing motor and sensory function in the feet

The motor function of the lower extremities is examined in a similar way. The Attendant should ask the patient to wiggle the feet or lift the legs at least one foot off the ground. The Attendant should specifically look for the presence of weakness and for any asymmetry between the strength of one leg compared to the other. In the patient with a decreased level of consciousness, a painful stimulus applied to the foot (pressure to the nail bed of the big toe)

usually elicits a motor response. The absence of response may indicate paralysis of that limb. Similarly, the response in one limb should be compared to the response in the other. Asymmetry of response or lack of any response, in the absence of a significant injury to the limb, is usually an indication of a neurological injury.

Sensory function may be tested by asking the conscious patient if there is numbness or tingling anywhere. Alternatively, the patient may be asked what is felt when the Attendant touches fingers or toes or any other part of the patient's body. In the comatose patient, sensory function is impossible to assess accurately. However, if the patient responds to a painful stimulus, it provides a clue that at least some sensory function is present. The absence of any response indicates that either sensory or motor function is absent but is not any more specific.

In summary, the neurological examination consists of three components:

1. Assessment of the level of consciousness using the Glasgow Coma Score (GCS)
2. Examination of pupils and their response to bright light
3. Determination of sensory and motor function of the face and all limbs

SUMMARY

This completes the secondary survey, a head-to-toe assessment of the patient as follows:

*   Vital signs
*   Chief complaint(s) and history of current injury or illness
*   Medications
*   Allergies
*   Head-to-toe examination
    *   Head
    *   Neck
    *   Chest
    *   Abdomen
    *   Pelvis and back
    *   Extremities
    *   Neurological examination

With the completion of the secondary survey, the Attendant can now proceed in a logical and systematic way to prioritize the patient's injuries and treat accordingly. At the beginning of this section we emphasized the importance of identifying serious injury and rapidly transporting these patients to hospital. With an understanding of basic anatomy and remembering the concept of energy transfer and injury potential, the presence of certain injuries must alert the Attendant to the presence of major trauma. Because of the reserve capacity of the circulatory and respiratory systems, the patient's vital signs may be normal initially in spite of serious injury. The Attendant is reminded of the importance of the Rapid Transport Criteria outlined on page 19.

PATIENTS WHO FALL INTO THE RAPID TRANSPORT CATEGORY REQUIRE CLOSE MONITORING WHICH INCLUDES REASSESSMENT OF THE VITAL SIGNS AT LEAST EVERY 10 MINUTES. IN THOSE TRAUMA PATIENTS WHERE A CRITICAL INTERVENTION WAS REQUIRED THE ABCs SHOULD BE REASSESSED EVERY 5 MINUTES.

This section covers all the essentials of trauma assessment outlining the Priority Action Approach. Following the methods outlined in this section allows the Attendant to focus on the patient rather than trying to figure out what to do next. However, practise makes perfect and optimal speed is achieved by team work. Plan regular exercises in patient evaluation to maintain your skills. Above all, remember the "golden hour".

Here is an outline of the Priority Action Approach for injured workers.

PRIORITY ACTION APPROACH

1. Scene assessment
2. Primary survey
   - Airway with C-spine control
   - Breathing
   - Circulation
3. Critical intervention/transport decision
4. Secondary survey
5. Treatment/transport decision

Part IV, Section A
Respiratory System Anatomy and Function

All living cells of the body extract energy from nutrients in a process called metabolism. In the course of metabolism, each cell uses oxygen and produces carbon dioxide as a waste substance.

Each living cell in the body requires a constant supply of oxygen, although some cells are more dependent than others. At normal temperatures, cells in the brain and central nervous system begin to die after four to six minutes without oxygen. Those cells can never be replaced and permanent disability may result from the damage.

RESPIRATORY SYSTEM (Figure IV-1)

The respiratory system supplies oxygen to the blood and removes the gaseous waste product carbon dioxide from it. Oxygen is obtained from the air, which is a mixture of oxygen, nitrogen, carbon dioxide and other gases. Air is delivered to the body through the respiratory system, which comprises:
- the airways (nose, mouth, pharynx, trachea, bronchi)
- the lungs (bronchioles, alveoli, pleura)
- thoracic muscles (intercostal, diaphragm)
- thoracic bones (ribs, sternum)

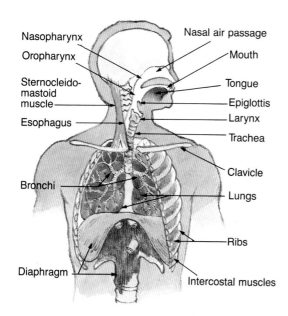

Figure IV-1 Respiratory System

AIRWAYS

Nose and Mouth

The upper airway is made up of the nose and mouth. Air is taken in through the nose or mouth. The lining of the nasal cavities contains many blood vessels, which heat and moisten the air.

Pharynx

The air passes into the back of the throat (pharynx). The muscular pharynx serves as a passageway for foods and liquids into the digestive system and for air into the respiratory system. The lower portion of the pharynx opens into two passageways:
1. anteriorly, the air pathway through the larynx (voice-box) down the trachea and into the lung;
2. posteriorly, the food pathway into the esophagus.

Guarding the opening of the larynx is a small, oval-shaped flap of tissue called the epiglottis. The epiglottis keeps food and foreign material out of the trachea, thus preventing choking. (See Section B, page 39, Airway Management Section.)

Trachea

The trachea is a tube that extends from the lower edge of the larynx to the centre of the chest behind the heart. It is a semi-rigid tube partially supported by rings of cartilage. These rings keep the trachea from collapsing when air is moved in and out of the lungs.

Bronchi

The trachea divides into the left and the right bronchus. These are the two main air tubes entering the lungs.

LUNGS

There are two lungs, one on each side suspended in the thoracic cavity.

Bronchioles

As soon as each bronchus enters the lung, it subdivides into branches which resemble those of a tree. Each individual bronchial tube subdivides again and again, forming progressively smaller divisions. The smallest are called bronchioles.

Alveoli

At the end of each bronchiole, there is a cluster of air sacs, resembling a bunch of grapes, known as alveoli. Each alveolus has a very thin wall, covered with many tiny capillaries. This arrangement provides an easy passage for oxygen and carbon dioxide entering and leaving the blood.

As the blood passes through the capillaries of the alveoli, gas exchange takes place. Oxygen leaves the air in the alveolus and passes into the blood in the capillary, while carbon dioxide passes in the opposite direction.

Pleura

Covering each lung is a doubled-walled sac of very smooth, slippery tissue called pleura. One layer of this sac lines the inside of the chest cavity and the other layer covers the lungs. Between these two layers is the "pleural space", which is, in fact, only a potential space, because the layers are in contact everywhere. Each layer is tightly sealed against the other by a thin film of fluid. When the chest wall expands, the lung is pulled with it and expands because of suction exerted by these closely applied pleural surfaces.

Any break in the sealed pleural space will permit air or blood to enter and separate the pleural surfaces, creating a space between the lung and the chest wall. Any collections of fluid, blood or air in this pleural space will interfere with efficient respiration.

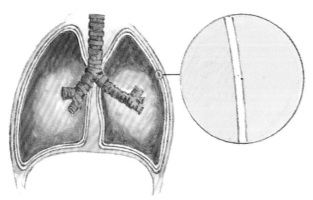

Yellow insert shows Pleural space

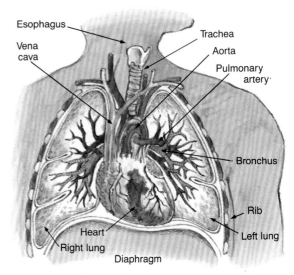

Organs of the chest cavity

THORACIC (CHEST) MUSCLES AND BONES

The thoracic cavity is a bony cage made up of the 12 thoracic vertebrae, 12 pairs of ribs and the sternum (breast bone). It is bounded below by the diaphragm. In the thorax are the lungs, esophagus, heart and major blood vessels.

The inner aspect of the thoracic cavity is also lined with pleura. Between the lungs is a space called the mediastinum which contains the heart, major blood vessels, trachea and esophagus.

MECHANICS OF BREATHING

There are two phases of breathing:
1. inhalation — air drawn into the lungs
2. exhalation — the expulsion of air from the lungs

During inhalation, the muscles of respiration (the diaphragm and intercostal muscles) contract to enlarge the thoracic cavity. When the muscles contract, pressure decreases in the sealed pleural spaces, causing a negative pressure within the chest. This causes a pull on the elastic lung tissue so that air rushes in to fill the air sacs.

During exhalation, the muscles of respiration relax, decreasing the size of the thoracic cavity. As the pressure in the chest is increased and becomes positive, air is pushed out through the trachea.

INHALATION

EXHALATION

Mechanics of breathing

RESPIRATORY CENTRE

Breathing is controlled by the respiratory centre in the brainstem (at the base of the brain). Breathing is involuntary, but it can be controlled to some extent.

The respiratory centre is governed by changes in the chemistry of the blood. If there is an increase in carbon dioxide or a decrease in oxygen (i.e. hypoxia), the respiratory centre is stimulated to increase the respiratory rate. The increase in respiratory rate will increase the level of oxygen and decrease the level of carbon dioxide in the blood.

Respiratory Rate

The normal rate of breathing varies from 12 to 20 times per minute, but it is normally higher in children.

The oxygen demand of the body depends upon the degree of activity in body cells. Some injuries and diseases affect the respiratory rate.

Part IV, Section B
Airway Management

PERSPECTIVE

There is little doubt that, of all the possible procedures performed by the IFA Attendant, securing and maintaining a "patent" (clear) airway in the injured patient is truly life saving and always the first priority. The IFA Attendant has limited techniques and equipment at his/her disposal. Therefore, basic airway management skills, as discussed in this section, must be perfected. Conversely, inability to recognize or failure to treat an unstable airway may be fatal.

Injuries occur in a multitude of settings: e.g. logging operations, construction sites and industrial plants. They occur at all times of the day and night with resultant extremes in lighting and temperature. We therefore need treatment options because what works in one setting may not succeed in another. For example, the IFA Attendant traditionally has been taught to manage the patient with a suspected airway problem in the ¾ prone position. In this section, you will learn that this is not always the best approach and, in certain settings, is detrimental to patient care.

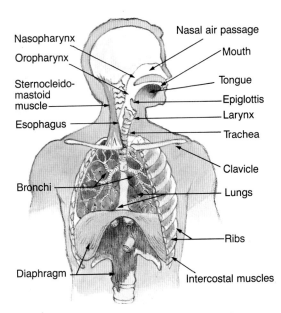

Anatomy of the respiratory system

ANATOMY

The various tissues of the body such as muscle, brain or heart require oxygen and other basic nutrients in order to perform their functions. Carbon dioxide (CO_2) is one of the waste products of tissue function. In order for tissues to function normally, the body must maintain a certain level of oxygen. Similarly, the level of carbon dioxide, a waste product, must also be kept near its normal level and not be allowed to rise significantly. The purpose of the respiratory system is to maintain adequate levels of oxygen and carbon dioxide in the body. The components of the respiratory system are:

- the airway
- the thorax
- the lungs

The airway is composed of the nose, mouth and throat (pharynx). The lower part of the pharynx divides into two passageways: the esophagus (through which food passes on the way to the stomach) and the trachea (which opens into the lungs). The trachea lies in front of (anterior to) the esophagus. The trachea is reinforced by hard cartilage rings. The trachea can be palpated in the midline, extending from the Adam's Apple to the sternum. The tracheal opening is protected by a small flap of tissue called the epiglottis. The muscles of the pharynx will cause the epiglottis to flip down and close the tracheal opening when swallowing. This prevents "choking on food". The airway acts only as a conduit, carrying air with oxygen *into* the lungs with inhalation and carbon dioxide from the lungs with exhalation. It is readily apparent why partial or complete obstruction of the airway is life threatening. This will be discussed in further detail below.

The voice box or larynx is located within the Adam's Apple at the opening of the trachea, below the epiglottis.

ASSESSMENT OF THE AIRWAY

It is absolutely essential that the Attendant learn to recognize the partially obstructed or completely obstructed airway. The IFA Attendant should be able to feel air passing in and out of the nose or mouth. If the conscious patient is able to speak clearly, even if the content of the speech is confused, then the airway is patent at that time.

An unstable airway is either partially or completely obstructed. The passage of air in and out of the airway (i.e. breathing) is normally silent. Noisy, congested or gurgling breathing may be the signs of a partially obstructed airway. The presence of hoarseness may be an indication of injury to the vocal cords located in the larynx. This is also a sign of an unstable airway. Stridor is a high-pitched noise that may be present in inspiration or expiration, or both. It results from a narrowing of the airway which creates a whistling noise to the passage of air. It represents constriction or narrowing of the airway and signals the presence of a partially obstructed airway that may completely close (occlude). Table IV-a below lists the signs of a compromised airway.

TABLE IV-a

Partial Obstruction	Complete Obstruction
1. noisy breathing	1. cyanosis
2. hoarseness	2. no movement of air in or out of the mouth or nose
3. stridor	3. chest wall does not rise with ventilations
4. possible cyanosis	4. if conscious, unable to vocalize

The patient with a completely obstructed airway will be cyanotic or ashen grey. With each attempt at respiration, the muscles of the neck and chest wall will be taut in an attempt to draw air into the lungs. If the obstruction has been present for some time, the patient may lose consciousness and cease making respiratory efforts. When an attempt is made to ventilate the patient, the chest wall will not rise because air cannot enter the lungs. Once the presence of a partially or completely obstructed airway is recognized, the Attendant must immediately begin the basic procedures to clear the airway.

CAUSES OF AIRWAY OBSTRUCTION

The most common cause of airway obstruction is the tongue. In the comatose patient who has lost voluntary control of the muscles of the mouth and throat, the tongue falls backwards (when the patient is supine) and obstructs the airway. Lifting the jaw by the recommended man-

oeuvres will cause the tongue to be pulled up and out of the way. Insertion of an oropharyngeal or oral airway will maintain the patency of the airway.

Foreign bodies or material are the next most common cause of airway obstruction. During assessment of the airway, foreign bodies such as loose-fitting dentures or broken teeth must be removed. Vomitus and blood can also obstruct the airway and must be removed, with body positioning, finger sweep or suction.

Swelling from injury to the soft tissue of the throat, neck or larynx can also cause airway obstruction. Some of the more common examples of tissue injury are direct blows to the anterior neck, facial fractures and smoke or chemical inhalation.

Often, the onset of airway obstruction is delayed and the Attendant must reassess these patients for the signs of airway compromise. There are many patients who are fine initially, only to deteriorate rapidly from delayed onset of airway obstruction.

BASIC TECHNIQUES OF AIRWAY MANAGEMENT

Airway assessment is the first priority for any patient. The treatment of airway emergencies must be guided by two concerns: (1) whether or not the patient is conscious, and (2) whether or not a cervical spine injury is suspected. As will be discussed in Part VI, Section D, page 141, a cervical spine injury must be suspected in any patient who has fallen from a height, who has been involved in a serious MVA, who has been injured while diving, or who has suffered any injuries involving the head or face.

In general, management of the airway in the absence of a suspected neck injury follows the current CPR guidelines outlined by the Canadian Heart Foundation.

THE FOLLOWING PROCEDURES DEAL SPECIFICALLY WITH AIRWAY MANAGEMENT IN TRAUMA PATIENTS OR WHENEVER A NECK INJURY IS SUSPECTED.

The first rule of first aid is: "Do no harm." The worst possible scenario would be to accidentally make the patient quadriplegic for life while clearing the airway. The following protocols will ensure that no harm will come to the patient.

Begin with the primary survey. Attendants should identify themselves in a reassuring manner, telling the patient to lie still, and asking a simple question like "What happened?" The patient's reply will give immediate information about the patency of the airway and level of consciousness. If the patient responds appropriately, with clear speech, it is now established that the airway is clear. The Attendant should then proceed with the remainder of the primary survey.

AIRWAY ASSESSMENT AND MANAGEMENT FOR THE CONSCIOUS PATIENT

The Attendant should use the LOOK, LISTEN AND FEEL approach to airway assessment. Often, conscious patients will be able to indicate, either by telling you or pointing, that an airway problem exists. The Attendant first "looks" at the patient and checks for the presence of cyanosis and/or evidence of respiratory distress. The patient may be able to open his/her mouth and the Attendant should perform a visual check for foreign bodies, bleeding, swelling or burns. "Listening" for air moving in and out of the mouth or nose is done best by placing one's ear next to the patient's face. Conscious patients with partial airway obstruction will often have stridor or hoarseness. Finally, the Attendant may "feel" for the movement of air with the cheek or bare hand. The rise and fall of the chest wall may also be assessed by "feel".

Conscious patients with partial or complete airway obstruction usually maintain a position that maximizes their ability to breathe and minimizes the degree of airway obstruction. These patients may be quite agitated and resistant to attempts to provide any treatment. For example, a hard cervical collar may not be tolerated. A face mask for providing supplemental oxygen may be "suffocating" to the patient.

The first step, however, is to provide supplemental high-flow oxygen by mask. The mask may be held by the Attendant as close as possible to the patient's face if wearing the face mask is intolerable. If the patient has blood, vomitus or other foreign material in the mouth, but is conscious, ask the patient to clear the airway by spitting or coughing the debris out. Assist if possible. Use a suction device if one is available but be very gentle. The Attendant should be careful not to cause any gagging. If a neck injury is suspected, the Attendant must stabilize the neck. If the patient is sitting upright, the Attendant should manually stabilize the patient's neck in a neutral position while encouraging the patient to clear the airway. If the patient is lying down, the Attendant should assist by rolling the patient into the lateral position to facilitate drainage. Once again, if a neck injury is suspected, the neck must be manually stabilized as the Attendant moves the patient. Do not insert an oral airway in a conscious patient with a partial airway obstruction as it may worsen the situation (e.g. completely obstructing the airway).

If a foreign body is suspected as the cause of the obstruction and the patient is unable to clear it, then abdominal thrusts (Heimlich manoeuvre), with the patient upright or in the supine position, would be of benefit.

Abdominal thrusts in either upright or supine position increase intra-abdominal pressure, which forcefully elevates the diaphragm. This, in turn, forces air out of the lungs, up the trachea and out the nose and mouth. It is thought that this force of air from the trachea may be strong enough to dislodge any foreign body obstructing the airway. For the trauma victim, one of the disadvantages of the Heimlich manoeuvre in the sitting position is the inability to stabilize the neck while doing it and, therefore, the supine position is preferred. On the other hand, the patient with a partial airway obstruction may resist the Attendant's attempts to lay the patient down. Ultimately, the Attendant must use common sense and good judgment when choosing either of the two positions. Finally, in the setting of blunt trauma to the anterior aspects of the neck and face, or in the case of smoke-inhalation injury, partial airway obstruction is usually due to swelling rather than a foreign body. In these situations, abdominal thrusts (Heimlich manoeuvre) will be ineffective and potentially harmful (i.e. it may induce vomiting).

The treatment protocol is essentially the same for patients with complete airway obstruction (except abdominal thrusts). Patients with complete airway obstruction usually lose consciousness rapidly and the Attendant should refer to the treatment protocols for the patient with a decreased level of consciousness.

If initial attempts to clear the airway fail, the Attendant repeats the cycle again and again as indicated in the flow chart. The Attendant must remember that patients with persistent partial airway obstruction are in the Rapid Transport Category.

AIRWAY ASSESSMENT AND MANAGEMENT FOR THE PATIENT WITH A DECREASED LEVEL OF CONSCIOUSNESS

THE PATIENT WITH A DECREASED LEVEL OF CONSCIOUSNESS IS BEST MANAGED IN THE SUPINE POSITION, ESPECIALLY IF THE PATIENT HAS RESPIRATORY DISTRESS OR A SUSPECTED AIRWAY OBSTRUCTION. THE ONLY EXCEPTIONS ARE THE PATIENTS WHO ARE ACTIVELY VOMITING OR WHO HAVE PROFUSE BLEEDING OF THE MOUTH OR NOSE. IN THESE CASES, THE PATIENT MUST BE TREATED IN THE LATERAL POSITION. IN ALL CASES, THE NECK MUST BE STABILIZED IN THE ANATOMICAL POSITION.

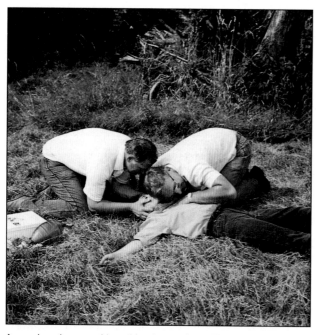

Assessing airway and breathing in a patient with a decreased level of consciousness

Once vomiting has stopped, the patient may be rolled to the supine position to complete the primary survey.

The patient with a decreased level of consciousness does not always vomit. Pooled secretions are not usually a problem in these patients. It is easier to assess the patient and provide airway management in the supine position.

THE PATIENT WITH A DECREASED LEVEL OF CONSCIOUSNESS MUST NEVER BE LEFT UNATTENDED IN THE SUPINE POSITION.

If for any reason the Attendant has to leave the patient's side, the patient should be moved to the lateral position until the Attendant returns.

If the patient's airway can be adequately assessed in the position found (i.e. look, listen and feel), the Attendant should proceed with the airway examination. If not, the patient must be log-rolled with careful C-spine control to the lateral or supine position in order to accurately assess the airway. The Attendant uses the "look, listen and feel" approach to assess the patient's airway. The Attendant observes whether or not the chest wall is rising, checking for the presence of cyanosis and looking for evidence of respiratory distress. The Attendant then listens for air moving in and out of the mouth or nose. Finally, the Attendant may feel the movement of air with a bare hand. Similarly, the rise and fall of the chest wall may be detected by feel. Unless the patient's collapse was witnessed and the Attendant can be assured that no significant injury occurred, all patients with a decreased level of consciousness must be treated as if they have a cervical spine injury. If unsure, it is always best to treat the patient as if there is cervical spine injury. The following procedures will provide safe, effective airway management in the trauma setting.

The Attendant should first attempt to open the airway with a jaw thrust manoeuvre. This is the method of choice because the Attendant can stabilize the neck at the same time. The Attendant can use an index finger to assess the carotid pulse. Never extend the neck of a trauma patient to open the airway. As illustrated in Figure IV-2, the thumbs are used to push the angles of the mandible forward. Because the tongue is attached to the jaw, it will be lifted forward and away from the posterior wall of the throat. This manoeuvre can also be performed if the patient is in the lateral position.

The Attendant should then attempt two ventialtions to see if the jaw thrust manoeuvre has cleared the airway. If the jaw thrust is successful, the patient's mouth should still be opened and a visual check of the oral cavity performed. Remove any loose-fitting dentures, foreign bodies or secretions from the oral cavity, using a finger sweep if necessary. A suction device would be helpful if available.

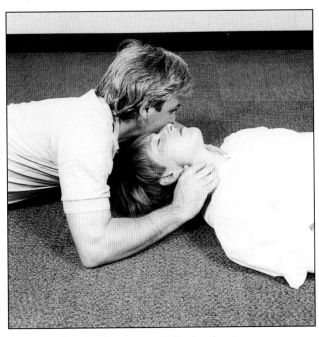

Figure IV-2 Opening the airway with the jaw thrust

An oral airway should then be inserted. Supplemental oxygen must be given and assisted ventilation may have to be provided if the patient's respiratory rate or depth of respirations are inadequate.

If the jaw thrust is unsuccessful and the airway remains partially or completely obstructed, the mouth should be opened and the pharynx cleared. Check for foreign material, dentures, teeth, etc. that may be present. Check the posterior throat carefully as this is often the location where foreign objects will obstruct the airway. Under poor lighting conditions, the pink colour of a denture plate at first glance will often be mistaken for normal tissue. At this point, reassess the airway.

If the combination of jaw thrust and clearing the airway is still unsuccessful at opening the airway, the Attendant must attempt to ventilate the patient with two slow, large forced breaths using mouth-to-mouth ventilations, a pocket mask or a bag-valve mask resuscitation device. If the chest wall rises with each breath, the airway is now patent. The Attendant should then insert an oral airway and ventilate the patient with a pocket mask or bag-valve mask device providing supplemental high-flow oxygen. The Attendant must frequently reassess the patient to ensure that the chest wall is still rising with each ventilation. Furthermore, the oral cavity may have to be cleared

of secretions often, using positioning, finger sweep or, if available, a suction device.

It is extremely difficult to assist ventilation in the lateral position as it is almost impossible to maintain a proper seal with the mask. Therefore, the supine position is preferred. As previously mentioned, the only exceptions are the presence of active vomiting or profuse bleeding of the mouth or nose. Therefore, in the absence of active vomiting or profuse bleeding of the mouth or nose, it is better to provide effective oxygenation and ventilation in the supine position than to be overly concerned about a potential risk (e.g. vomiting) and provide ineffective ventilation in the lateral position. The preferred position is the supine position.

AT ANY TIME, IF THE PATIENT RETCHES/ VOMITS:

1. LOG-ROLL THE PATIENT TO THE LATERAL POSITION, MAINTAINING STABILITY OF THE NECK
2. RAPIDLY CLEAR THE AIRWAY OF VOMITUS
3. AFTER THE PATIENT HAS STOPPED RETCHING OR VOMITING, REPOSITION SUPINE
4. RESTART ASSISTED VENTILATION

If the chest wall does not rise with forced breaths, a complete airway obstruction is present. The jaw thrust is attempted again. The mouth must be opened and the pharynx carefully rechecked for foreign debris. In this second attempt to clear the airway, an oral airway is inserted and then ventilation with two breaths is attempted. If the airway remains blocked, a series of abdominal thrusts (6-10) in the supine position should be attempted. If fewer attempts are successful, no further abdominal thrusts would be required.

However, if an oral airway had already been inserted, it must be removed prior to the abdominal thrusts. The presence of the oral airway could prevent the foreign body from being dislodged. Abdominal thrusts in the supine position are preferred because the patient does not have to be lifted (the patient is already supine) and there is no additional risk to the cervical spine. Following the abdominal thrusts, the oral cavity is again inspected for foreign bodies with a direct visual check and a finger sweep. Abdominal thrusts are not recommended unless a foreign body or debris is obstructing the airway. In the case of blunt neck trauma or smoke inhalation, where swelling is the usual cause of airway obstruction, abdominal thrusts should not be performed. Ventilation is again attempted. The sequence is repeated until successful. Once the airway is cleared, an oral airway should be inserted and the patient given assisted ventilation supplemented with high-flow oxygen. The primary survey is then completed. PATIENTS WITH A DECREASED LEVEL OF CONSCIOUSNESS, AND A PARTIAL OR COMPLETE AIRWAY OBSTRUCTION, EVEN AFTER THE AIRWAY IS CLEARED, ARE IN THE RAPID TRANSPORT CATEGORY. The secondary survey and any additional treatment must be done en route or while waiting for transport to arrive.

The patient with an airway that remains partially or completely obstructed requires immediate transport to hospital. The Attendant must continue attempts to clear the airway repeating the above procedures. At the same time, the patient must be prepared for rapid transport to hospital.

AIRWAY ASSESSMENT AND MANAGEMENT FOR THE PATIENT WITH A DECREASED LEVEL OF CONSCIOUSNESS AND VOMITING OR PROFUSE BLEEDING IN THE UPPER AIRWAY

Patients with a decreased level of consciousness, and active vomiting or profuse bleeding of the mouth or nose are the most difficult cases that the IFA Attendant will ever face. These patients must be initially assessed and treated in the lateral position. The same sequence of manoeuvres as previously described are used in this situation to open the airway. Repeated attempts however must be made to clear the oral cavity — drainage, finger sweeps and/or suction (if available). An oral airway is usually required to keep the mouth open to facilitate drainage. The oral cavity must be cleared as much as possible before the oral airway is inserted. The oral airway should not be inserted in the presence of large pieces of vomitus, broken teeth or blood clots, as it may push them back into the throat and cause a complete airway obstruction. One suggestion is to initially insert the oral airway only part way — just enough to keep the teeth and mouth open (thereby permitting drainage) but not far enough to precipitate airway obstruction. Once the oral cavity has been

cleared, the oral airway can then be fully inserted properly. Furthermore, the oral airway may become clogged with debris and must be frequently cleaned or changed.

If the airway has been cleared and the bleeding or vomiting has ceased, the patient should be rolled supine and assisted ventilation with high-flow oxygen should be provided to correct the patient's hypoxia. The primary survey is then completed. The patient's airway must be reassessed frequently. If bleeding or vomiting recurs, the patient is again rolled to the lateral position and the sequence is repeated.

If the airway remains partially obstructed by ongoing bleeding or active vomiting, the Attendant must repeat attempts to clear the oral cavity, maintaining the patient in the lateral position. At this point, the Attendant is faced with the following dilemma: despite the presence of the debris in the airway, the patient requires oxygen. The patient may also require assisted ventilation. How is this provided best in the setting of ongoing bleeding or vomiting in the upper airway?

If the patient with a decreased level of consciousness is breathing adequately despite the presence of foreign debris (i.e. the chest wall is rising and falling appropriately, air can be heard or felt moving in and out of the mouth), the Attendant must provide supplemental high-flow oxygen by hand-held mask without assisted ventilation. A tight-fitting mask may fill up with blood or vomitus. This may be prevented with a hand-held mask. The primary survey is then completed. Additional critical interventions are performed only if required and the patient is rapidly transported to hospital.

If the patient with a decreased level of consciousness is not breathing adequately because of blood or vomitus in the mouth, supplemental high-flow oxygen *with* assisted ventilation must be provided. However, the airway must first be cleared as well as possible. The positive pressure supplied with each assisted ventilation can force vomitus or blood into the trachea, worsening the degree of obstruction or causing aspiration. Despite these risks, the patient with a decreased level of consciousness who is not breathing adequately must be ventilated with high-flow oxygen.

In the lateral position, it is extremely difficult to achieve a good seal between the face and the mask. If possible, use two hands to hold the mask and ask an assistant to compress the ventilation bag. Furthermore, an oral airway must be inserted because the mouth is usually closed in the comatose patient in the lateral position. Brain tissue can only survive four to six minutes without oxygen before it is permanently damaged. Therefore, the Attendant cannot allow the patient with a decreased level of consciousness who is not breathing adequately to lie there waiting for the blood or vomitus to drain away. Assisted ventilation with high-flow oxygen must be provided.

The Attendant should provide two ventilations every 10 seconds. In between ventilations, the sequence of jaw thrusts and clearing of the oral cavity is continued. The oral airway and mask may have to be cleared or replaced because of bleeding or vomiting. The primary survey is completed and preparation is made to transport the patient rapidly to hospital.

FLOW CHART IV-a

AIRWAY MANAGEMENT FOR THE CONSCIOUS PATIENT

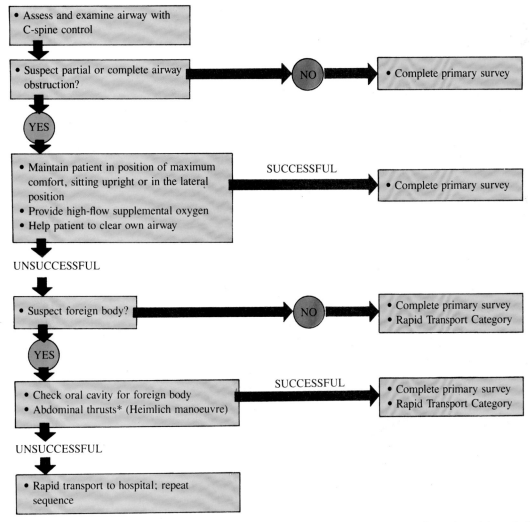

SPECIAL CASE: Profuse bleeding or vomiting in upper airway. Maintain patient in the lateral position. Stabilize C-spine. Suction aggressively, if available.

---

* Not recommended for smoke inhalation, neck or facial injuries.

FLOW CHART IV-b

AIRWAY MANAGEMENT FOR THE PATIENT WITH A DECREASED LEVEL OF CONSCIOUSNESS

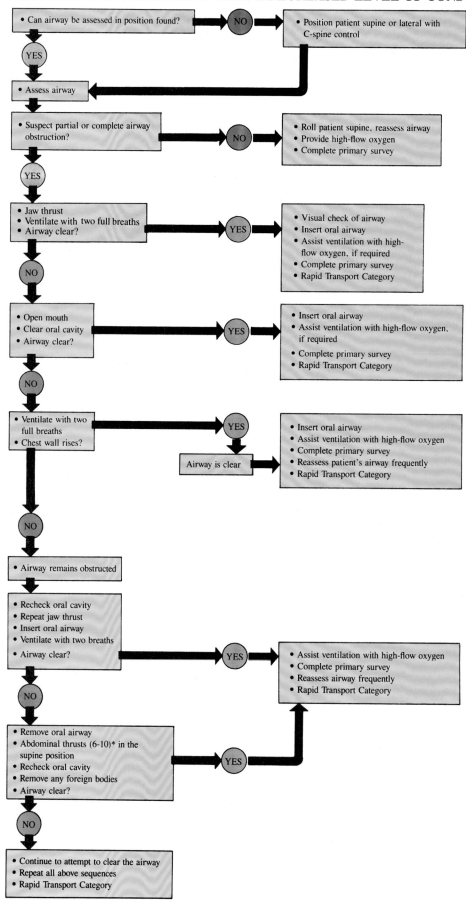

* Not recommended for smoke inhalation or blunt neck trauma.

FLOW CHART IV-c

SPECIFIC AIRWAY MANAGEMENT FOR THE PATIENT WITH A DECREASED LEVEL OF CONSCIOUSNESS, AND VOMITING OR PROFUSE BLEEDING IN UPPER AIRWAY

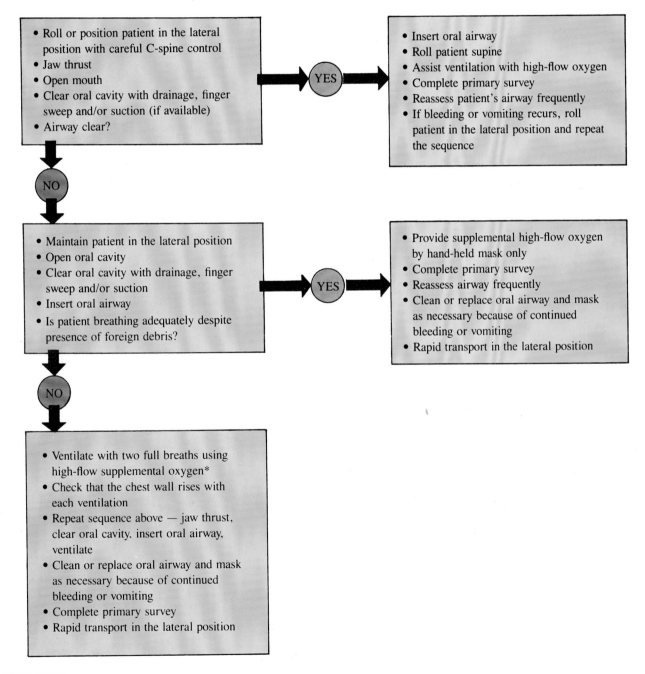

* NOTE: It is extremely difficult to assist ventilation in the lateral position. If possible, use two hands to maintain a good seal and ask an assistant to compress the ventilation bag.

TECHNIQUES FOR OPENING THE AIRWAY

1. Never extend or tilt the head to open the airway on a trauma victim. Head tilting is the basic technique taught in all CPR courses for the management of a cardiac arrest patient. However, the trauma patient must be treated differently. Tilting or extending the head of a patient with a cervical spine fracture may result in permanent spinal cord injury (quadriplegia).

2. **Modified jaw thrust.** This is the best procedure for the trauma patient. This method requires only one rescuer. It also allows the use of the index finger to check the carotid pulse at the same time. As illustrated in Figure IV-2, use the thumbs to push up or forward on the angles of the jaw. This has the effect of pushing the tongue forward and opening the airway.

   An alternative method is illustrated in Figure IV-3. Position three fingers behind the angle of the jaw with your thumbs on the cheekbones. Lift both hands, lifting the mandible upward as you push down on the cheekbones with the thumbs. For both methods, it is best to anchor the elbows on a stable surface. Do not extend or tilt the neck as you push or pull up on the jaw.

3. **Heimlich manoeuvre** (abdominal thrusts). This method is only to be used on a patient with a suspected foreign-body obstruction of the upper airway. It is ineffective for partial or complete airway obstruction due to swelling, secretions or bleeding (i.e. smoke inhalation, blunt neck or facial trauma).
   a) Patient in Sitting Position
      - From behind the victim, the Attendant wraps both arms around the patient's waist.
      - Make a fist with one hand and hold the fist (thumb side) against the victim's abdomen at a point midway between the lower tip of the sternum (breastbone) and the navel.
      - Grasp the fist with the other hand and press into the patient's abdomen with a quick, forceful thrust, directed upwards.
      - Repeat the thrusts until the foreign body is expelled (maximum 10 thrusts) or the patient collapses.

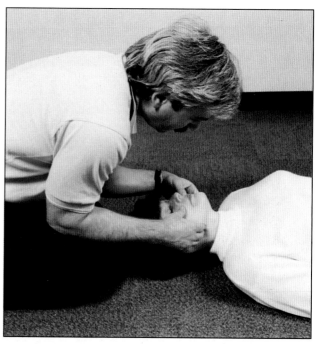

Figure IV-3 Alternative method placing thumbs on cheekbones and fingers behind the jaw

      - Reassess the patient's airway, remove foreign bodies.
      - Repeat all above sequences, if necessary.
   b) Patient Supine
      Have an assistant stabilize the neck to prevent it from flopping to the side. This method is not effective for partial or complete airway obstruction caused by swelling, secretions or bleeding (i.e. smoke inhalation, blunt neck or facial trauma).
      - The hands are positioned the same as for external chest compressions except that they are located well below the lower tip of the sternum (breastbone) but above the navel.
      - Compress the abdominal wall with a quick forceful thrust directed upwards.
      - Repeat the thrusts until the foreign body is expelled (up to a maximum of ten thrusts). The Attendant must then reassess the patient's airway and remove any foreign bodies.
      - Repeat all above sequences, if necessary.

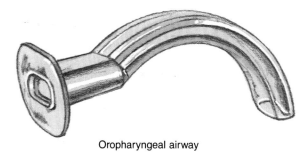

Oropharyngeal airway

4. **Oral airway.** The oral airway is a semi-circular hollow plastic device that, when inserted in the proper position, will maintain patency of the airway. It also has the advantage of keeping the mouth open to enable one to clear the airway with the index finger or with a suction device. For the patient who must be managed in the lateral position because of profuse bleeding or vomiting, it will permit drainage. Remember, the lateral and ¾ prone positions are only effective for drainage if the patient's mouth is open. If the victim is clenching the teeth or does not keep the mouth open, these positions will not permit drainage of blood or vomitus. THE INSERTION OF AN ORAL AIRWAY MUST BE ATTEMPTED ON ALL PATIENTS WHO ARE UNRESPONSIVE TO VERBAL STIMULATION.

There are two ways to insert an oral airway, once the correct size has been determined (see Figures IV-4a and IV-4b).

- The more common method is to insert the oral airway upside down sliding along the roof of the mouth. When almost completely inserted, rotate the airway 180° so that it slips into position behind the tongue.
- Open the mouth with a tongue depressor and push the tongue out of the way, then under direct vision insert the oral airway directly into position.

If the patient does not tolerate the oral airway, it must be removed because it may cause retching and vomiting. HOWEVER, THE ATTENDANT MUST REASSESS THE PATIENT'S AIRWAY FREQUENTLY. IF THE PATIENT'S CONDITION DETERIORATES, INSERTION OF THE AIRWAY MUST BE ATTEMPTED AGAIN.

Remember the following key points:

- The flange of the airway **must not** be allowed to slip inside the teeth or gums.
- An **incorrectly** inserted oral airway will cause complete airway obstruction.
- Do not use **excessive** force.

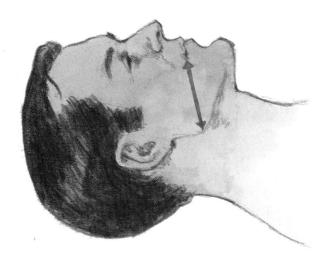

Figure IV-4a Measurement for airway size

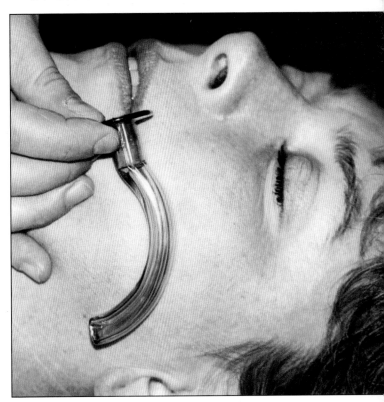

Figure IV-4b Measurement for airway size

- The oral airway **may become obstructed** with **dried foreign matter or blood clots;** therefore, movement of air should be monitored regularly. The airway should be cleaned or replaced as necessary.

AN ATTEMPT MUST BE MADE TO INSERT AN ORAL AIRWAY IN THE FOLLOWING CASES:
- ALL PATIENTS WHO ARE UNRESPONSIVE TO VERBAL STIMULATION
- ALL PATIENTS WHO REQUIRE ASSISTED VENTILATION
- ALL PATIENTS WITH A PARTIALLY OR COMPLETELY OBSTRUCTED AIRWAY THAT HAS BEEN CLEARED WITH ONE OF THE MANUAL MANOEUVRES

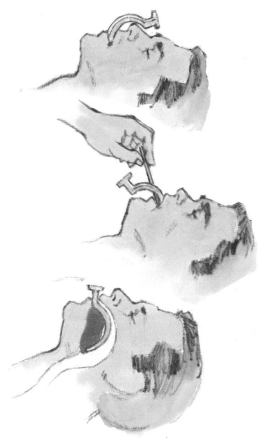

Inserting the oral airway

SUCTIONING AND SUCTION DEVICES

Patients with a decreased level of consciousness have usually lost voluntary control of their neck muscles. For the same reasons that allow the tongue to fall back and obstruct the airway, the epiglottis, which protects the opening to the trachea and the lungs, cannot function properly. Therefore, any foreign material in the mouth — such as blood, vomitus, teeth, etc. — may be inhaled into the lungs. Stomach acid present in vomitus is highly damaging to lung tissue, causing an extensive inflammatory response. This is called aspiration pneumonia. Similarly, the bacteria mixed with oral secretions or blood, when inhaled into the lungs, may ultimately cause pneumonia, further complicating the patient's treatment. Foreign objects such as teeth or gravel may also be inhaled and obstruct some of the larger airways within the lungs, thereby interfering with respiration. Conscious patients are usually able to clear the oral cavity on their own by spitting or coughing up the material. The patient with a decreased level of consciousness cannot do this and therefore it is the responsibility of the Attendant to try and keep the airway clear. Drainage positions such as the lateral position are helpful; therefore, patients with profuse bleeding of the mouth or nose, or who are actively vomiting, should be managed in the lateral position. However, more often than not, the material is too thick and tenacious to drain away by gravity alone.

Therefore, the Attendant should check the oral cavity frequently and clear it using a finger. Noisy breathing is often an indication that secretions are piling up in the back of the throat or in the plastic oral airway device.

Although drainage position and finger sweeping is helpful, it is not always effective. The best method is to use one of the portable suction devices that are now commercially available. All industrial ambulances and/or first aid rooms should have one of these suction units available. ATTENDANTS MUST FAMILIARIZE THEMSELVES WITH ITS USE AND MUST PERIODICALLY CHECK THE DEVICE TO ENSURE PROPER FUNCTIONING.

There is nothing more frustrating than having a non-functioning suction unit while treating a patient with a decreased level of consciousness who is vomiting. To operate the device properly, follow these steps:

1. Attach a clean suction tip and tubing to the machine. The preferred suction tip should be transparent, non-flexible and wide calibre (e.g. tonsil suction, Yankeur suction).

2. The suction tips should have a venting hole which must be covered by the thumb or finger to ensure adequate suction at the tip. See Figure IV-5. Turn the device on and test it. With the fingers off the venting hole, insert the suction into the mouth and then activate the suction by sealing the venting hole with a finger. The suction tips that do not have a venting hole are not recommended.

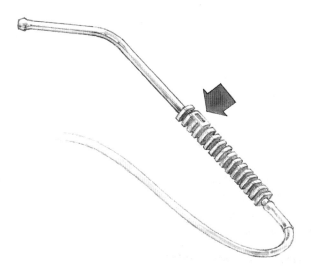

Figure IV-5 Rigid suction tip with a venting hole

3. Turn suction on to see if it works. In the presence of thick secretions — clotted blood, etc. — the suction tip may partially clog, reducing its effectiveness. The suction tip may be cleared easily by dipping it into a small container of water or saline solution (if available) while the suction is on.

4. In the presence of profuse bleeding or vomitus, the large-calibre suction tube may have to be used directly without a suction tip in order to clear the oral cavity.

5. LIMIT SUCTIONING TO 20 SECONDS AT A TIME. Remember that the device is also suctioning away oxygen. The patient becomes relatively hypoxic during the procedure. Administer oxygen and/or assisted ventilations for 20 seconds between suctioning attempts.

6. Be gentle — aggressive suctioning at the back of the throat may stimulate retching, vomiting or cause injury.

7. Repeat the procedure as often as necessary to maintain a clear airway.

VENTILATION TECHNIQUES

Assisted Ventilation

The Attendant may have to treat a patient with profound respiratory failure for which assisted ventilation is required. It is often difficult to determine which patient requires assisted ventilation: THE FOLLOWING CRITERIA OUTLINE THE SITUATIONS WHERE ASSISTED VENTILATIONS MUST BE INITIATED IMMEDIATELY UPON RECOGNITION, USING ANY OF THE TECHNIQUES DESCRIBED BELOW.

Criteria for Assisted Ventilation

1. Partial or complete airway obstruction
2. Absent or slow respirations (respiratory rate less than 10 per minute)
3. Presence of cyanosis
4. Shallow, ineffective respirations
5. Severe respiratory distress
6. Head injury (Glasgow Coma Score less than 10)

Mouth-to-Mouth

This traditional method remains the most effective; it needs no special equipment and requires a minimum of training. One disadvantage is that, in the presence of secretions, bleeding or vomitus, the Attendant may be reluctant to do it. There is also a small risk of communicable disease transmission (e.g. AIDS or hepatitis) (see Part XIII, page 320). Effective mouth-to-mouth ventilation requires that the Attendant make a good seal over the patient's mouth and hold the patient's nostrils closed at the same time. Remember, do not extend the neck of a trauma patient to ventilate. Despite the possible hazards, mouth-to-mouth resuscitation may be life-saving in the absence of airway and ventilation equipment. It should therefore be initiated as soon as possible.

Pocket Mask Ventilation

Commercially designed pocket masks are particularly well suited for ventilation in the field. There is an oxygen inlet through which high-flow oxygen can be provided. They overcome most of the disadvantages of mouth-to-mouth ventilation. Finally, the pocket masks are easier to use than the bag-valve mask system. Pocket masks are equipped with one-way valves to prevent contamination

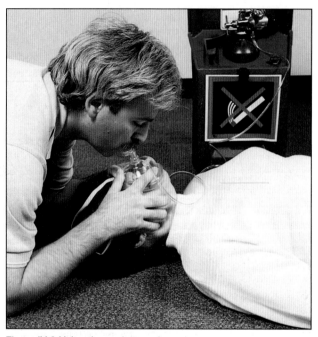

Figure IV-6 Using the pocket mask

of the Attendant with the patient's secretions. Pocket masks not equipped with one-way valves are not recommended. Follow the steps outlined below and refer to Figure IV-6.

1. The neck must be stabilized in a neutral position. The patient cannot be effectively ventilated in the ¾ prone or lateral position, and must be log-rolled to the supine position. The Attendant is usually able to manually stabilize the neck while holding the pocket mask in proper position. Alternatively, an assistant can hold the neck in a neutral position.

2. Connect one end of the oxygen tubing to the inlet valve on the pocket mask and the other end to the oxygen cylinder.

3. Open the oxygen cylinder and set the flow rate to 10 litres per minute.

4. Insert an oral airway as described previously.

5. Place the mask in the proper position over the patient's nose and mouth and establish a good seal. USE TWO HANDS!

6. Ventilate at 16-20 breaths per minute with enough volume (a large deep breath every 3 seconds is usually sufficient). Ensure that the chest wall rises with each ventilation. If it doesn't, check the following:
   • Clear airway of foreign bodies or debris.
   • Open airway by jaw thrust.
   • Reposition oral airway.
   • Reposition pocket mask to ensure a good seal.
   If the Attendant develops symptoms of hyperventilation (dizziness, numbness, tingling), the ventilation rate should be slowed.

7. If the patient is breathing spontaneously, the Attendant should time the ventilations to match the patient's inspirations. If the patient is breathing at a rate less than 10 breaths per minute, the Attendant should interpose additional ventilations between the patient's own breaths, to a combined total of 16-20 breaths per minute (one breath every three to four seconds).

Bag-valve mask Ventilation

The bag-valve mask system is the one most commonly used by ambulance and hospital personnel. The system requires considerable expertise, training and practise to use it effectively. That simple fact is often not recognized by first aid personnel. In less experienced hands, the pocket mask method is preferred.

Figure IV-7 illustrates two typical models. The mask is triangular in shape with the apex fitting over the bridge of the nose and the base just above the chin. The Attendant must ensure a tight seal for its effective use. Unless the IFA Attendant has an assistant, he/she must be able to hold the mask in proper position (as shown) and provide an effective seal, all with one hand. The other hand is needed to compress the bag and ventilate the patient. This is not as easy as it looks and requires considerable practise! Inability to maintain the seal will result in oxygen

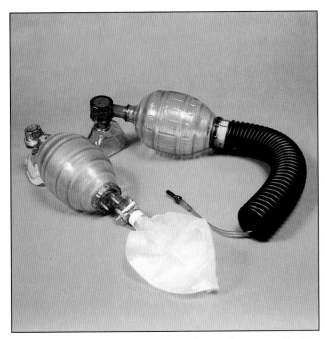

Figure IV-7 Two typical models of bag-valve mask systems. On the left the O_2 reservoir is a bag, on the right the reservoir is a snorkel.

leaking out the side and not going into the lungs — the major disadvantage of the system. The mask should also be transparent to enable the Attendant to monitor for vomitus or bleeding.

The bag is self-inflating and is supplied with an oxygen inlet to which the oxygen cylinder must be connected. The delivered oxygen concentration is approximately 35-40%. The addition of an oxygen reservoir to the bag (Figure IV-7) will increase the delivered oxygen concentration to 90%. For that reason, a bag-valve mask without an oxygen reservoir is not recommended.

Connected to the bag is the "valve". This is a one-way valve allowing oxygen to flow into the mask when the reservoir bag is compressed. When the bag is let go, the bag self-inflates with oxygen from either the oxygen reservoir or directly from the oxygen cylinder. The valve closes when the patient exhales and the carbon dioxide vents to the atmosphere, not back into the bag. Some systems are not equipped with a valve and the bag is connected directly to the mask. These systems are not recommended.

Follow these steps when using the bag-valve mask system.

1. The neck must be stabilized in a neutral position. The patient cannot be effectively ventilated in the ¾ prone or lateral position and, unless there are contraindications, must be log-rolled to the supine position. A simple technique is to stabilize the patient's head and neck between the knees while kneeling. This method frees up both hands to ventilate the patient. Alternatively, an assistant can hold the neck in the neutral position while the Attendant ventilates the patient.

2. Connect the oxygen tubing to the oxygen reservoir at one end and the oxygen cylinder at the other end.

3. Open the oxygen cylinder and set the flow rate to 15 litres per minute.

4. Attach the mask to the bag-valve device. The mask should be transparent so the Attendant can monitor for blood or vomitus.

5. Insert an oral airway into the patient as previously described.

6. Place the mask in proper position on the patient's face — the apex over the bridge of the nose and the base below the lower lip against the chin. Maintain a good seal. Hold the mask snugly against the patient's face. Use two hands if necessary.

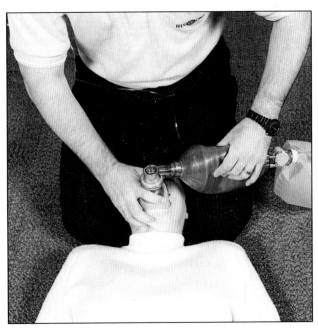

Using the bag-valve mask system

7. Ventilate with enough volume. This is difficult and tiring with one hand. An assistant may be asked to fully compress the bag while the Attendant uses two hands to maintain the seal. Ensure that the chest wall rises with each ventilation. THE TWO MOST COMMON REASONS FOR INADEQUATE VENTILATIONS WITH THIS DEVICE ARE FAILURE TO MAINTAIN A PROPER JAW POSITION AND FAILURE TO MAINTAIN AN EFFECTIVE SEAL. These are corrected by pulling up on the mandible and repositioning the mask.

8. Do not tilt the head of a trauma patient during ventilation. Remember to maintain the neck in a neutral position. In non-trauma patients, the head may be tilted, if necessary.

9. Time the ventilation to match inspiration if the patient is breathing spontaneously.

10. All trauma victims requiring assisted ventilation should be ventilated at a rate of 16-20 breaths per minute (about one breath every three to four seconds).

11. Ensure that the chest wall rises with each ventilation. If not, check the following:
    - Clear airway of foreign bodies or debris.
    - Open airway by jaw thrust.
    - Reposition oral airway.
    - Reposition mask to ensure a good seal.

Part IV, Section C
Traumatic Respiratory Emergencies

DYSPNEA

Dyspnea may be defined as difficult or laboured breathing. The patient with dyspnea feels short of breath. *This is a serious condition and is often terrifying for the patient.*

Dyspnea can be due to several causes (traumatic and non-traumatic):

1. Inadequate oxygen in the air breathed.
2. An obstruction to the flow of air in the upper airway, trachea or the bronchi. It may occur in cases of trauma, aspiration of vomitus or blood, or when there is a foreign body.
3. Air may not pass easily in or out of the air sacs in the lung, as with patients suffering from a number of conditions (e.g. inhalation injury or asthma, etc.).
4. Injury to the chest wall may impair the normal mechanics of breathing (e.g. flail chest or multiple rib fractures).
5. A lung may be collapsed and unable to expand (e.g. spontaneous or traumatic pneumothorax or hemothorax).
6. The lung tissue may be directly damaged (e.g. bruising, laceration).
7. The lung tissue may lose its elasticity and no longer respond to the normal motions of breathing (e.g. emphysema).
8. The lungs may be filled with fluid because the heart muscle has failed and is no longer able to circulate blood properly (e.g. heart failure).
9. Infection in the lung tissue (e.g. pneumonia).

Management of Dyspnea

The dyspneic patient may be terrified and become exhausted from the effort of breathing. The Attendant must use the Priority Action Approach to assess and treat the dyspneic patient.

1. Begin the primary survey.
2. Ensure an open airway with cervical spine control.
3. If a cervical injury is suspected, with C-spine control, position the patient supine or in the lateral position (see Part VI, Section D, page 147). If there is no concern for cervical injury, position the patient for comfort (e.g. in a semi-sitting, sitting upright or a lying position with the injured side of the chest down).
4. Expose the chest to assess for adequate breathing.

AN OPEN AIRWAY DOES NOT ENSURE ADEQUATE VENTILATION. Look for open wounds or other signs of chest injury (e.g. inadequate and/or asymmetrical chest movements, the use of the accessory muscles of respiration, overexpanded chest, etc.).

5. Assess for respiratory distress or signs of oxygen deficiency (e.g. dyspnea, gasping, cyanosis or rapid breathing). If necessary (respiratory rate less than 10 per minute), provide assisted ventilation. A bag-valve mask and supplemental oxygen at 10 Lpm or pocket mask is the preferred method. Time the assistance to the victim's breathing pattern.
6. Administer high-flow oxygen by mask (at 10 Lpm).
7. Control life-threatening external bleeding.
8. Using the Priority Action Approach, attempt to determine the cause of the patient's dyspnea. In the absence of injury, a history may identify the cause of dyspnea (e.g. asthma, heart disease, allergy, infection).

CHEST TRAUMA

Injuries to the chest are of major importance because they may impair the body's ability to receive an adequate supply of oxygen.

Major chest injury occurs in half the multiple trauma deaths in British Columbia each year. No other pre-hospital emergency situation requires more urgent treatment than a patient with a chest and/or airway injury.

The magnitude of injury to the intrathoracic organs cannot be determined by external appearance alone. Blunt trauma may leave only a few external marks of injury and yet there may be extensive internal damage. Unless suspected and properly treated, these injuries may be rapidly fatal. The body lacks the capacity to store oxygen. Any injury that interferes with normal breathing must be treated without delay, to prevent permanent damage of cells which are critically dependent on a constant oxygen supply (e.g. brain and spinal cord).

Chest injuries may appear minor initially but rapidly prove to be major and potentially fatal. Victims with potential chest trauma should receive careful and repeated assessments. Using the mechanism of injury (e.g. MVA associated with a bent steering wheel), the Attendant may identify patients with potentially serious internal chest injuries that require rapid transport.

CHARACTERISTIC SIGNS AND SYMPTOMS

Not all of the following signs and symptoms may be present or evident in a patient with a chest injury. They are listed as general signs and symptoms that the patient may exhibit or feel.

Sign or Symptom	Indication
• PAIN AT THE SITE OF INJURY	• Pain in the chest at the site of an obvious fracture or bruise indicates injury of the chest wall. It may also indicate injury to the lung or heart.
• PLEURITIC PAIN (PAIN THAT IS AGGRAVATED BY BREATHING BUT IS NOT REPRODUCED BY DIRECT PRESSURE ON THE CHEST WALL AT THE SITE OF INJURY)	• Indicates irritation of pleural surfaces of the lung or chest wall. Lacerations of pleural surfaces by fractured ribs can result in pleuritic pain.
• SHORTNESS OF BREATH OR DIFFICULTY BREATHING (DYSPNEA) (page 55)	• Any change in the normal breathing pattern is an important sign.
• FAILURE OF ONE OR BOTH SIDES OF THE CHEST TO EXPAND NORMALLY	• Direct chest wall injury, such as flail chest or splinting from multiple rib fractures.
	• Over-inflation of chest wall, as with tension pneumothorax.
	• Bilateral injury to nerves supplying the respiratory muscles (e.g. spinal cord injury).
• COUGHING UP BLOOD (HEMOPTYSIS)	• May indicate that the lung or airway has been lacerated or bruised. If the alveoli are injured, frothy red blood may pass into the bronchial passages and be coughed up as the patient attempts to clear the airways.
• RAPID AND WEAK PULSE. COOL AND/OR MOIST SKIN	• Signs of shock resulting from insufficient circulating, oxygenated blood. It usually indicates a loss of blood, most often from internal bleeding.
• CYANOSIS (BLUE COLOUR OF THE LIPS, FINGERNAILS OR EAR LOBES)	• Blood is insufficiently oxygenated.
• SUBCUTANEOUS EMPHYSEMA	• When a lung laceration from a fractured rib has allowed air to escape into the tissues of the chest wall. This condition can be detected by a crackling sensation under the fingertips (like rice crispies) as the Attendant feels the area of the fracture. Sometimes the crackling can be heard. It can become extensive. The crackling is an indication that air is being forced out of the lung into the tissues.

Chest Injury Classification

There are two types of chest injuries: closed (blunt) and open (penetrating).

Closed

The skin is intact in a closed chest injury; therefore, the danger of such injuries may be underestimated. Even when a wound is not open, the heart, vessels and lungs may have lacerations and contusions. Blunt trauma and crush injuries cause closed chest injuries.

Open

Open chest injuries are those in which the chest wall has been penetrated, as by a knife, bullet or the patient falling on a sharp object. Open chest injuries may also be associated with severe rib fractures, where the broken end of the rib has lacerated the chest wall and the skin. As with closed chest injuries, there may also be contusions or lacerations of the heart, lungs or major blood vessels. To avoid aggravating existing injury, protruding objects such as knives and sticks must not be removed from the wound.

GENERAL PRINCIPLES OF MANAGEMENT OF CHEST INJURIES

The evaluation and management of the injured worker with chest injuries follows the Priority Action Approach outlined in Part III, page 20.

1. Begin the primary survey.
2. Ensure an open airway with cervical spine control.
3. If a cervical injury is suspected with C-spine control, position the patient supine, or the lateral position (see Part VI, Section D, page 147). If there is no concern for cervical injury, position the patient for comfort (e.g. in a semi-sitting or lying position with the injured side of the chest down).
4. Expose the chest to assess for adequate breathing. AN OPEN AIRWAY DOES NOT ENSURE ADEQUATE VENTILATION. Look for open wounds or other signs of chest injury (e.g. inadequate and/or asymmetrical chest movements, bruising, abrasions or paradoxical movement). The chest injuries that most often compromise breathing are: a large flail chest with pulmonary contusion, tension pneumothorax and open pneumothorax. An open chest wound should be temporarily sealed at this time.

5. Assess for respiratory distress or signs of oxygen deficiency (e.g. dyspnea, gasping, cyanosis or rapid breathing). If necessary, provide assisted ventilation. A bag-valve mask and supplemental oxygen or pocket mask is the preferred method. Time the assistance to the victim's breathing pattern.
6. Administer high-flow oxygen by mask (at 10 Lpm).
7. Control life-threatening external bleeding.
8. ALL PATIENTS WITH CHEST INJURIES ASSOCIATED WITH RESPIRATORY DISTRESS FALL INTO THE RAPID TRANSPORT CATEGORY. Following the primary survey and initial management of life-threatening injuries, the patient must be transported rapidly to the nearest hospital.
9. Treat flail segments as outlined below. Seal any open chest wound with an airtight dressing as described below. Watch for the development of a tension pneumothorax and be prepared to unseal the dressing briefly to release the air under tension.
10. Stabilize impaled objects in the chest with appropriate dressings.
11. If there are secretions in the airway, encourage the patient to cough, which will help to clear the airway.

TYPES OF CHEST INJURIES AND THEIR SPECIFIC MANAGEMENT

RIB FRACTURES

Fracture of the ribs is a common chest injury.

Rib fractures are usually caused by direct blows or compression injuries of the chest. The trauma victim with rib fractures may have associated injuries. They may have associated pneumothorax, hemothorax and/or lung contusions. Upper ribs are fractured less often than lower ribs because they are protected by the shoulder girdle. Upper rib fractures may be associated with injuries in the mediastinum. Lower rib fractures may be associated with underlying liver, spleen or kidney damage.

Recognition of Rib Fractures

All the general signs and symptoms of chest injuries as previously described may be present. In addition, patients with rib fractures may demonstrate the following:

- History of a blow or compression injury to the chest.
- Pain at the fracture site or localized tenderness to palpation.
- Deep breathing, coughing or movement usually increases the pain at the fracture site (pleuritic pain).
- The patient may often lean toward the injured side, holding the affected area to keep it immobilized.
- The patient usually wishes to remain still.
- There may be a rib deformity, chest wall bruising or laceration.
- If any of the following general signs and symptoms (as previously described) are present, i.e. moderate/severe respiratory distress, cyanosis, hemoptysis, shock, more serious chest injuries must be suspected.

Management of Rib Fractures

The Attendant must follow the Priority Action Approach and treatment protocols outlined under the general management of chest injuries. As mentioned, the trauma patient with rib fractures often has associated internal injuries. Consequently, the Attendant must regularly reassess the patient. If the lungs, heart or vessels have not been damaged, the patient usually breathes without much difficulty and colour remains normal. Simple rib fractures are not wrapped, strapped or taped. If there is no concern for associated injuries (e.g. neck, back or internal bleeding), the patient should be positioned to maximize comfort for transport to a hospital.

Fractured ribs often cannot be diagnosed without x-ray.

STERNAL FRACTURES

A fractured sternum is a rare condition and usually indicates severe trauma to the anterior chest. Sternal injuries may be associated with injuries to the chest or under-lying injuries to the neck, lungs, heart or other mediastinal structures. Patients in respiratory distress with sternal injuries fall into the Rapid Transport Category. The patient with sternal injuries without obvious deformity or dyspnea should be treated as for a simple rib fracture.

FLAIL CHEST

When two or more consecutive ribs are fractured in two or more places, or detached from the sternum, a segment of the chest wall may become disconnected from the rest of the bony thorax.

The segment of the chest wall floating between the fractures is called the "flail" segment.

The movement of the flail area is opposite of the remainder of the chest. When the patient inhales, the flail does not expand; when he/she exhales, it protrudes while the rest of the chest wall contracts (see Figure IV-8). This is called "paradoxical movement".

Flail chest is a particularly serious injury. The patient with a flail chest may be breathing without difficulty or may be severely dyspneic. It depends on the size of the unstable chest wall segment and on the magnitude of the underlying injury to the lung or other intrathoracic organs. The degree of respiratory distress may also depend on the presence of shock. When the patient inhales, the paradoxical movement of a large flail segment reduces the volume of air entering the lungs. A force sufficient to cause a flail segment is usually severe enough to produce bleeding of the lungs.

All cases of flail chest should be considered life-threatening emergencies. Even patients who appear stable may rapidly develop shock and severe respiratory distress.

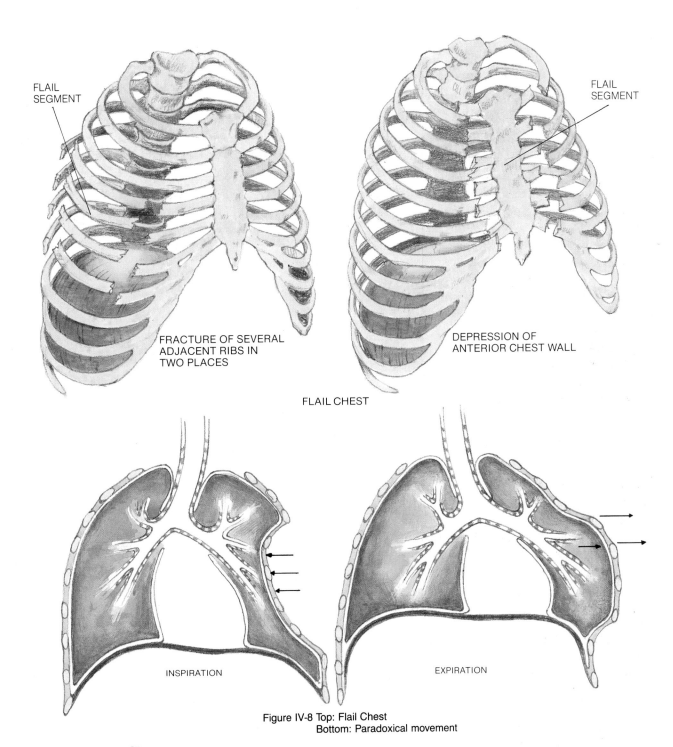

FLAIL
SEGMENT

FLAIL
SEGMENT

FRACTURE OF SEVERAL
ADJACENT RIBS IN
TWO PLACES

DEPRESSION OF
ANTERIOR CHEST WALL

FLAIL CHEST

INSPIRATION

EXPIRATION

Figure IV-8 Top: Flail Chest
Bottom: Paradoxical movement

Recognition of Flail Chest

The patient with a flail chest will have some or all of the general signs and symptoms of chest injury and rib fractures. They may also have some or all of the following:

- history of blunt trauma to the chest;
- paradoxical movement or deformity, visible on observing the naked chest;
- marked shortness of breath and/or respiratory distress;
- anxiety and fear;
- pain in the fracture area.

If the lungs are damaged, the patient may:

- cough up blood or frothy, bloody sputum;
- collapse or show signs of shock;
- show signs of tension pneumothorax.

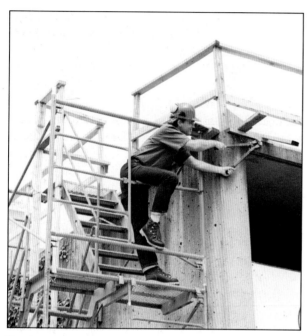

Unsafe work practices

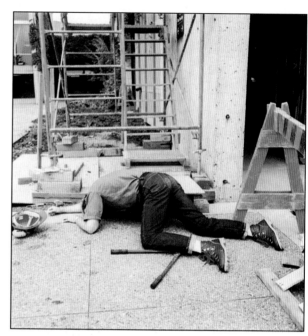

Mechanism of injury

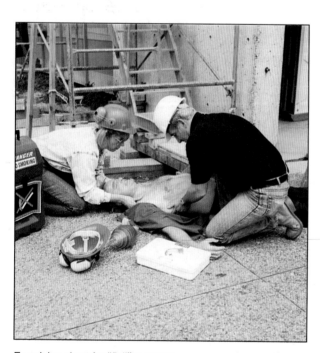

Examining chest for "flail" segment

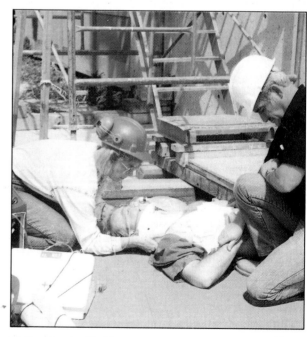

Pad taped to the "flail" segment while waiting for transportation vehicle

Management of Flail Chest

The assessment and management of victims with a flail chest should follow the Priority Action Approach to the injured patient (Part III, page 20) and the general principles of management of chest injuries as outlined above.

ALL PATIENTS WITH FLAIL CHEST FALL INTO THE RAPID TRANSPORT CATEGORY.

Specific Treatment of the Flail Chest

THE SPECIFIC TREATMENT OF THE FLAIL CHEST IS AIMED AT:
- PROVIDING OPTIMAL OXYGENATION;
- RESTORING AND MAINTAINING STABILITY OF THE CHEST WALL. There are several techniques that can be used to stabilize the flail segment, depending upon the size and location of the flail segment and the presence of associated injuries (particularly of the head and neck).

For flail segments located on the anterior and anterolateral chest wall, a pad, large enough to cover the flail segment and no larger, should be taped over the segment firmly enough to stop the paradoxical movement. Place the pad when the flail segment is sucked into its lowest point — when the chest is in full inspiration. Adhesive tape, 6.5 - 8 cm (3″ or 4″) wide, should be applied over a thick, firmly rolled pad, a towel or similar available material of the size and shape of the flail segment. The taping should be horizontal and vertical and applied generously so that it is anchored to the stable chest wall. The flail segment may be temporarily controlled by holding the hand firmly over the segment to control the paradoxical movements. Do not apply any fully encircling tapes or ties around the chest of an injured patient, as this will make it hard for the patient to breathe.

DO NOT DELAY TRANSPORT FOR THE PURPOSE OF TAPING A PAD IN PLACE. STABILIZING A FLAIL SEGMENT IN THIS MANNER CAN BE DONE EN ROUTE.

Alternative Method

Where circumstances allow (lateral flail segment, supine patient), a securely taped sandbag may be substituted for the tape bandage method. If there are no contraindications, the patient may be turned to lie on the affected side. Prior to turning, the flail segment should be treated with a taped pressure dressing as described above. In this position, the flail segment is effectively splinted and the uninjured chest wall moves freely.

In the absence of a decreased level of consciousness, neck injury or shock, position the patient for ease of breathing, semi-sitting.

All injured victims with a flail chest must receive high-flow (10 Lpm) oxygen. It should be administered by mask if breathing is adequate. If necessary, the Attendant must provide assisted ventilation timed to the patient's breathing pattern. Complications can arise from assisted ventilation in such patients, as the oxygen administered under pressure may cause a pneumothorax (see below) by forcing air into the pleural cavity through damaged lung tissue. The risk created by assisted ventilation must be taken if the victim is not breathing adequately. Without assisted ventilation, the patient may not survive.

Because of the seriousness of these injuries, the patient may deteriorate despite the assisted ventilation provided by the Attendant. In this situation, the patient must be transported rapidly to hospital. The Attendant must persevere and continue to provide assisted ventilation.

CLOSED PNEUMOTHORAX

Pneumothorax occurs when lung tissue is torn and air leaks from the lung into the pleural space. Air is therefore contained within the thoracic cavity but outside the lung. The lung collapses, its volume reduced, thereby diminishing the amount of air that can be inhaled. As the degree of pneumothorax increases, hypoxia ensues and respiratory distress becomes evident. The patient's condition may range from a complete absence of symptoms to severe dyspnea.

A closed pneumothorax is usually caused by rib fracture(s). Torn lung tissue may result, permitting air to enter the pleural space. Patients with suspected pneumothorax should be assessed at a hospital.

Recognition of a Closed Pneumothorax

Signs and symptoms may include:
- history of chest trauma;
- pain at the site of injury;
- increased pain upon inspiration (pleuritic pain);
- difficulty breathing (dyspnea);
- cyanosis;

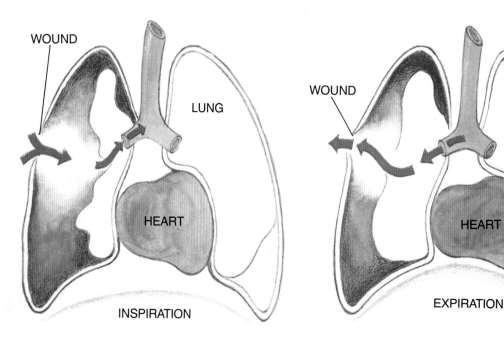

Pneumothorax with punctured lung

- rapid, weak pulse;
- subcutaneous emphysema at the site of injury, over the chest or in the neck.

Management of a Closed Pneumothorax

The management of the victim with a pneumothorax should follow the Priority Action Approach for the injured patient as outlined in Part III, page 20. ALL PATIENTS WITH A SUSPECTED CLOSED PNEUMOTHORAX SHOULD BE UPGRADED TO THE RAPID TRANS-PORT CATEGORY. In managing the victim with a suspected closed pneumothorax, the Attendant should also follow the general principles of management of chest injuries as outlined above.

OPEN PNEUMOTHORAX

In penetrating wounds of the chest wall, air enters the pleural space from outside the chest wall, thereby collapsing the lung.

Air passes back and forth through the wound on inspiration and expiration. Because this often creates a sucking sound, these wounds are sometimes referred to as open, sucking chest wounds.

Depending on the size of the opening in the chest wall, damage to underlying structures and the pre-existing condition of the lung, the patient may have no symptoms or may be severely dyspneic. Small sucking wounds of the chest in patients with normal lungs may not cause dyspnea.

Recognition of an Open Pneumothorax

A patient with an open pneumothorax may have some or all of the general signs and symptoms of chest injury. Specific signs and symptoms of this condition may also be present, including:
- a sucking sound as air passes through the opening in the chest wall;
- an open chest wound;
- blood or blood-stained bubbles may be expelled from the wound on exhalation;
- coughing up blood (hemoptysis);
- possible exit wound.

Management of an Open Pneumothorax

The management of an open pneumothorax should follow the Priority Action Approach for the injured patient as outlined in Part III, page 20. All patients with an open pneumothorax fall into the Rapid Transport Category. In managing this condition, the Attendant should follow the general principles of management of chest injuries as outlined above.

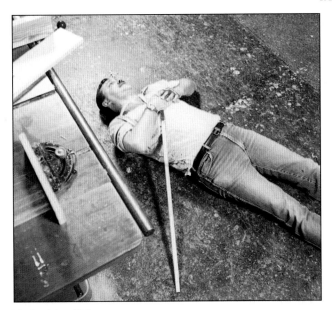

Mechanism of injury

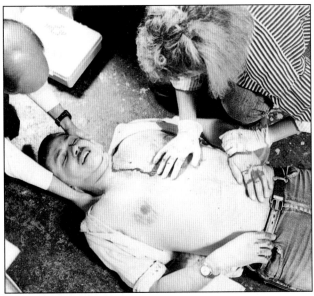

Temporarily sealing open wound with the hand

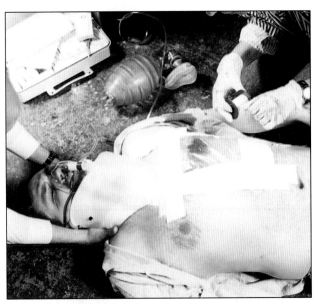

All four sides sealed with occlusive dressing

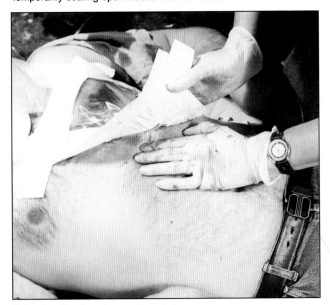

Releasing the dressing to allow air to escape

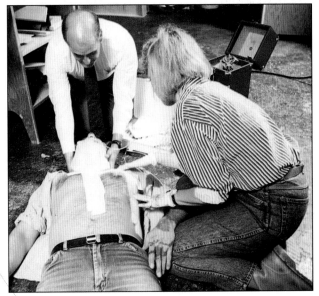

Alternative method of sealing three sides

Specific Treatment of an Open Pneumothorax

The Attendant should seal the open chest wound as quickly as possible. Seal the wound with a hand if necessary. Do not delay sealing the wound while searching for an occlusive dressing. To effectively seal the wound, apply an occlusive dressing. Any piece of airtight material such as an Esmarch bandage, piece of plastic bag, aluminum or aluminum foil may be taped firmly over the wound. It must be large enough (e.g. 5 - 6.5 cm (2"-3") wider than the wound), so that it is not sucked into the wound. Use adhesive tape to fasten all sides of the airtight seal. The patient's skin must be clean and dry for the tape to stick. If the tape will not adhere to the skin due to the presence of perspiration, blood or other liquids, place thick dressings over the occlusive dressing and hold in place with tape across the chest, but not circumferentially around the chest. In the presence of an open pneumothorax, always check the posterior chest for an exit wound. It also must be treated with an occlusive dressing.

The risk of placing an occlusive dressing over an open sucking wound in the chest wall is that the patient may subsequently develop a tension pneumothorax (see below). Signs of a developing tension pneumothorax include: increasing respiratory difficulty, increasing signs of shock and uneven chest wall movement.

If a tension pneumothorax develops, unseal the occlusive dressing by lifting a corner of the seal for three to four seconds in order to let the air under tension escape. The patient's condition should improve almost immediately as pressure is relieved from around the uninjured lung and heart. Reseal the wound and continuously monitor the patient. This procedure may have to be repeated several times.

An equally acceptable method of treating open pneumothorax is to apply the occlusive dressing with all but one side taped down. By leaving one side unsealed, air under tension within the chest cavity will escape when the patient exhales. When the patient inhales, the negative pressure inside the chest will cause the occlusive dressing to seal the wound preventing air entry, thus creating a "flutter valve".

If a "flutter valve" dressing is used, the Attendant must still carefully monitor the patient for the development of a tension pneumothorax or other complications, because the free corner of the dressing may become stuck to the chest wall or the dressing may be drawn into the wound with consequent flutter valve failure.

ON INSPIRATION, DRESSING SEALS
WOUND, PREVENTING AIR ENTRY

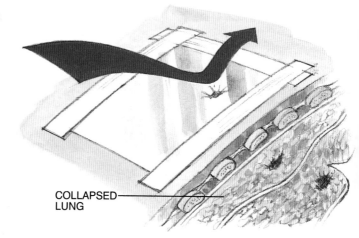

COLLAPSED
LUNG

EXPIRATION ALLOWS TRAPPED AIR TO ESCAPE
THROUGH UNTAPED SECTION OF DRESSING

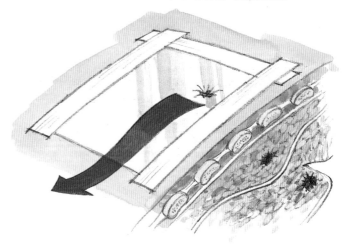

Pneumothorax dressing

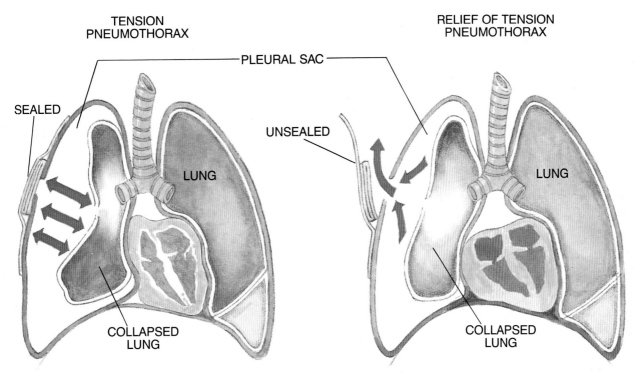

TENSION
PNEUMOTHORAX

RELIEF OF TENSION
PNEUMOTHORAX

PLEURAL SAC

SEALED

UNSEALED

LUNG

LUNG

COLLAPSED
LUNG

COLLAPSED
LUNG

IF PATIENT'S CONDITION DECLINES
AFTER SEALING PUNCTURE WOUND,
OPEN THE SEAL IMMEDIATELY

TENSION PNEUMOTHORAX

Tension pneumothorax is the accumulation of air in the pleural space under pressure. The air under tension collapses the lung on the side of the injury and then displaces the mediastinum away from the air-filled pleural space, partially collapsing the other lung. Tension pneumothorax can occur from either penetrating or blunt chest trauma when the injury creates a one-way valve, so that air can enter but not leave the pleural space. In blunt trauma, the lung may be torn (most commonly by a rib fracture). The site of lung injury acts as the one-way valve. It allows air into the pleural space during inspiration but prevents its return to the lung during expiration. Air under increasing pressure consequently collects in the pleural space. The resulting collapse of the lung and, particularly, the displacement of the heart towards the unaffected lung precipitates severe dyspnea and shock. The shift of mediastinal structures compresses the heart and great vessels and markedly reduces the venous return to the right atrium,

all of which may rapidly lead to shock. The collapse of the injured lung, the shift of the trachea and the compression of the good lung, combined with the increasing intrathoracic pressure, cause impairment of ventilation and the patient becomes severely short of breath.

Recognition of Tension Pneumothorax

All the general signs and symptoms of chest injuries may be present.

In addition, a patient with a tension pneumothorax may demonstrate the following:

- severe progressive respiratory distress;
- distended neck veins due to an obstruction of the superior vena cava;
- marked over-expansion on the affected side of the chest;
- agitation and restlessness;
- a deviation or shift of the trachea away from the side of the tension pneumothorax.

Management of Tension Pneumothorax

Management of a tension pneumothorax should follow the Priority Action Approach to the injured patient as outlined in Part III, page 20. All patients with a suspected tension pneumothorax are in the Rapid Transport Category because this condition may be rapidly fatal. In managing the patient with a tension pneumothorax, the Attendant should follow the general principles of management of chest injuries as outlined above.

Specific Treatment of Tension Pneumothorax

The patient requires expert and immediate treatment at a hospital. Management must include high-flow oxygen by mask (10 Lpm) and, if required, assisted ventilation.

Tension pneumothorax is not limited to a closed chest injury. A patient with a sucking chest wound may also have a lung laceration. If the external wound is effectively bandaged and the lung continues to leak, a tension pneumothorax may develop. Intermittent removal of the airtight dressing releases air pressure built up inside the chest cavity. Tension pneumothorax is often a complication of flail chest.

IT MUST BE EMPHASIZED THAT TENSION PNEUMOTHORAX IS ONE OF THE VERY IMMEDIATE LIFE-THREATENING EMERGENCIES. DEATH MAY OCCUR WITHIN MINUTES OF THE INJURY.

Because of the seriousness of these injuries, the patient may deteriorate despite the assisted ventilation provided by the Attendant. In this situation, the patient must be transported rapidly to hospital. The Attendant must persevere and continue to provide assisted ventilation.

SPONTANEOUS PNEUMOTHORAX

A pneumothorax may develop without injury and is called a spontaneous pneumothorax. Lungs can develop a weak area on their surface, either from a developmental birth defect or because of underlying disease (e.g. emphysema, see Section D, page 70). The weak area ruptures and air leaks into the chest cavity causing the pneumothorax. As the affected lung collapses, symptoms of dyspnea may appear.

Recognition of Spontaneous Pneumothorax

When a patient has no apparent chest injury or airway obstruction but is obviously in respiratory distress, spontaneous pneumothorax should be considered. The patient experiences a sudden sharp pleuritic chest pain with varying degrees of dyspnea.

Management of Spontaneous Pneumothorax

Some patients notice no particular discomfort or difficulty in breathing. However, in cases of respiratory distress, the patient should be placed in the Rapid Transport Category. Management should include high flow oxygen by mask (10 Lpm). Transport the patient to hospital in a sitting position, which is usually the most comfortable position. All cases of suspected pneumothorax must be referred to a hospital. If there is marked respiratory distress, assisted ventilation as outlined in the protocol for the general management of chest injuries should be instituted.

HEMOTHORAX

Hemothorax occurs when blood collects within the pleural space. It may be caused by open or closed chest injuries and is frequently associated with pneumothorax. The bleeding may come from lacerated vessels in the chest wall, from lacerated major vessels within the chest cavity itself or from a lacerated lung. Bleeding within the thoracic cavity is hidden and often severe. Because of the capacity of the thoracic cavity to accommodate large volumes of blood (1-3 litres), the patient may exhibit signs of shock from blood loss.

Recognition of Hemothorax

Patients will exhibit many of the general signs and symptoms of chest injuries outlined above. Of special concern with this condition are signs of increasing respiratory distress and/or shock.

Management of Hemothorax

The management of the patient with a hemothorax should follow the Priority Action Approach to the injured patient, Part III, page 20. All patients with a suspected hemothorax fall into the Rapid Transport Category. In managing such patients, the Attendant should follow the general principles of management of chest injuries as outlined above.

PULMONARY CONTUSION

A pulmonary contusion is a bruise of the lung. It is almost always associated with blunt injuries to the chest (e.g. automobile accidents and serious falls). It is similar to a bruise of any other tissue. The blood vessels in the lung are injured and a considerable amount of blood may be lost into the lung tissue. The patient may or may not be in respiratory distress, depending on the extent of the contusion. Patients with significant pulmonary contusions frequently cough up blood. The signs and symptoms of pulmonary contusion may develop 12 to 24 hours after the injury. Some pulmonary contusions are so severe that the patient is in respiratory distress almost from the moment of injury.

Recognition of Pulmonary Contusion

Patients with pulmonary contusions may demonstrate any or all of the general signs and symptoms of chest injuries described above.

Management of Pulmonary Contusion

The management of patients with suspected pulmonary contusions should follow the Priority Action Approach to the injured patient as outlined in Part III, page 20. All patients with this condition fall into the Rapid Transport Category. In managing patients with pulmonary contusion, the Attendant should follow the general principles of management of chest injuries as outlined above.

BLAST INJURIES

An explosion creates sudden extreme changes in the air pressure in the lungs. This can damage the air sacs and produce widespread bleeding. The alveoli become filled with blood and edema, preventing the normal exchange of gases. As fluid accumulates in the lungs, it interferes with the movement of oxygen from the alveoli into the bloodstream. The victim becomes hypoxic. Changes in lung function may not occur immediately. The process of bleeding into the lung may occur over several hours.

Pressure waves may also strike the outside wall of the body, causing pressure changes that damage the lungs and the contents of the abdominal and cranial cavities. Heart damage is a common complication associated with blast injuries.

Recognition of Blast Injuries

Blast injuries vary in severity and can be fatal without any evidence of external damage to the body.

In addition to the general signs and symptoms of chest injury, the Attendant should be aware of these indications of a blast injury:
- history of an explosion;
- pain in the chest and/or abdomen;
- respiratory distress;
- coughing — frothy sputum which may be blood-stained;
- nausea or vomiting;
- shock — mild to severe;
- decreased level of consciousness;
- bloodshot eyes, minute red or blue spots on the face, neck or upper chest (caused by microhemorrhage);
- abdominal tenderness and/or rectal bleeding;
- possible delayed onset of dyspnea, headache, chest pain or shock.

Management of Blast Injuries

The management of victims of a blast injury should follow the Priority Action Approach for the injured patient found in Part III, page 20. These patients may develop life-threatening complications and fall into the Rapid Transport Category. In managing blast injuries, the Attendant should follow the general principles of management of chest injuries as outlined above.

TRAUMATIC ASPHYXIA

Traumatic asphyxia is a rare condition, caused by blunt trauma to the chest. An injury of this type forces the anterior chest wall back, compressing the heart against the vertebral column. This sudden compression of the heart, especially of the thin-walled right atrium, forces the blood back into the valveless veins of the upper chest, neck and head. The force is so great that multiple tiny hemorrhages occur in the minute veins of the skin and mucus membranes. The patient will often have bluish mottled skin on the head, neck and upper thorax and may have subconjunctival hemorrhages. The lips and tongue may be swollen and cyanotic. This alarming appearance may or may not reflect the presence of serious underlying chest injuries (e.g. hemopneumothorax, flail chest, cardiac injury, etc.).

Recognition of Traumatic Asphyxia

In addition to the general signs of chest injury, the patient may demonstrate any or all of the following:
- purple face, neck and shoulders;
- bloodshot eyes, which may bulge;
- stove-in chest;
- cyanotic and swollen tongue and lips.

Management of Traumatic Asphyxia

The management of the patient with traumatic asphyxia should follow the Priority Action Approach for the injured patient outlined in Part III, page 20. All patients with traumatic asphyxia fall into the Rapid Transport Category as they can rapidly develop life-threatening complications. In managing traumatic asphyxia, the Attendant should follow the general principles of management of chest injuries as outlined above.

SMOKE INHALATION

Respiratory injury from smoke inhalation is a major cause of death in patients with or without body surface burns. Smoke is a combination of suspended particles and gaseous products of combustion. The particulate matter (soot) does not cause major respiratory problems. These problems may be caused by: gases from burned plastics, sulphur and nitrogen compounds, carbon monoxide, heat and lack of oxygen.

Smoke inhalation may affect the upper airway, causing inflammation and swelling in the mouth, larynx and trachea. It may also affect the more distal portions of the lung, causing generalized inflammation and fluid formation (pulmonary edema) in the lower airways and alveoli.

Respiratory distress may be immediate or delayed. Upper airway obstruction from tissue fluids may not occur for several hours. Furthermore, pulmonary edema, which may be rapidly fatal, may not be evident for many hours. It usually occurs 8 to 36 hours after the inhalation. All patients suspected of smoke inhalation must be transported to a hospital as rapidly as possible.

The following information concerning smoke inhalation should be obtained:
- Location of the victim when exposed to the smoke — a patient found in an enclosed space is likely to suffer significant inhalation injury.
- Duration of exposure — a victim with very brief exposure is less likely to suffer significant injury.
- Presence of toxic substances — alerting the Attendant to possible respiratory irritation.
- Decreased level of consciousness — may be due to hypoxia, carbon monoxide or other toxic gases.
- Any other information that might be a factor, such as head injury or alcohol abuse.

Recognition of Smoke Inhalation

- Sore throat, hoarseness, shortness of breath, swallowing difficulties and pain on deep inspiration.
- Cough, especially when it produces soot-tinged sputum.
- Headache or dizziness, restlessness, confusion, comatose, possible convulsions.
- Respiratory distress with noisy, rapid respiration or a barking cough.
- Cyanotic or pale. NOTE: The cherry-red appearance formerly thought to be associated with all carbon monoxide poisoning is, in fact, rarely seen.
- Facial burns, especially about the mouth and nose.

Management of Smoke Inhalation

THE ATTENDANT SHOULD NOT ENTER AN AREA THAT MAY HAVE A TOXIC ATMOSPHERE OR INADEQUATE OXYGEN CONTENT WITHOUT WEARING THE PROPER RESCUE BREATHING APPARATUS. The patient should be removed from the contaminated atmosphere to fresh air before the primary survey is conducted.

The management of the patient with smoke inhalation should follow the Priority Action Approach to the injured patient found in Part III, page 20. VICTIMS OF SMOKE INHALATION MUST ALWAYS BE ASSESSED FOR ASSOCIATED INJURIES. All victims suspected of smoke inhalation fall into the Rapid Transport Category. In managing this condition, the Attendant should follow also the general principles of management of chest injuries as outlined above.

Part IV, Section D
Non-Traumatic Respiratory Emergencies

ASTHMA

The term "asthma" is derived from a Greek word meaning breathlessness. The chief symptom of asthma is dyspnea or difficulty breathing (see Section C, page 55). It is a disease characterized by attacks of widespread narrowing of the airways that occur intermittently and may range from mild attacks of shortness of breath to profound respiratory failure and death. The asthma attacks are interspersed with symptom-free periods. It is the narrowing of the airways (bronchospasm) that produces the typical wheezing, whistling noises of breathing during an asthmatic attack.

Asthma affects approximately 5% of adults and up to 10% of children in the United States and Canada. Although the mortality is relatively low, the disability it causes is very great. It accounts for a significant amount of lost days from work or, alternatively, restricted activity.

The chief characteristic of asthma is its periodic reversible acute attacks of bronchospasm. The bronchospasm is caused by the contraction of the smooth muscles of the walls of the airways (bronchi and bronchioles), which leads to their constriction. Narrowing of the airways in this fashion impairs ventilation.

In addition to the widespread bronchial constriction, edema forms in the mucous membrane of the airways and the numerous glands in this membrane produce copious amounts of very sticky secretions. These changes result in further narrowing of the airways and interference with ventilation. The greatest interference with air flow is during expiration. Consequently, air enters the alveoli and becomes trapped. The volume of air in the lungs builds up progressively and the patient works increasingly harder to push each breath out. As the disturbance progresses, both inspiration and expiration become increasingly difficult. The sensation that the patient's air supply is being shut off frequently induces a state of apprehension and anxiety, which may progress to panic. This disturbed mental state generally aggravates the respiratory attack. The failure of proper air exchange causes reduced oxygen in the blood. If the attack progresses, carbon dioxide will also begin to accumulate in the blood.

The bronchial smooth muscles in asthmatics are sensitive to various stimuli. Acute asthmatic attacks are precipitated by different factors for different individuals, but may include:

- allergic reactions to pollens, animal dander, dust, smoke, sawdust, etc.;
- respiratory infections (e.g. cold viruses);
- cold air;
- medication (e.g. aspirin);
- emotional distress;
- exercise;
- some other irritant.

Asthmatic attacks may be part of a serious allergic reaction (e.g. following a bee sting) and may progress rapidly to anaphylactic shock (see Part V, Section B, page 101). Therefore, it is important to find out what precipitated the attack and whether the patient has a history of recurrent attacks of a similar kind but can breathe normally in between.

To reverse the bronchoconstriction of the attack, many patients with asthma have their own prescription medications (bronchodilators), often in the form of sprays or inhalers. There may be oral medications as well. The medications may be administered with the Attendant's assistance. If possible, a history of all medications and the amount used for the current attack should be provided to hospital staff.

Status Asthmaticus

Status asthmaticus occurs when the patient has a severe, prolonged asthmatic attack that has not responded to the usual medications. The history will reveal that the attack has persisted for several hours. The patient is usually exhausted and dehydrated. The chest is usually very overinflated and exhibits minimal movement with respiratory effort. Even wheezing may not be heard (silent chest) because there is virtually no air moving through the swollen narrowed airways. The patient may appear sleepy, as the accumulated carbon dioxide in the blood will sedate the patient.

PATIENTS WITH STATUS ASTHMATICUS — AS EVIDENCED BY:

- DROWSINESS,
- EXHAUSTION, and
- SILENT NON-MOVING OVERINFLATED CHEST ARE A LIFE-THREATENING MEDICAL EMERGENCY AND FALL INTO THE RAPID TRANSPORT CATEGORY.

Recognition of the Acute Asthmatic Attack

History

- Precipitating factors (e.g. cedar dust, pollens)
- Previous attacks
- Medication (inhaler or pills)
- Dyspnea

Physical Findings

- Respiratory distress (the patient sits upright and may lean forward, fighting for breath).
- A non-productive cough but may produce scant amounts of very thick whitish-yellow mucus.
- Overinflated chest with prolonged expiration, and the movement of the chest wall may diminish as the attack becomes more severe.
- Whistling, wheezing breathing, usually more evident on expiration. (NOTE: A silent chest in a distressed patient means danger.)
- Anxiety — some patients may be very frightened and struggling for breath.
- The respiratory rate and pulse rate are usually increased.

Management of the Asthmatic Attack

1. Calm and reassure the patient.
2. Maintain and support the patient in the most comfortable sitting position.
3. Always apply oxygen at a high flow (10 Lpm) and humidify the oxygen if possible.
4. Help the patient to take the medication.
5. Assist ventilation with a bag-valve mask and high-flow oxygen if the patient is sleepy or unresponsive.
6. ALL ASTHMATIC PATIENTS IN RESPIRATORY DISTRESS FALL INTO THE RAPID TRANSPORT CATEGORY. AN ASTHMATIC WHO IS DROWSY, EXHAUSTED OR EXHIBITS A SILENT CHEST WITH A PROLONGED ATTACK IS A LIFE-THREATENING MEDICAL EMERGENCY.

CHRONIC OBSTRUCTIVE PULMONARY DISEASE (COPD)

Chronic obstructive pulmonary diseases (COPD) are long-standing obstructive airway diseases characterized by diffuse obstruction to air flow within the lungs. The most common forms of COPD are emphysema and chronic bronchitis. Individuals with chronic obstructive lung disease are usually older and have a long history of respiratory problems. These diseases affect more than one-fifth of all North American adults and account for a great many lost work days. COPD involves destruction of lung tissue with diffuse obstruction of air flow and progressive dyspnea. THE MOST IMPORTANT CAUSATIVE FACTOR IN PRODUCING COPD IS CIGARETTE SMOKING. Most sufferers have a combination of both emphysema and chronic bronchitis and may also have some superimposed asthma.

EMPHYSEMA

Emphysema refers to the chronic permanent destructive change in the alveoli, resulting in loss of their elasticity. The alveoli become distended with trapped air and cease to function. The walls of such affected alveoli often break down to produce larger air-containing sacs with thickened walls that do not participate in oxygen or carbon dioxide transfer. Consequently, over time, there is a dramatic decrease in the total number of alveoli, making it more difficult for the patient to breathe and reducing their respiratory reserve significantly. Less oxygen is able to travel through the alveolar walls and, hence, into the blood, greatly diminishing the patient's exercise tolerance. The bronchioles are also destroyed in the same fashion as the alveoli, causing further air trapping and dyspnea.

Recognition of the Patient with Emphysema

History

- Usually a long history of cigarette smoking or exposure to other respiratory irritants (e.g. hard-rock mining, asbestos).
- Usually thin, with a history of weight loss.
- History of increasing dyspnea on exertion over months or years.
- May have a history of sudden increasing shortness of breath which may be associated with a recent chest cold, and the sputum may have recently changed colour to grey, green or yellow.
- Medications (inhalers and/or pills).

CHRONIC BRONCHITIS

This condition is characterized by recurrent infections involving the bronchial tree. Usually, the history of heavy cigarette smoking for many years produces inflammation, swelling and excessive mucus in the airways. The airway changes predispose the individual to recurrent infections. Typically, the patient with chronic bronchitis has a productive cough for at least three months per year over two consecutive years. Because of the airway disease, air flow to the alveoli is impaired, which impairs ventilation. Commonly, the patient with chronic bronchitis often has an associated heart disease and may develop congestive heart failure.

Recognition of the Patient with Chronic Bronchitis

History

- Often, a long history of cigarette smoking and recurrent respiratory infections.
- History of productive cough for several months in each of the two previous years.
- There is an aggravation of cough and dyspnea with exertion (i.e. walking up stairs).
- May have a history of sudden increasing shortness of breath, which may be associated with a recent chest cold, and the sputum may have recently changed colour to grey, green or yellow.
- Medications in the form of inhalers and/or pills.

Physical Findings

- Respiratory distress.
- Often, cyanosis.
- Individuals may appear overweight and out of shape and, because of the cyanosis, are often called "blue bloaters".
- There may be an audible wheezing respiration with prolonged expiration and recurrent productive cough.
- Respiratory rate is increased and there is usually tachycardia with increased heart rate greater than 100 per minute.
- The neck veins may be distended.

NOTE: It is very important for the Attendant to remember that the "pink puffer" and the "blue bloater" descriptions represent the two extremes of patients with COPD. Most patients with COPD have some history and

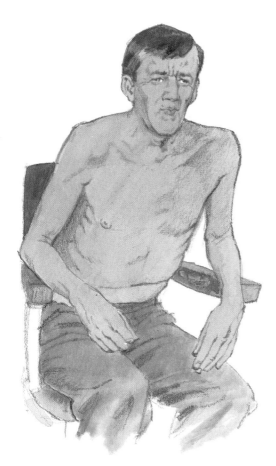

Emphysemic Patient

Physical Findings

- Respiratory distress, with the patient hunched forward in a sitting position.
- Often, an overinflated barrel chest in a thin individual.
- Little chest movement with respiration and the patients are often using accessory muscles of respiration, involving the neck, clavicles and shoulders.
- Prolonged expiration with audible wheezing, and the patient may purse the lips during exhalation.
- Increased respiratory rate and tachycardia with a heart rate of greater than 100 per minute.
- May be drowsy from hypoxia or CO_2 retention.
- Often, patients are not cyanotic and tend to pink up with the administration of oxygen, consequently called "pink puffers".

physical findings of both conditions. The patient with established COPD is prone to recurrent bouts of decompensation, which is usually precipitated by an additional stress, such as a superimposed cold or flu and will present with acute respiratory distress.

Management of Patients with COPD Who are Decompensating

Field management of COPD patients with acute respiratory distress is aimed at relieving hypoxia and transporting rapidly to medical aid. As discussed in the "Respiratory System" section, the main stimulus to take a breath for normal individuals is only small increases of carbon dioxide in the blood. Falling oxygen levels are not the primary stimulus until they have dropped to a considerably lower level. See Section A, page 37.

HOWEVER, *A VERY SMALL MINORITY OF PATIENTS WITH ADVANCED COPD* LOSE THEIR SENSITIVITY TO CO_2 AND BREATHE AS A CONSEQUENCE OF LOW BLOOD OXYGEN LEVELS (I.E. BY A HYPOXIC DRIVE). Because of the destruction in the lung tissue, carbon dioxide does not readily diffuse out of the blood into the lung alveoli. Over the years, such patients develop increasing amounts of carbon dioxide in the blood, desensitizing the respiratory centre in the brain to its presence. The condition also hampers the diffusion of oxygen into the blood and these patients usually have below normal blood oxygen levels. The low oxygen level triggers each breath in these patients, but this hypoxic drive is not nearly as sensitive as the carbon dioxide stimulus to breathe in normal people. The oxygen level in their blood must fall to almost half the normal amount before such COPD patients are stimulated to take another breath.

If such a COPD victim breathes high levels of oxygen, the only drive to breathe is removed and the ventilation rate slows. In fact, the patient may not take another breath for some time and this is called *oxygen apnea*. The decrease in breathing causes the carbon dioxide to accumulate to even higher levels, leading to central nervous system depression. If the high oxygen treatment is continued, the patient will become confused, then lapse into coma and, ultimately, die of a respiratory arrest. The process is called *carbon dioxide narcosis*. As mentioned,

this condition is found in a relatively small number of patients with advanced chronic obstructive lung disease. Such patients are very unlikely to be able to hold down any type of job, owing to their complete lack of exercise tolerance. Consequently, they are unlikely to be found in the workplace.

HOWEVER, THIS CONDITION IS NOT A JUSTIFICATION TO WITHHOLD OXYGEN FROM A COPD VICTIM, BECAUSE THEY MAY DIE. THE ATTENDANT MUST WATCH FOR ANY EVIDENCE OF RESPIRATORY DEPRESSION IN THE PATIENT'S RESPIRATORY EFFORT AND BE PREPARED TO ASSIST VENTILATION WITH A BAG-VALVE MASK.

Treat COPD patients as follows:

1. Calm and reassure the patient.
2. Ensure that there is an adequate airway.
3. Maintain and support the patient in the sitting position of greatest comfort.
4. Administer oxygen at a 1-2 Lpm flow in most circumstances for the patient with suspected advanced chronic obstructive lung disease. THE EXCEPTION TO THIS RULE IS THE PATIENT WHO HAS SUFFERED MULTIPLE TRAUMA. THE PATIENT SHOULD BE GIVEN HIGH-FLOW OXYGEN EN ROUTE TO THE HOSPITAL. ASSIST VENTILATION WITH BAG AND MASK IF NECESSARY. OXYGEN PROVIDED SHOULD BE HUMIDIFIED IF POSSIBLE.
5. Assist the patient in taking prescribed medications.
6. Check the vital signs every 15 minutes. Of most importance are the respiratory rate and level of consciousness. The slowing of respiratory rate and/or decrease in awareness are usually early signs of impending carbon dioxide narcosis.
7. If a COPD patient's respiratory condition deteriorates and the patient shows increasing dyspnea despite 1-2 litre flow of oxygen, increase the concentration gradually at a rate of 1 litre every 5 minutes. Continue to monitor the patient's respiratory rate and depth. Be prepared to assist ventilations if respirations become depressed or level of consciousness deteriorates.
8. NEVER stop oxygen therapy abruptly once it has been initiated; it should be tapered off. If it is stopped

abruptly, the oxygen levels in the blood will drop below pre-treatment levels and may induce respiratory arrest.

9. If the patient is suspected of developing carbon dioxide narcosis, oxygen should not be completely removed. Decrease the flow rate and be prepared to assist breathing.

10. The patient should be encouraged to cough and clear secretions.

11. Patients with decompensating COPD fall into the Rapid Transport Category.

PNEUMONIA

One of the most common diseases affecting the respiratory tract is pneumonia. Although this is frequently thought of as a single disease, it is actually a group of diseases affecting the lung, sometimes in different ways. There are many varieties of the disease: lobar pneumonia, bronchopneumonia and viral pneumonia are among them.

The principle characteristic in all the pneumonias is an *exudation* of serum and cells into the alveolar spaces and small bronchioles. Associated with the infection is the slowing down of the blood supply surrounding the alveoli and a thickening of the alveolar walls by fluid and cells which escape from the capillaries.

It is not difficult to see how such changes in the tissue of the lung will result in very serious changes and derangement of its functions. *Narrowing* of the bronchioles results from secretion interfering with the free passage of air. There is *exudate* in the air spaces, which prevents the entrance of air and hinders the passage of oxygen through the walls of the alveoli into the blood, and there is *thickening* of the alveolar wall itself, causing further interference of gas exchange. In addition, the fluid causes the lung to lose elasticity, which is necessary for proper ventilation. It follows that ventilation in these areas is very much affected and becomes much more work for the patient. Pneumonia therefore produces hypoxia in all cases. If enough lung is involved, cyanosis is produced and accompanied by rapid and shallow respiration, weakness and symptoms of oxygen deficiency.

Prior to the advent of antibiotics, pneumonia was one of the most common causes of death. Although the course of the disease varies with the type of pneumonia, with the

drugs currently available, the severe disturbance, generally speaking, does not last very long. However, very aggressive and virulent organisms can produce pneumonias that cause death, even today. Formerly, pneumonia was a process that dragged on for one to three weeks and recovery depended upon the patient's ability to survive a severe respiratory handicap. Today, the course of the illness is usually much shorter and with an excellent outcome, providing appropriate care is given. Serious cases require admission to hospital and aggressive treatment with intravenous antibiotics, physiotherapy, oxygen therapy and, at times, mechanical respiratory support. It is important that the Attendant refer any individual with a suspected pneumonia for medical attention.

Lobar pneumonia was once the most common of all pneumonias but is much less common today. The reason for the decrease in incidence is probably due to the use of new drugs. Lobar pneumonia is primarily caused by the pneumococcus organism and the disease process involves an entire lobe of the lung. It usually presents very suddenly with the patient developing a high fever, pleuritic pain on the affected side, weakness and productive cough of a rusty sputum. In more serious cases, the patients may be very dyspneic and cyanotic. Such patients are usually hypoxic and benefit greatly from oxygen therapy. Patients suspected of having a lobar pneumonia should be rapidly transported to hospital.

Bronchopneumonia, on the other hand, is a disease that involves the lung tissue diffusely and frequently involves both lungs. The very diffuseness of the disease creates quite a severe hypoxia. These patients usually produce purulent greenish-yellow sputum with cough. They may be very ill, with marked respiratory distress and require urgent medical attention. They will benefit from oxygen therapy en route.

Viral pneumonia may be caused by a variety of viruses. The patient has fever, weakness and may demonstrate some of the findings of asthma, as the bronchioles and other airways may be inflamed and narrowed owing to the inflammatory process. They usually have a dry cough but may have quite profound dyspnea and cyanosis. Such patients will benefit from supplemental oxygen and should also be referred for medical attention.

HYPERVENTILATION SYNDROME

Dyspnea may occur in patients without any lung abnormalities or medical problems. Often, anxious people or individuals with unusual stress may unconsciously start to breathe at a rate and depth greater than needed physiologically. The patient is often unaware that he/she is breathing abnormally, deeply or rapidly. The phenomenon causes a lowering of the normal carbon dioxide levels in the blood which, if it continues, causes an alteration in the body chemistry (alkalosis). This alkalosis produces a number of characteristic signs and symptoms and is known as the hyperventilation syndrome. All or only some of these findings may be found in any one patient.

Symptoms of Hyperventilation

- Marked shortness of breath or dyspnea, often with a feeling that the individual cannot take or get a deep enough breath.
- Marked anxiety and even panic (e.g. feeling as though they are going to die).
- Feelings of dizziness or that their eyes are not quite in focus.
- A feeling of depersonalization (feeling detached, "unreal" and not fully in control of their body).
- Variable pressure across the chest or stabbing, fleeting chest pain.
- Numbness or tingling, or needles and pins about the mouth, over the scalp and in the fingertips and toes.
- No history of significant cardiac or respiratory disease.

Physical Findings

- Rapid respirations or occasional deep sighing respirations.
- Tachycardia.
- A brief faint but no seizure activity or postictal phase.
- Carpopedal spasm may occur in advanced attacks where the fingers and wrists become stiff and flexed like claws, with the thumb held stiffly across the palm.

Management of Hyperventilation Syndrome

Not all patients who are breathing deeply or rapidly are hyperventilating. The term "hyperventilation" means breathing at a depth or rate greater than needed to control normal levels of carbon dioxide in the blood. Consequently, as a result of hyperventilation, the CO_2 level in the arterial blood falls. On the other hand, a diabetic with acidosis will appear to be hyperventilating but, in fact, the CO_2 levels in the blood are not reduced. This may also be true for certain poisonings. THEREFORE, BEFORE MAKING THE DIAGNOSIS OF HYPERVENTILATION, THE ATTENDANT MUST RULE OUT A DISEASE PROCESS CAUSING THE PATIENT'S CLINICAL PICTURE.

In a young patient, it is important to rule out asthma, spontaneous pneumothorax or diabetic acidosis. The patient's age and lack of cardiac history will usually rule out the diagnosis of heart attack. Therefore, the diagnosis of hyperventilation syndrome is one of exclusion. Once other causes have been ruled out, the following protocol may be instituted for managing this condition:

1. Treatment is aimed at calming the patient in order to restore the patient's carbon dioxide levels to normal. Therefore, the Attendant should remain calm, listen carefully and show understanding.
2. The Attendant should briefly explain to the patient the nature of the process and that their symptoms will abate if they hold their breath and slow their breathing rate down.
3. DO NOT USE A REBREATHING PAPER BAG. Formerly, it was recommended to have the patient breathe in and out of a paper bag, tightly sealed over the mouth and nose. This was to enable the patient to rebreathe the exhaled carbon dioxide and help return the blood level to normal. The practice is no longer recommended as it lowers the oxygen level in the blood to a dangerous degree.
4. If in doubt about the cause of symptoms, administer oxygen at 10 Lpm, as it will not make the hyperventilation worse.
5. If the attack does not resolve spontaneously within 15 minutes, transport the patient to medical aid.

PULMONARY EDEMA

Dyspnea can be caused by acute pulmonary edema. Pulmonary edema is the accumulation of fluid within the alveoli, causing impairment of the flow of oxygen from the alveoli into the blood. With the presence of fluid in the alveoli, the lung tissue becomes stiffer and the patient must work harder to breathe. Similarly, the fluid collection is not limited just to the alveoli but may also occur in the walls of the smaller bronchioles, causing them to become narrower. This process is often associated with bronchospasm as described in "Asthma", with further impairment of the ventilation. It also accounts for the wheezing respiration that may occasionally be present in some patients with pulmonary edema.

The most common cause of pulmonary edema is left ventricular failure. It is discussed under "Congestive Heart Failure", Part V, Section E, page 118. Several other causes of pulmonary edema have been referred to in other sections, including inhalation of noxious gases (e.g. chlorine gas) (Part XII, Section A, page 312), near-drowning (Part XI, Section F, page 301), smoke inhalation (Section C, page 68). Other less common causes of pulmonary edema include acute altitude sickness, and overdose with some poisons (e.g. heroin or aspirin).

The most common symptom of pulmonary edema, regardless of cause, is dyspnea. This symptom may range from a mere heaviness of the chest to a desperate struggle for breath in a terrified patient. The onset of respiratory distress may be dramatically sudden or may develop over a period of several hours. Lying down aggravates the dyspnea. In its most advanced form, cough productive of white to pink foamy sputum is typical. Severe agitation is associated with advanced hypoxia, as the patient "drowns" in his/her own secretions, if the course of the disease is not altered.

Recognition of Acute Pulmonary Edema

History

- If it is caused by left heart failure, there may be chest pain with an associated heart attack, history of high blood pressure or history of previous attacks.
- Exposure to other precipitating factors listed.
- Dyspnea, often severe, with inability to lie down.

Physical Findings That May Be Present

- Increasing respiratory distress and the patient may be agitated, restless or confused.
- May have cold, clammy skin and distended neck veins if there is a cardiac origin.
- Cyanosis.

- Tachycardia with pulse usually greater than 100 beats per minute.
- Cough with frothy white or pink sputum.
- Wheezing respirations.

Management of Pulmonary Edema

1. Calm and reassure the patient.
2. Position patient sitting upright in the position of comfort, with the legs dangling, if possible.
3. Periodic rapid suctioning of the airway may be necessary for accumulated secretions, if the patient cannot clear them.
4. If the patient is becoming drowsy or is extremely dyspneic, assisted ventilation timed to the patient's breathing, with a bag-valve mask and high-flow oxygen, should be instituted.
5. The comatose patient with acute pulmonary edema will require suctioning and assisted ventilation with high-flow oxygen.
6. Patients with pulmonary edema fall into the Rapid Transport Category.

Part IV, Section E
Oxygen Therapy and Equipment

INTRODUCTION

The purpose of this section is to provide the Industrial First Aid Attendant with a convenient reference for the use of oxygen therapy equipment.

This section will discuss safe handling practices, cylinders, regulators, gauges, accessory equipment, operating procedures, adaptors, patient application and special considerations of oxygen use.

SAFE HANDLING PRACTICES

1. Oil or grease should NEVER be used on any device that will be attached to an oxygen cylinder.
   Grease or oil can violently explode if it comes in contact with high-pressure oxygen. If grease or oil is noted around or on the regulator, do not try to clean it but return the regulator to the nearest supplier for cleaning and repair before being used. If grease or oil is noted on or around the cylinder valve or aperture, do not use the cylinder and immediately inform the oxygen supplier of this condition.
2. Do not allow smoking around oxygen equipment that is operating and never use oxygen around an open flame.
   Although oxygen will not explode or burn by itself, it does support combustion and will cause burning objects to flame vigorously. The area where oxygen is in use must be clearly marked with signs that read "Oxygen — No Smoking".
3. Oxygen cylinders should always be well secured, preferably supported by a case in the upright position or lying horizontally. This will prevent damage to the valve assembly. Since oxygen cylinders when full contain between 2,000 to 2,200 pounds per square inch (PSI) of pressure, breaking of the valve assembly could turn the cylinder into a jet-propelled missile.
4. Store cylinders that are not in use in a cool, well-ventilated room and away from any corrosives.
5. Use only regulators and gauges intended for use with oxygen.
6. When opening the cylinder, stand so that the cylinder valve is between you and the regulator; this could prevent injury if the regulator should explode.

7. Ensure the valve seat insert and gasket are in good condition before assembling equipment; this will prevent dangerous leaks. (See Figure IV-9.)

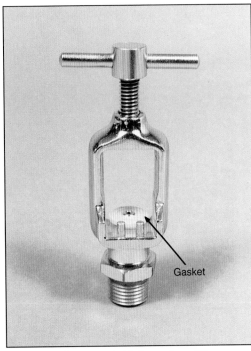

Figure IV-9 Ensure gasket is in good condition.

8. The Attendant should NEVER attempt to tighten the cylinder valve or any parts of the valve.
   If the cylinder valve is leaking, it should be placed well away from hazards and the oxygen supplier notified immediately.
9. Oxygen cylinders are NOT to be refilled by unauthorized personnel. Always return empty cylinders to qualified plants for refilling.

CYLINDERS

Oxygen cylinders come in various sizes. There are three sizes that the Attendant is most likely to use: the "D" (14.5 cubic ft.), "E" (26 cubic ft.) and the 17 cubic ft. cylinder. The Attendant may also have occasion to use the "K" size (244 cubic ft.) industrial cylinder (to be discussed later).

Oxygen cylinders are usually made of seamless steel, although there are some lightweight aluminum cylinders in use. There are two systems used to connect the valve to the top of the cylinder. These can be either the medical post type (Figure IV-10) or the threaded type with a hand valve (Figure IV-11).

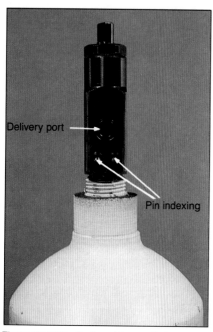

Figure IV-10 Medical post type cylinder

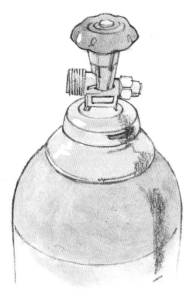

Figure IV-11 Threaded type cylinder

Oxygen cylinders must be tested for structural weakness by hydrostatic testing every five years in accordance with WCB regulations. Whenever sending oxygen cylinders out for refilling, check the date of the last hydrostatic test that is stamped on the cylinder (see Figure IV-12). If it is over five years, inform supplier that additional testing is required.

Oxygen cylinders being sent for refilling should have some residual pressure left in them. It is recommended that at least 100 PSI be left but never any less than 50 PSI.

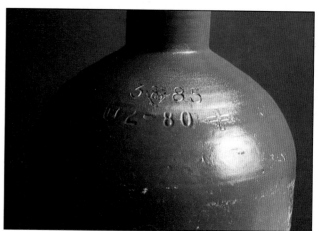

Figure IV-12 Hydrostatic test date

Cylinder Duration

There are several methods of calculating how long the oxygen in the cylinder will last. Whatever method is used, the Attendant must ensure that arrangements are made to switch to a new cylinder before the one in use is empty. The Attendant must also be sure that there is a sufficient supply of oxygen to complete the trip to hospital. It may be good practice to secure the appropriate table from the following chart to the oxygen container for quick easy reference.

OXYGEN CYLINDER DURATION

TANK SIZE — "D" CYLINDER — 14.5 CU. FT.

LBS. PRESSURE	6 LPM	8 LPM	10 LPM
2,000	63 min.	47 min.	38 min.
1,500	47 min.	35 min.	28 min.
1,000	31 min.	24 min.	19 min.
500	16 min.	12 min.	9 min.

TANK SIZE — "E" CYLINDER — 26 CU. FT.

LBS. PRESSURE	6 LPM	8 LPM	10 LPM
2,000	113 min.	83 min.	68 min.
1,500	85 min.	63 min.	51 min.
1,000	56 min.	42 min.	34 min.
500	28 min.	21 min.	17 min.

TANK SIZE — 17 CU. FT.

	2 LPM	4 LPM	6 LPM	8 LPM	10 LPM
FULL	240 min.	120 min.	80 min.	60 min.	48 min.
3/4	180 min.	90 min.	60 min.	45 min.	36 min.
1/2	120 min.	60 min.	40 min.	30 min.	24 min.
1/4	60 min.	30 min.	20 min.	15 min.	12 min.

TANK SIZE — "K" CYLINDER — 244 CU. FT.

LBS. PRESSURE	6 LPM	8 LPM	10 LPM
2,000	1,050 min.	780 min.	630 min.
1,500	780 min.	590 min.	470 min.
1,000	525 min.	390 min.	365 min.
500	260 min.	195 min.	155 min.

REGULATORS

Regulators can be either one or two stage. This refers to the number of steps required to reduce the cylinder pressure to a safe working pressure. Most regulators, currently in use, are two stage.

Regulators are connected to oxygen cylinders by two methods:

1. On "D" and "E" cylinders, the regulator is connected to the cylinder by a yoke assembly. The yoke is provided with pins that match the corresponding holes on the medical post. This aligns the regulator

inlet with the delivery port on the medical post (see Figure IV-13). This pin indexing prevents the yoke assembly from being connected improperly or to a cylinder of another type of gas.

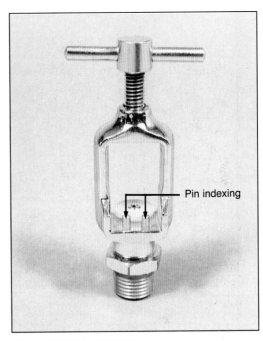

Figure IV-13 Yoke assembly

2. On the 17 cubic ft. or "K" cylinders, there is a hand valve assembly with a threaded outlet; the standard 540 thread has been adapted to avoid connecting the regulator to any other gas.

GAUGES

There are usually two gauges attached to the regulator: a pressure gauge and a flow meter. The pressure gauge indicates the amount of oxygen available in the cylinder in pounds per square inch. The flow meter indicates the flow rate of oxygen to the patient in litres per minute.

MODIFICATION OF STANDARD CYLINDERS AND REGULATORS

Adaptors for "D" and "E" Size Units

At times, in isolated areas, where large volumes of oxygen may be required, a commercial oxygen cylinder (244 cubic feet size "K") may be used. A larger-type regulator and gauges with female 540 thread (see Figure IV-14) fit directly onto the male cylinder threads.

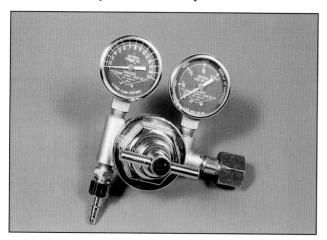

Figure IV-14 Regulator and gauges with female 540 thread

It is important to remember that each type of regulator fits only one type of cylinder. In order to connect different cylinders to a non-matching regulator (e.g. 540 thread), the appropriate adaptor is required.

540 thread (on cylinder) to pin indexed regulator and gauges

In order to fit the smaller-type pin indexed regulator and gauges to the large 540 thread commercial cylinder, the adaptor illustrated in Figure IV-15 is used. The final assembly is shown in Figure IV-16.

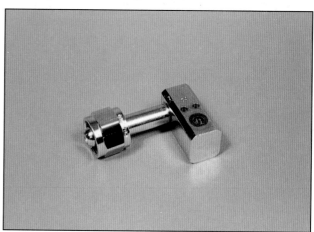

Figure IV-15 Adaptor for a commercial cylinder

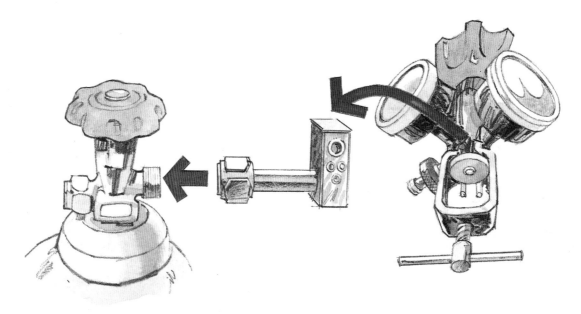

Figure IV-16 Assembly using the adaptor

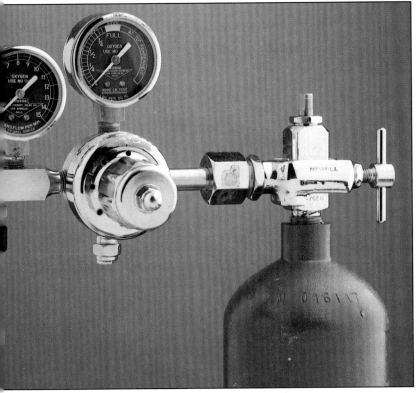

Figure IV-17 540 thread regulator and adaptor yoke connected to oxygen bottle

Pin indexed medical post (on cylinder) to 540 thread regulator and gauges

In order to fit the larger 540 thread regulator and gauges onto the pin indexed medical cylinders, the illustrated adaptor yoke (Figure IV-13) is needed. The final assembly would connect as in Figure IV-17.

It is not necessary to use both types of adaptors. Either type is effective and the choice is up to the company providing the first aid services.

ACCESSORIES

Pocket Mask

Commercially designed pocket masks are particularly well suited for ventilation in the field. There is an oxygen inlet through which high-flow oxygen can be provided. They overcome most of the disadvantages of mouth-to-mouth ventilation. Finally, the pocket masks are easier to use than the bag-valve mask system. Pocket masks are equipped with one-way valves to prevent contamination of the Attendant with the patient's secretions. Pocket masks not equipped with one-way valves are not recommended.

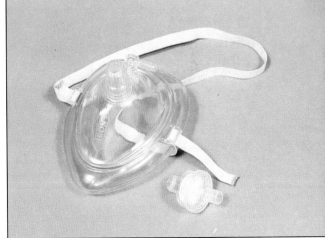

Pocket mask with valve

Bag-Valve Mask Resuscitator

All bag-valve mask resuscitators have several common components:
- An inflatable bag has an oxygen inlet at one end. A one-way valve is connected between the face mask and the bag.
- Most bag-valve mask resuscitators currently on the market are provided with an OXYGEN RESERVOIR to permit delivery of oxygen concentrations approaching 100%. Without the oxygen reservoir, it is difficult to achieve oxygen concentrations above 50%. To achieve this concentration, an O_2 flow of 15 Lpm is required to inflate and maintain the reservoir. It is recommended that all bag-valve mask resuscitators have this O_2 reservoir accessory.

The plastic tube that is connected to the oxygen cylinder is attached to the bag-valve mask resuscitator. Bag-valve mask resuscitators are used to assist ventilations in patients who are breathing inadequately. See Section B, page 52 for a more detailed description.

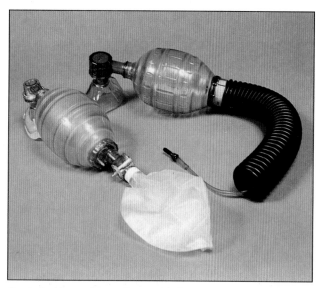

Two typical bag-valve mask systems. On the left the O$_2$ reservoir is a bag; on the right the reservoir is a snorkel.

Simple Face Mask

The simple face mask is a formed clear plastic unit with soft sides that conforms to the patient's face. An elastic strap fastened to the mask holds it on. Perforations in the mask allow excess oxygen and the patient's exhaled carbon dioxide to escape to the atmosphere. These masks are inexpensive and disposable, and eliminate the need for cleaning and sterilization.

Simple face masks are used when moderate concentrations of supplemental oxygen are required. Oxygen concentrations will vary between 30% at a 6-litre flow and 50% at a 10-litre flow. You cannot provide 100% oxygen to a patient with a simple face mask, because the perforations allow atmospheric air to enter the facepiece with each inhalation.

Partial Rebreathing Mask

This mask combines a face mask with a reservoir bag, which allows part of the patient's exhaled air to enter the reservoir bag where it is enriched with oxygen from the supply system. Each time the patient inhales, the enriched mixture from the reservoir bag plus pure oxygen from the cylinder is supplied. Increased concentrations of oxygen can be delivered with the partial rebreathing mask ranging from 30% to 60% when flow rates are between 6 and 10 litres per minute. The partial rebreathing mask must be well fitted so that the bag does not deflate completely when the patient inhales. When increased oxygen concentrations are required, the non-rebreathing mask is preferred.

Non-Rebreathing Mask

As the name of this mask implies, it does not allow the patient to rebreathe any of the exhaled air. The main feature of this mask is a one-way valve placed between the mask and the reservoir bag. During expiration, carbon dioxide vents to the atmosphere. On inspiration, the patient receives high concentrations of oxygen from the reservoir bag and the cylinder. The one-way valve prevents exhaled air from entering the reservoir bag during exhalation.

The non-rebreathing mask is a very effective means of delivering high concentrations of oxygen to the spontaneously breathing patient. Concentrations of as much as 100% can be provided as long as there are no leaks and the mask is properly fitted.

Venturi Mask

This type of mask is preferred when precise lower concentrations of oxygen are required. The oxygen is delivered through a jet at a velocity that draws air from outside through holes in the sides of the mask. These masks are disposable and are available to deliver the following levels of concentration: 24%, 28%, 35%, 40% and 50%.

The venturi masks are designed to supply a constant concentration of oxygen over a wide range of flow rates. These masks have little application in the industrial setting. They are designed for patients with severe chronic respiratory disease.

Humidifier

Oxygen that is delivered from a cylinder is completely free of water vapour and will dry the mucus membranes of the nose, throat and lungs.

A humidifier is a receptacle of water which is attached on line from the oxygen supply (see Figure IV-18). The operation is quite simple. The oxygen becomes humidified as it bubbles through the water, picking up moisture en route to the patient. It is preferred, if practicable, that all first aid rooms and transportation vehicles be equipped with a humidifier.

OPERATING PROCEDURES

1. Setting Up the Equipment
   - Inspect the cylinder and regulator for dirt, dust, oil and grease, especially around areas where high-pressure oxygen can come into contact with it. Inspect the regulator inlet for damage. Check the threads of the cylinder outlet and internal surfaces for damages, especially those surfaces that are in contact with oxygen under high pressure.
   - Inspect the rupture disk on the cylinder valve assembly for damage.
   - Secure the cylinder in an upright position. Remove the dust cover from the cylinder if one is present, then "crack" the cylinder valve to blow any dust or dirt from the cylinder outlet.

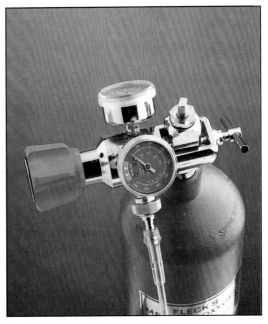

Regulator attached to oxygen bottle

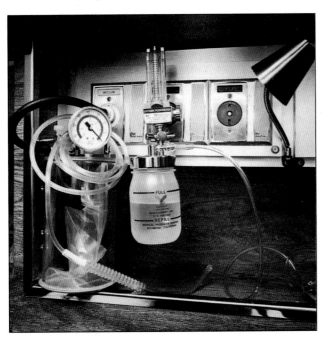

Figure IV-18 Humidifier on the right, suction unit on the left

2. Installing the Regulator
   - If the regulator has a YOKE-TYPE INLET connection:
     i) Remove the tape which may be covering the cylinder outlet and "crack" the cylinder valve to blow any dirt or dust from the cylinder outlet.
     ii) Make sure the sealing washer is in place on the yoke inlet.
     iii) The yoke should be slipped over the cylinder medical post and the yoke's index pins fitted into the holes in the cylinder valve. Caution should be taken to make sure the pins fit properly into the connection holes; they are not to be forced into the holes.
     iv) Turn the "T" handle to tighten the regulator securely for a leak-proof seal.
   - If the regulator has a NUT GLAND INLET connection:
     i) Remove the protective dust cover from the cylinder outlet and "crack" the cylinder valve to blow any dust or dirt from the cylinder outlet.
     ii) Fit the regulator to the cylinder connection and thread the nut on the regulator connection to the cylinder valve connection.
     iii) With a suitable wrench, tighten the nut to secure the regulator and make a leak-proof seal.

- If the regulator has a HANDTIGHT INLET connection:
  i) Remove the dust cover from the cylinder outlet and "crack" the cylinder valve to blow any dirt or dust from the cylinder outlet.
  ii) The regulator inlet connection is fitted to and threaded onto the cylinder valve connection.
  iii) Tighten the regulator hand nut to secure it to the cylinder and make a leak-proof seal.

3. Connecting Oxygen Delivery Equipment to the Regulator's Outlet Connection

   The connection of the tubing from the regulator outlet nipple to the face mask is made by hand. These connections should not be forced nor should they be so loose that they fall off. In order to protect the patient from injury, the connection will blow apart whenever flow exceeds 15 litres.

4. Opening the Cylinder Valve
   - Be sure the regulator has been shut off before opening the cylinder valve.
   - Open the cylinder valve counter-clockwise slowly and carefully until the regulator high-pressure gauge indicates pressure in the regulator. Wait for the regulator pressure to stabilize and then open the cylinder valve one full turn.
   - To check the cylinder valve, inlet fitting, high-pressure gauge or regulator seat, close the cylinder valve and observe the regulator's high-pressure gauge for five minutes. If there is any drop in the pressure gauge reading, retighten the regulator to cylinder connection and repeat the test. Should there still be a drop in the high-pressure gauge, the regulator MUST BE REMOVED FROM SERVICE.

5. Adjusting Regulator Flow
   - For flow-gauge regulators:
     The litre flow adjusting knob on the regulator should be turned clockwise until the flow gauge reads the rate of oxygen flow desired.
   - For the flow-meter-equipped regulator:
     The flow adjusting valve is opened until the centre of the ball is aligned with the line indicating the rate of flow desired.

6. Closing the Cylinder Valve
   - Close the cylinder valve, then open the regulator and allow the gas pressure in regulator to escape. The gas will cease to flow and the two needles on the regulator gauges will drop to zero if a flow gauge is being used. When a regulator equipped with a flow meter is being used, the high-pressure gauge needle will fall to zero and the ball float will fall to the bottom of the flow meter flow scale when the gas ceases to flow.
   - The regulator valve should be closed after all the pressure has been relieved. Excessive force must not be used to close the regulator valve; it could result in damage.

7. Removing the Regulator from the Cylinder

   The regulator does not have to be removed unless the cylinder is nearly empty (i.e. 100 PSI or less).

   IF THERE IS ANY PRESSURE SHOWING ON THE HIGH-PRESSURE GAUGE, NEVER ATTEMPT TO REMOVE THE REGULATOR FROM THE CYLINDER. FOLLOW THESE STEPS:
   - CLOSE THE CYLINDER VALVE.
   - OPEN THE FLOW VALVE TO BLEED THE RESIDUAL PRESSURE FROM THE GAUGES.
   - REMOVE REGULATOR.

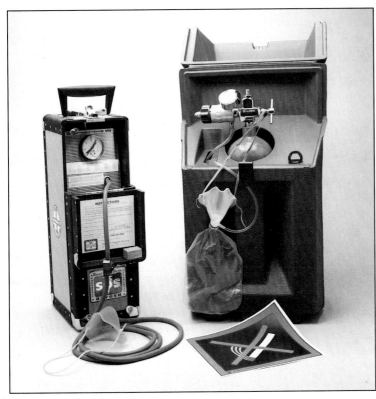
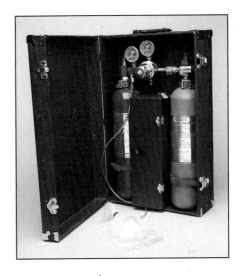

Typical oxygen therapy units

If a humidifier is being used during therapy, disconnect it from the regulator before removing the regulator from the cylinder. This will prevent water from entering the regulator and damaging it.

- The nut-and-gland-type inlet connection is removed by loosening the nut with a wrench and turning the nut counter-clockwise until free. The regulator should be well supported during removal.
- The "T" handle on the yoke-type inlet connection is turned counter-clockwise until the yoke connection can be slipped up over the cylinder valve (medical post) and removed.
- To remove the handtight connection, loosen the inlet connection nut by hand. A wrench may be carefully used to initially loosen the seal. The regulator should be well supported during the removal.

PATIENT APPLICATION

Indications for the Use of Oxygen

- Respiratory and/or cardiac arrest
- All trauma victims in the Rapid Transport Category
- Shortness of breath — acute or chronic
- Shock
- Cardiovascular or respiratory illness
- Inadequate respirations (e.g. drug overdose)

- Decreased level of consciousness
- Pregnant patients
- All medical air evacuation patients

Basic Principles of Oxygen Therapy

- Hypoxia should be suspected in all patients who are confused, restless or excessively drowsy.
- The body is unable to store oxygen. If oxygen is required, administer it continuously.
- Supplemental oxygen is no substitute for a clear airway.
- Never leave a patient with a decreased level of consciousness alone with an oxygen mask secured to the face, even in the lateral position. If the patient vomits, he or she will aspirate.
- If a patient is showing marked respiratory distress, provide supplemental oxygen at a 10-litre flow. If there is a limited supply of oxygen and the patient becomes less distressed, reduce the flow accordingly. Assisted ventilations may also be required.
- If possible, never leave a patient with advanced chronic obstructive pulmonary disease (COPD) alone while receiving oxygen. Watch for signs of impending carbon dioxide narcosis, slowing of the respiratory rate, sleepiness, confusion and decreasing level of consciousness (see Section D, page 70).

Applying Oxygen to the Patient

Attach the tubing from the face mask to the oxygen cylinder, open the flow valve and initiate the flow of oxygen as previously explained. Turn the regulator litre flow valve clockwise to the desired flow and allow the oxygen to flow through the tubing for a few seconds before placing the mask on the patient's face. This is necessary to clear out any fluid or dust that may have lodged in the tubing.

Many patients have never seen oxygen equipment and it may cause some uneasiness or alarm. To minimize this, it is sometimes reassuring to allow the patient to hold the mask to his/her own face with the oxygen flowing. Once the patient has become accustomed to the mask and oxygen flow, you can slip the elastic strap on the mask over the head to hold the mask in position. The oxygen should always be flowing when you are applying the face mask to the patient. Reassure the patient about the use of oxygen and its benefits. Explain what you are doing and answer questions the patient may have about it.

Signs of the beneficial effects of oxygen:

- improvement in skin colour and condition
- quieter, easier breathing
- less pain
- less restlessness or improved level of consciousness
- decrease in an abnormally rapid pulse rate

GENERAL OXYGEN THERAPY TREATMENT FOR CHRONIC OBSTRUCTIVE LUNG DISEASE VICTIMS

- Administer oxygen at a one-to-two-litres-per-minute flow in most circumstances for the suspected COPD patients (see Section D, page 72). The only EXCEPTION to this rule is if the patient has suffered MULTIPLE TRAUMA. In that case, *FULL* DOSES OF O_2 should be given en route to the hospital. Assist ventilation with bag-valve mask if necessary.
- Allow the patient to assume the position of most comfort unless contraindicated (e.g. cervical injury, shock).
- Check the vital signs every 15 minutes. Of most importance are the respiratory rate and level of consciousness. The slowing of respiratory rate and/or decrease in awareness are usually early warning signs of impending carbon dioxide narcosis.
- If a COPD patient's condition deteriorates and the patient shows increasing dyspnea despite a one- or two-litre flow, increase the concentration gradually. Be prepared; you may have to assist ventilations.
- If respiratory efforts are failing and the patient becomes unresponsive, ventilate either by mouth-to-mouth, bag-valve mask or pocket mask.
- Never stop oxygen therapy abruptly once it has been initiated; it should be tapered off. If it is stopped abruptly, the oxygen levels in the blood will drop below pre-treatment levels and may induce respiratory arrest.
- If the patient is suspected of developing carbon dioxide narcosis, oxygen should not be completely removed. Decrease the flow rate and be prepared to assist breathing.

SPECIAL CONSIDERATIONS

Special consideration should be given to victims with advanced chronic obstructive pulmonary disease (COPD) such as emphysema and chronic bronchitis.

Normally, breathing is stimulated by the carbon dioxide levels in the blood. Only slight increases in the CO_2 tension of the blood stimulate an increased respiratory effort. Over the years, people with advanced chronic obstructive pulmonary disease develop increasing amounts of carbon dioxide in their blood, desensitizing the brain cells to its presence. The condition also hampers diffusion of oxygen into the blood and causes below normal blood oxygen levels. It is the low oxygen level in the blood that stimulates these people to breathe but this hypoxic drive is not nearly as sensitive as the carbon dioxide stimulus. The oxygen levels in the COPD patient must fall to almost half of that in a normal person before he is stimulated to take another breath.

If oxygen is administered to these patients at a high level, it can remove their only drive to breathe and their ventilation rate will slow. As the respirations decrease, higher and higher levels of carbon dioxide begin to accumulate, causing central nervous system depression. If the oxygen treatment is continued, the patient may become confused then lapse into a coma and may die of respiratory arrest.

NOTE: PATIENTS WITH ADVANCED COPD WHO HAVE DEVELOPED THIS SEVERE CONDITION ARE *NOT* FOUND IN THE WORK SITE. THEY WOULD BE TOO BREATHLESS TO WORK.

The COPD patient can usually be recognized by the presence of all or a few of the following characteristics.

- History of being a heavy smoker for many, many years (e.g. usually more than 30 years at 1-2 packages per day).
- Admission to hospital on *numerous* occasions for chest infections or episodes of shortness of breath.
- An established medical history of emphysema or chronic bronchitis.
- Progressive breathlessness which has developed over several years.
- Barrel-like or over-expanded chest with minimal movement on breathing.
- The patient may breathe through pursed lips.
- Patients with asthma that usually responds to treatment in the emergency ward are not COPD patients and should be given oxygen at high flow and concentration. For shortness of breath caused by an asthmatic attack, see Section D, page 69.

DIVING EMERGENCIES

Diving accidents may cause a variety of complex medical problems. Immediate and proper attention must be given to the victim at the accident site, but the Attendant must not delay transport to a hyperbaric facility. In diving accidents, treatment actions must be initiated immediately. They include: recognition, maintenance of vital signs, administration of oxygen and arranging immediate evacuation to a hyperbaric facility.

All of these actions are important. The most critical is the delivery of high percentages of oxygen. Oxygen delivery will ensure that those tissues which are hypoxic will receive the benefit of high oxygen concentrations. Increased oxygen concentrations may also help to alleviate some symptoms of decompression sickness.

Oxygen must be started as soon as possible, at the highest percentage possible, i.e. non-rebreathing mask at 10 litres per minute. The delivery of oxygen should not be discontinued for any reason.

CLEANING, CARE AND STORAGE

When the Attendant has finished using the equipment, ensure that the cylinder is shut off and the oxygen "bled" out of the gauges so that they read zero. If the gauges are left under pressure, they can be damaged. Check the cylinder, gauges and regulator over for any damage that may have occurred during use. Be sure to check the amount of oxygen left in the cylinder to ensure an adequate supply for almost any further emergency. The face mask and delivery tubing can be cleaned with soap and water. Be sure to rinse the tubing and face mask well (see Part IX, Section E, page 213). The face mask can be wiped with an antiseptic (not alcohol) after rinsing. The plastic face mask or tubing should not be autoclaved or boiled. The cylinders when not in use should be stored in an upright position and secured firmly in place. Store them away from any corrosives and in a well-ventilated area that is not subject to high temperatures.

AUTOMATIC MECHANICAL VENTILATORS

Automatic mechanical ventilators are covered by Industrial First Aid Regulation 1.110, which reads as follows:

The use of automatic mechanical ventilators shall be permitted only in circumstances where workers could be subjected to injury and entrapment in toxic atmospheres.

These automatic mechanical ventilators shall:

a) *Be of a standard acceptable to the Board.*

b) *Be maintained and operated in accordance with the manufacturer's specifications, and*

c) *Be operated only by qualified operators specifically trained in the equipment to be used.*

The intent of the above regulation includes only those oxygen therapy devices with resuscitation capabilities. Those devices depend on manual triggering of an auxiliary valve to provide a controlled positive pressure for inflating the lungs. These devices are commonly referred to as "portable gas-powered manually activated mechanical resuscitators" and must conform to the following criteria:

- They should not contain an active negative pressure phase.
- They should be volume limited, not pressure limited.
- They should meet the requirements found in the National Standard of Canada, under the title "Lung Ventilators", Can3-Z168.5 -M78, Section 4.7. This standard covers both ventilators used in operating rooms and emergency resuscitators.

Part V, Section A
Circulatory System Anatomy and Function

The circulatory system is the transportation system of the body. It provides a continuous supply of nutrients and oxygen to the cells and rids them of carbon dioxide and other waste products.

The circulatory or cardiovascular system is a complex arrangement of tubes called arteries, arterioles, capillaries, venules and veins. Through these tubes, blood is circulated throughout the entire body under pressure from the pumping mechanism — the heart.

The circulatory system is made up of two separate systems. One provides circulation through the lungs (pulmonary circulation) and the other provides circulation through the rest of the body (systemic circulation).

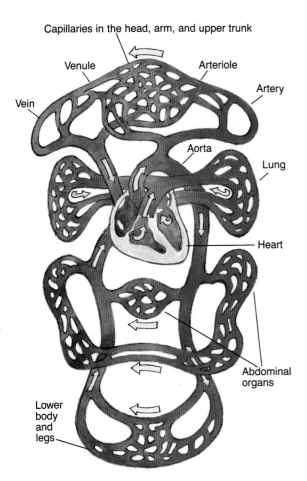

Circulatory System

BLOOD

Blood is a thick fluid which varies in colour from bright red (oxygenated) to a dark, brownish red (less oxygenated).

The blood has two main components:

- **Plasma** The liquid that carries the blood cells and transports nutrients to all tissues. It also transports waste products to the organs of excretion.
- **Blood cells** Red cells give colour to the blood and carry oxygen. White cells help defend the body from infection. Platelets promote clotting, which is necessary to stop bleeding.

The three main functions of blood are:

1. **Transportation**

   Oxygen from the air in the lungs is absorbed by the hemoglobin in the red blood cells, and carried to all the tissues of the body. Carbon dioxide, a waste product of all metabolism, is carried by the plasma from the tissues to the lungs, where it is exhaled. The blood carries nutrients from the intestine to all body tissues. Waste products are transported by the blood to the liver and the kidneys for excretion.

   Special secretions called hormones, which regulate growth and normal body functions, are transported by the blood from their organs of origin to their various destinations. The blood also transmits heat from the muscles to other parts of the body.

2. **Combatting infection**

   Certain white cells and proteins in the blood defend the body from disease-causing organisms.

3. **Coagulation (process of clot formation)**

   Cellular and protein elements in the blood stop bleeding when a blood vessel is damaged.

HEART

The heart is a hollow muscular organ, slightly bigger than a fist. It is located between the lungs in the centre and just to the left of the midline of the body.

A wall (septum) divides the heart down the middle. Each side of the heart is divided into an upper receiving chamber (atrium) and a lower chamber (ventricle). The

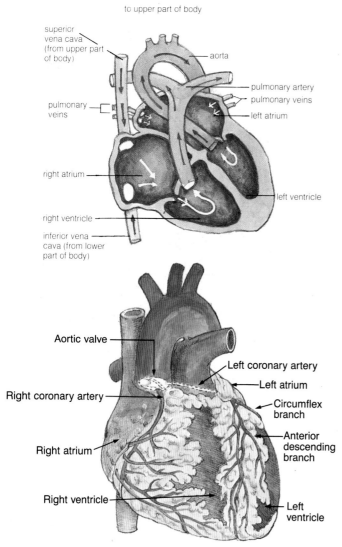

Figure V-1 Arteries and Valves

the left atrium. The left atrium then delivers this oxygenated blood to the left ventricle. The left ventricle has much thicker muscular walls than the right ventricle as it must pump the oxygenated blood to all parts of the body. There are two openings in each heart chamber, guarded by one-way valves. The valves prevent back flow of blood and keep it moving through the arteries and veins in the proper direction. (See Figure V-1.)

When a ventricle (lower chamber) contracts, the valve to the artery opens and the valve between the ventricle and the atrium (upper chamber) closes. Blood is forced from the ventricle into large arteries (on the right side into the pulmonary arteries and on the left side into the aorta). At the end of the contraction, the ventricle relaxes. The valve to the artery closes, the valve to the atrium opens, and blood flows from the atrium to fill the ventricle. When the ventricle is stimulated, the pumping cycle repeats itself.

The rhythmical sequence of the pumping action of the different chambers of the heart is initiated by the heart's intrinsic pacemaker. Impulses generated in the pacemaker are carried over complex nerve pathways to all parts of the heart.

The contraction of the right and left ventricles is called systole; the relaxation of the heart while the ventricles fill with blood is called diastole. Therefore, within the arteries, there is a continuous variation between maximum pressure (systolic) to minimum pressure (diastolic).

SYSTEMIC CIRCULATION

Arteries

Arteries carry blood away from the pumping chambers of the heart (ventricles) to the organs and other parts of the body. The walls of arteries are thicker and more muscular than those of veins.

The aorta is the major artery leaving the left side of the heart. The aorta has many branches, supplying the head and neck, arms, thoracic and abdominal organs. In the lower abdomen, it divides into the two main arteries which lead to the lower extremities. Each artery divides into smaller and smaller branches (arterioles), finally forming the thin-walled tiny capillaries.

heart is really a double pump with both the right ventricle and left ventricle acting as the pumps. The right atrium receives the venous blood returning from the body tissues. The right atrium then delivers this venous blood to the right ventricle which pumps it to the lungs. The venous blood is pumped into the capillary network of the lungs. The capillaries are in close contact with the air sacs of the lung. At this point, oxygen passes into the blood and carbon dioxide passes from the blood into the alveoli. This blood, rich in oxygen, then flows from the lungs into

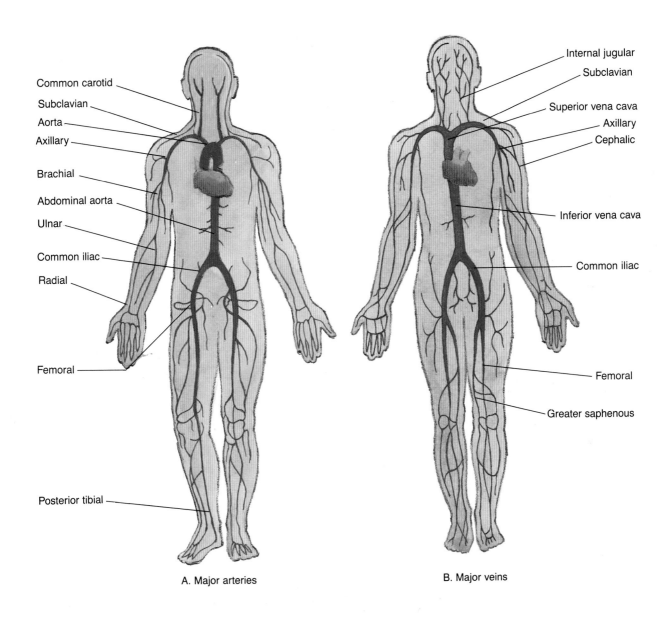

A. Major arteries

Common carotid
Subclavian
Aorta
Axillary
Brachial
Abdominal aorta
Ulnar
Common iliac
Radial
Femoral
Posterior tibial

B. Major veins

Internal jugular
Subclavian
Superior vena cava
Axillary
Cephalic
Inferior vena cava
Common iliac
Femoral
Greater saphenous

Capillaries and Cells

The capillaries have the thinnest walls of any vessel, as they are only one cell thick. The fine capillary walls readily allow exchanges between the blood and body cells. Oxygen, water and other nutrients pass from the blood cells and plasma in the capillaries through their walls to the cells of the body tissues.

Carbon dioxide and other waste products pass from the tissue cells to the blood to be carried away. Blood in the arteries is bright red because it is rich in oxygen. Blood in the veins is a dark brownish red colour because it is low in oxygen. Capillaries connect at one end with the arterioles and at the other with venules. By the time the arteriolar blood reaches the capillaries, the blood pressure is very low, just enough to keep the blood flowing through the capillary beds.

Veins

Blood from the capillary system returns to the heart through the veins. The smallest veins, called venules, are formed by the union of capillaries. These join to form larger veins. The veins of the entire body ultimately join to form two major veins, the superior vena cava and the inferior vena cava.

Blood returning from the head, neck, shoulders and upper extremities passes through the superior vena cava. Blood from the abdomen, pelvis, and lower extremities passes through the inferior vena cava. Both the superior and inferior vena cava empty into the right atrium. Veins are equipped with one-way valves that permit the blood to flow in only one direction. There is little pressure from the capillaries to force the blood back to the heart, so the return is aided by the activity of the skeletal muscles, particularly in the lower limbs.

As described above, the right ventricle receives blood from the right atrium and pumps it into the lungs through the pulmonary arteries.

LUNG CIRCULATION

Blood vessels from the right side of the heart branch and re-branch, finally forming the pulmonary capillaries. These capillaries form an extensive network over the surface of each alveolus (small air sac) in the lung tissue. Oxygen from the alveoli and carbon dioxide from the blood exchange in opposite directions between the alveoli and the blood. The oxygenated blood from the lungs returns to the heart and enters the left atrium. It then passes to the left ventricle and is pumped into the arterial circulation again.

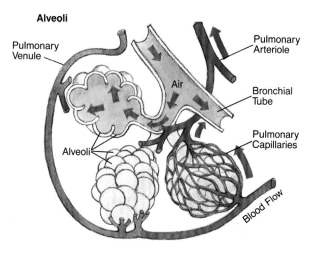

Lung circulation

PULSE AND BLOOD PRESSURE

Pulse

The ventricles pump blood into the arteries about 60 to 80 times a minute. The force of ventricular contraction starts a wave of increased pressure which begins at the heart and travels along the arteries. This wave is the pulse. It can be felt in the arteries that are relatively close to the surface, particularly if the vessel can be pressed against a bone. The carotid artery pulse can be felt in the anterior neck adjacent and just lateral to the thyroid cartilage (Adam's apple). The radial artery pulse is felt at the wrist on the flexor surface at the base of the thumb. The femoral artery pulse is felt in the groin in the anterior crease between the leg and abdomen at a point approximately at the middle of the crease.

Blood Pressure

Blood pressure is the force exerted by the blood against the walls of the arteries as it passes through them. The repeated ejection of blood from the left ventricle of the heart into the aorta is transmitted through the arteries as a series of pressure waves. This serves to keep the blood moving through the body. The arterial blood pressure can be measured with a blood pressure cuff. The two measurements are of:

- systolic pressure: the maximum pressure occurring at the peak of the left ventricular contraction
- diastolic pressure: the minimum pressure during relaxation of the left ventricle

Several factors control arterial blood pressure — the blood volume itself, the state of the arteries and arterioles (dilated or constricted) and the capacity of the heart muscle to contract normally.

The pressure of the blood in veins is much less than that of the blood in arteries. Two factors control the pressure of the venous blood: blood volume and the capacity of the veins.

The average adult body has approximately 6 litres of blood. However, the capacity of all the body's blood vessels is much larger than 6 litres. When a person is healthy, the difference between the blood volume and the capacity of the blood vessels is constantly adjusted by a complex auto-regulation system.

This system matches the fluctuating blood needs of the various organs and other parts of the body. Thus, when the body is exercising, more blood flow will be directed to the muscles from the organs that do not have as high a metabolic need, i.e. the gastrointestinal tract. Conversely, when the individual has a meal, more blood will be directed to the gastrointestinal tract and away from the muscles.

The change in the size of the arteries and veins is governed by muscles in their walls. These muscles can contract or relax in response to changes in blood volume, heat, cold, injury or an infection. Contraction or relaxation of the muscle fibre causes changes in the diameter of the artery or vein. These muscles do not act as pumps, but change the diameter of the vessels. If the muscles of the arteries and veins contract, the vessel diameters decrease and the system holds less fluid. But if these muscles relax, then the vessels dilate and the system can hold a larger volume of blood.

Loss of normal blood pressure is one indication that the blood cannot circulate efficiently to the body organs. There may be many reasons for the loss of blood pressure. The end result in each case is the same — body organs are no longer adequately perfused! This means that the cells in these organs are not receiving sufficient oxygen or nutrients and that waste products of cell function, carbon dioxide and acids, are not being removed. Without adequate perfusion, the cells will die. This state of inadequate perfusion is called shock. (This topic is fully discussed in the section on Shock, see page 95.)

Part V, Section B
Shock

INTRODUCTION

CIRCULATORY SHOCK IS AN EMERGENCY THAT, IF NOT RECOGNIZED AND TREATED EARLY, MAY CAUSE THE DEATH OF THE PATIENT. EARLY RECOGNITION AND TREATMENT ARE ESSENTIAL.

CELLULAR FUNCTION

Shock is a disorder of the body cells. The smallest complete unit of life is the cell. Cells with similar functions are grouped together into tissues. Tissues with similar functions are then grouped together into individual organs.

The heart and brain, which are the "vital" organs, are much more important for the moment-to-moment existence of the body than others. Should they fail suddenly, the body will die very quickly.

The cells of tissues and organs have specific functions. To function properly, each cell requires energy and a system of waste removal. The cells use oxygen and sugar to make energy. When the cell is getting little or no oxygen, there is an alternative method by which it can make energy; this method is very inefficient and generates a large amount of waste (mostly acids).

Oxygen is important to the body cells because the lack of oxygen will affect:
1. energy production
2. accumulation of harmful waste products

Perfusion

Perfusion is the flow of blood to and from the body cells. As blood flows to the cells, it carries life-giving oxygen and nutrients. As the blood flows by the cells, it gives up oxygen and nutrients in exchange for carbon dioxide, acid and other wastes. The blood then carries these wastes away from the cell.

Proper cell function requires adequate perfusion. The body achieves this with the cardiovascular or circulatory system by:
1. the blood (fluid transport of fuels and wastes)
2. the heart (pump)
3. the blood vessels (the system of arteries, veins and capillaries which transport blood to and from all the individual cells)

In order to ensure that there is an adequate supply of oxygen to the cells, the body must also have an intact respiratory system.

DEFINITION OF SHOCK

Shock is the state of inadequate perfusion of the cells.

The ultimate result of inadequate perfusion for each cell will be that it has too little oxygen and too much acid. This will cause a series of changes:
1. cell function stops
2. cell dies
3. tissue dies
4. organ dies
5. body dies

The aim is to interrupt the series of changes before cell death begins. The fundamental problem in shock, regardless of cause, is a marked reduction in blood flow through the tissues. Initially, that results in cellular hypoxia (low oxygen) and, ultimately, acidosis (accumulation of acids). The body tries to control the metabolic consequences of impaired tissue perfusion. After a certain point, all control is lost and shock becomes *irreversible*. The primary aim in the treatment of shock is to increase tissue perfusion and, unless this is done quickly, the patient will die. There may be only a short time between the onset of shock and the point when it becomes irreversible. It is essential that the cause of the problem be identified promptly and the patient transported to hospital as soon as possible.

Among injury victims, shock is almost always caused by blood loss (hypovolemic shock). It is often made worse by any condition impairing adequate air exchange (i.e. chest injury). RECOGNIZING SHOCK IN THE *EARLY* STAGES AND PROMPTLY TRANSPORTING THE VICTIM TO HOSPITAL IS *ONE* OF THE MOST IMPORTANT FUNCTIONS OF THE FIRST AID ATTENDANT. ANY PATIENT IN SHOCK FALLS INTO THE RAPID TRANSPORT CATEGORY. Since most First Aid Attendants are unable to use intravenous fluids or advanced airway techniques to treat shock, they must be even more alert to the early evidence of shock.

Normal system (6 liters)

Blood reservoir

Blood vessels

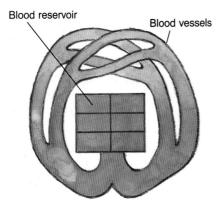

**Constricted system
(Hypovolemic shock)**

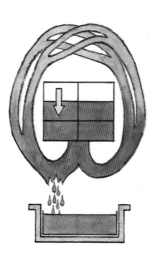

**Dilated system
(Anaphylactic septic and spinal shock)**

Inadequate blood supply

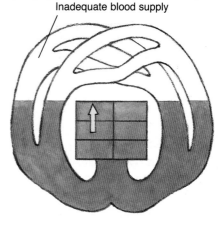

CAUSES OF SHOCK

1. The volume of blood in circulation becomes inadequate (hypovolemic shock) through loss of blood or fluid loss, i.e.:
   - blood loss: bleeding
   - fluid loss: burns
2. The pump (heart) is damaged and fails to function properly, i.e.:
   - cardiogenic shock: myocardial infarction (heart attack)
3. The blood vessels dilate excessively. In this situation, the normal volume of blood is insufficient to fill the dilated blood vessels to capacity. This leads to inadequate tissue perfusion, i.e.:
   - anaphylactic shock
   - septic shock
   - spinal shock

Any combination of problems with the heart, blood volume or blood vessels may cause inadequate perfusion of the cells leading to the state of shock, for example: an injured worker with internal bleeding whose hypovolemic shock is complicated by a heart attack.

Any condition that impairs adequate air exchange and oxygen transfer in the lungs, such as airway obstruction, pneumothorax or flail chest, will worsen the patient's shock state.

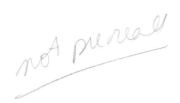

THE BODY'S RESPONSE TO SHOCK

The autonomic nervous system regulates the cardiovascular system to provide adequate perfusion. The tissues of the body require much more blood when they are active than during rest. Without the autonomic nervous system regulating the flow of blood, it would be necessary to continuously supply all of the tissues at the maximum rate. This would take much more blood and a much larger heart. However, the arterioles leading to tissues that are at rest constrict, and those supplying active tissues dilate. The blood is distributed according to need.

The blood pressure depends upon: 1) the volume of blood pumped by the heart into the systemic circulation, and 2) the resistance to flow of the circulating blood by the arterioles. Arteriolar resistance refers to back pressure exerted by the arterioles on the blood flow. The concept of arteriolar resistance (also called peripheral resistance) is best illustrated by the example of the adjustable nozzle at the end of a hose. Without a nozzle, a fully open tap may not produce sufficient pressure. With a suitably adjusted nozzle, even a small flow from a tap may produce pressure that propels the stream of water forcefully.

The arterioles' muscular walls are constantly receiving nerve impulses from the autonomic nervous system. This keeps them in a state of partial contraction. Just as the pressure in the hose depends on the amount of water flowing from the tap and the adjustment of the nozzle, so the blood pressure depends upon the cardiac output and the degree of constriction of the arterioles in the arteriolar system. The autonomic nervous system matches cardiac output to peripheral resistance to maintain the blood pressure and ensure adequate perfusion of the cells as their needs change.

Any reduction in cardiac output will tend to cause a reduction in systolic pressure. This change in pressure is detected by special pressure receptors. The receptors trigger the autonomic nervous system, which attempts to restore cardiac output and blood pressure to normal. The two key hormones in this system are adrenalin and noradrenalin.

Adrenalin and noradrenalin cause:

1. An increase in heart rate and a more forceful heart contraction. These actions will increase cardiac output and increase blood pressure.
2. Constriction of the arterioles (vasoconstriction) in non-vital organs (skin, kidneys, liver, gut, etc.) which decreases the blood flow to these areas. This action redistributes blood flow to the vital organs (brain, heart).
3. Sweating (diaphoresis). This is not a useful response by the body to shock, but it is a key sign in the detection of shock. The Attendant must watch for this effect.

Figure V-2 illustrates how the various causes of shock may act on the three major parts of the circulatory system: the blood, pump and blood vessels. THIS ILLUSTRATED CYCLE MUST BE INTERRUPTED BY EARLY VIGOROUS MEDICAL THERAPY.

The body has a great ability to compensate for bleeding by using the same mechanisms that operate in normal situations. The body compensates for the decreased circulating blood volume by releasing large amounts of adrenalin and noradrenalin. Consequently, most of the remaining blood volume is redistributed to the vital organs (heart and brain) (see Figure V-2).

This vasoconstrictive response attempts to maintain blood pressure and perfusion of the vital organs until blood loss can be replaced. However, it deprives the other tissues of blood they need to maintain their metabolic activity.

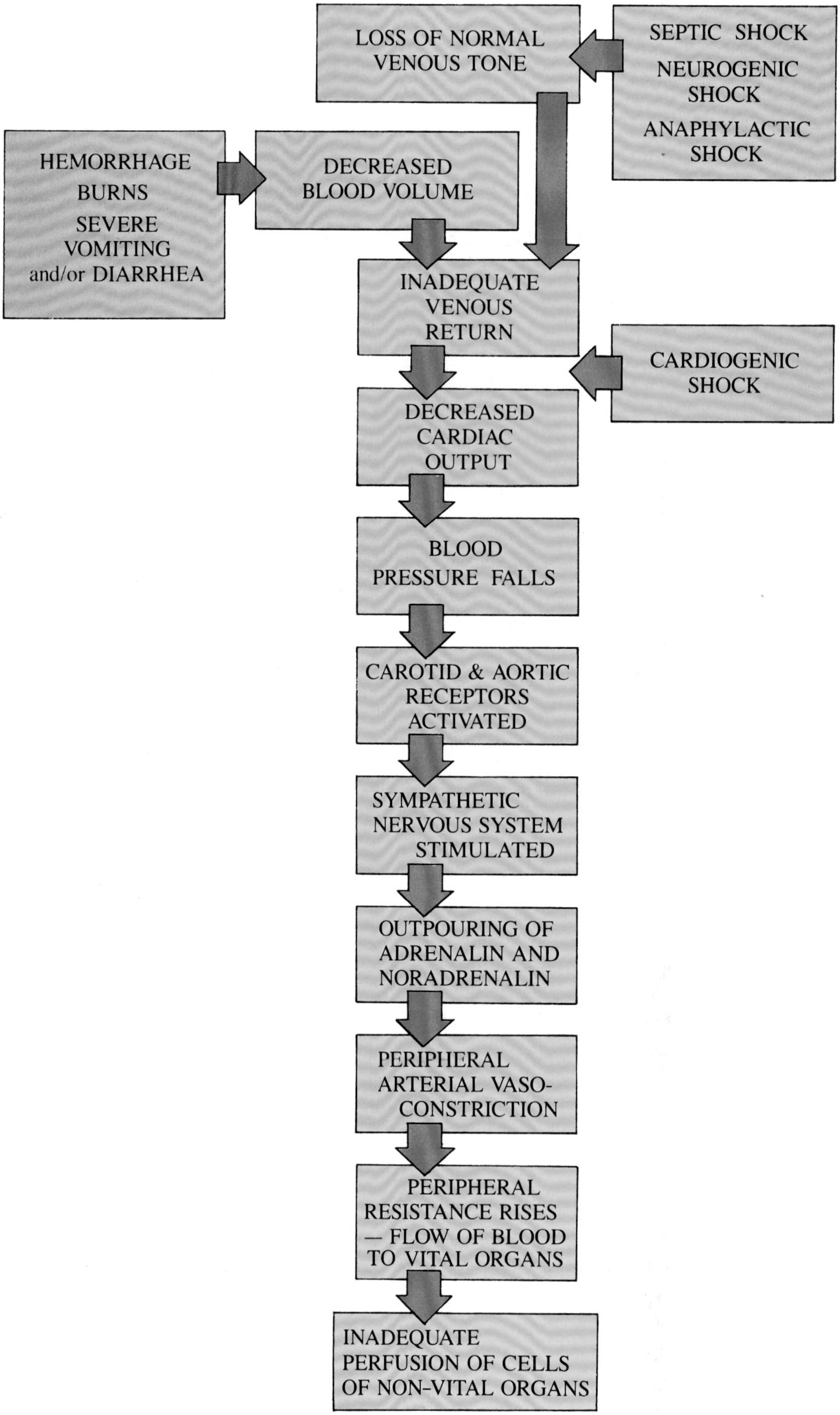

LOSS OF NORMAL
VENOUS TONE

SEPTIC SHOCK

NEUROGENIC
SHOCK

ANAPHYLACTIC
SHOCK

HEMORRHAGE

BURNS

SEVERE
VOMITING
and/or DIARRHEA

DECREASED
BLOOD VOLUME

INADEQUATE
VENOUS
RETURN

CARDIOGENIC
SHOCK

DECREASED
CARDIAC
OUTPUT

BLOOD
PRESSURE FALLS

CAROTID & AORTIC
RECEPTORS
ACTIVATED

SYMPATHETIC
NERVOUS SYSTEM
STIMULATED

OUTPOURING OF
ADRENALIN AND
NORADRENALIN

PERIPHERAL
ARTERIAL VASO-
CONSTRICTION

PERIPHERAL
RESISTANCE RISES
— FLOW OF BLOOD
TO VITAL ORGANS

INADEQUATE
PERFUSION OF CELLS
OF NON-VITAL ORGANS

Figure V-2 Body's compensation in shock

If blood volume loss continues or if shock is not reversed by early medical treatment, the perfusion of body organs will eventually become insufficient to maintain normal cell function. As the condition worsens, the cells die with subsequent tissue and organ dysfunction. As the shock state progresses, the cardiac output cannot be maintained, blood pressure falls, and death becomes inevitable. (see Figure V-3)

Patients with early signs of shock will demonstrate signs of increased autonomic nervous system activity, especially the effects of increased adrenalin and noradrenalin. The earliest signs of hypovolemic shock are coolness of the skin followed by sweating.

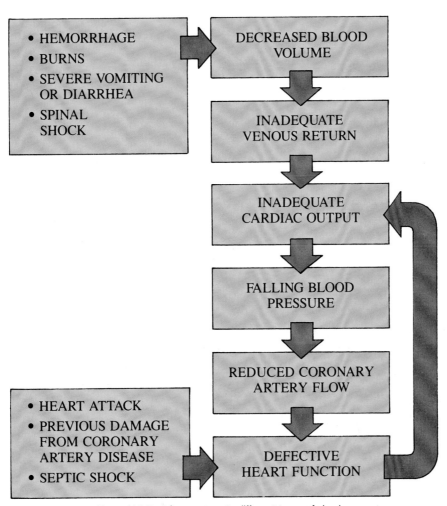

Figure V-3 Body's response to different types of shock

TYPES OF SHOCK

This section discusses the following types of shock:
1. Hypovolemic Shock
2. Cardiogenic Shock
3. Anaphylactic Shock
4. Bacteremic or Septic Shock
5. Spinal Shock (Neurogenic)

HYPOVOLEMIC SHOCK

Excessive blood loss, as from injury, leads to inadequate circulating blood volume. As a result of the decrease in circulatory blood volume, there is inadequate perfusion and a state of shock ensues.

A similar effect may occur because of fluid loss, either through the gastrointestinal tract, such as with profound diarrhea or vomiting, or from the body surfaces, as when a patient has extensive burns.

Signs and Symptoms of Hypovolemic Shock

Many of the signs and symptoms of shock are caused by the body's vasoconstrictive response. The following signs and symptoms are provided in the order in which they tend to occur as the shock state progresses.

- Cool skin: Often, an early sign of shock and detected best in the extremities. It occurs when warm blood is rerouted from the skin as a consequence of the vasoconstrictive response.
- As shock deepens, the capillary refill test will become delayed. This test is performed by depressing the victim's fingernail and releasing quickly. The normal response is for the colour to return within two seconds. If it takes longer than two seconds, the test is delayed and provides strong evidence of shock. However, if the capillary refill is normal, shock may still be developing and the patient should be reassessed frequently. The capillary refill test cannot be interpreted in the hypothermic patient because the skin is already vasoconstricted due to the cold.
- Sweating: This develops as a direct effect on the sweat glands of the autonomic nervous system's response to shock. It suggests that the shock state is more advanced. The skin may be cold and clammy.
- Pallor: With vasoconstriction, blood is no longer flowing to the surface; consequently, the skin loses its colour.

- Increased heart rate (usually greater than 100/min.): This reflects the heart's response to adrenalin and noradrenalin. A more rapid heart rate usually indicates a more severe state of shock.
- Low blood pressure (hypotension): This is defined as a systolic pressure reading less than 100 mm Hg. Alternatively, the absence of the radial pulse indicates a blood pressure reading of less than 90 mm Hg. Hypotension indicates either: 1) a rapid massive loss of blood volume (e.g. internal hemmorhage) with the body unable to compensate, or 2) a late sign of shock occurring when the body's vasoconstrictive response fails. Regardless of the cause, the patient is in very urgent need of medical attention.
- Alteration of behaviour and/or Level of Consciousness (LOC): In its early stages, shock is often associated with anxiety, restlessness or combativeness. This is due in part to the release of adrenalin. As shock increases and hypoxia becomes more pronounced, the patient may become very agitated and restless, sometimes gasping for breath with "air hunger". The agitation may be more pronounced with an associated head injury. As the perfusion to the brain decreases, the LOC decreases.
- Tachypnea (increased respiratory rate between 20-30 breaths/min.): Usually a patient in shock breathes more rapidly as a consequence of hypoxia and acidosis. This sign may also be present with associated chest injuries. The Attendant must be very concerned about an associated chest injury if the respiratory rate is greater than 30 breaths/min.
- Thirst: Owing to a reduced blood volume, patients in shock often complain of intense thirst. The victim should be given nothing by mouth in the event that surgical treatment may be required.

Victims of Hypovolemic Shock Who Must Receive Special Consideration

- **Athletes**

  The trained athlete has a well-conditioned heart muscle and cardiovascular system. The normal resting heart rate may be below 50 beats per minute. As a consequence, despite significant blood loss, the athlete may adequately compensate for shock. Therefore, they may not exhibit an increased heart rate or diminished blood pressure until either a large volume of blood has been lost or the shock state has become advanced.

- **Pregnancy**

  During pregnancy, a women will have up to a 20% increase in blood volume. Consequently, following trauma, she may not initially exhibit signs of shock owing to her increased blood volume. The fetus, however, will experience profound shock as the maternal vasoconstrictive response to shock shunts the blood from the fetus to the maternal vital organs. ANY PREGNANT WOMAN WHO HAS RECEIVED TRAUMA, EVEN IF INSIGNIFICANT (E.G. A FALL ON A STAIR), SHOULD BE REFERRED TO A PHYSICIAN FOR ASSESSMENT. Any pregnant woman who has received significant trauma (e.g. major limb fractures, chest or abdominal trauma) or exhibits any signs of shock falls into the Rapid Transport Category. (See Part VIII, Section E, page 191.)

- **Cardiac Patients**

  There are two major complications with cardiac patients:

  i) Cardiac patients are at a higher risk of developing shock from trauma because of their weaker heart. Furthermore, they may also develop chest pain and/or shortness of breath.

  ii) Patients on heart medication may not exhibit the signs of shock because these medications may dampen the body's normal vasoconstrictive response.

      Any cardiac patient who has received significant trauma must be watched closely and put into the Rapid Transport Category if the Attendant suspects impending shock.

CARDIOGENIC SHOCK

In cardiogenic shock, the heart muscle does not pump enough blood and oxygen to peripheral tissues. The most common cause of cardiogenic shock is acute myocardial infarction (AMI). The strength and force of the left ventricular contraction is reduced because of extensive structural damage to the ventricle wall. Other conditions that can cause cardiogenic shock include: valvular heart dis-ease, congestive heart failure and trauma (e.g. contusion of the heart, pericardial tamponade or tension pneumothorax).

The signs and symptoms of cardiogenic shock are essentially the same as seen with hypovolemic shock.

ANAPHYLACTIC SHOCK

This condition is caused by a severe allergic reaction. It may be caused by the injection, ingestion or inhalation of a foreign protein substance into a person sensitized to it. The allergic reaction may lead to a loss of the normal tone of the blood vessels. The shock state is caused by abnormal dilatation of the blood vessels, causing inadequate perfusion of the cells.

Agents that may commonly cause anaphylactic shock include: insect stings, antibiotics, seafoods and blood or other transfusions. Some individuals susceptible to severe allergic reactions wear Medic Alert bracelets or necklaces. This form of shock is distinguished by its rapid onset. One cannot predict how severe the allergic reaction is likely to be in susceptible individuals. Severe reactions may occur immediately or be delayed for half an hour or more. There may be constriction of the upper airway and the bronchioles, with impaired breathing. The impairment of breathing and of proper circulation prevent the normal supply of oxygen from reaching the cells. Patients undergoing a suspected anaphylactic reaction fall into the Rapid Transport Category.

Signs and Symptoms of Anaphylactic Shock

Patients experiencing anaphylactic shock may develop any of the following signs and symptoms:

- Generalized itching
- Numbness and tingling, especially about the face and mouth
- Blotchy areas of raised reddish-pink swelling of the skin which are very itchy (hives)
- Swelling of the tongue and face
- Tightness in the throat or upper airway
- Breathing difficulty with possible wheezing
- A tight discomfort across the chest
- General weakness, restlessness, dizziness or anxiety
- Abdominal cramps, diarrhea or vomiting
- A rapid, weak pulse

Bacteremic or Septic Shock

Profound circulatory collapse may result when certain bacteria invade the bloodstream. It is believed that these bacteria produce toxins. They ultimately affect the blood vessel walls, causing generalized vasodilatation and, ultimately, diminished tissue perfusion. This type of shock is seen most often in the hospital setting. Recently, it has been recognized in women as toxic shock syndrome associated with the use of tampons.

Signs and Symptoms of Septic Shock

* Confusion is often the earliest sign
* High fever with warm flushed skin that later becomes cool and pale
* Increased pulse rate
* Increased respiration

NEUROGENIC SHOCK (SPINAL SHOCK)

In neurogenic shock, the blood vessels to the lower extremities, abdomen, trunk and sometimes part of the upper extremities suffer impairment of their autonomic nerve control. As a consequence, the blood vessels dilate markedly, increasing their capacity. The patient's blood volume becomes pooled in the dilated blood vessel system, resulting in a reduced return to the heart. Although there is no actual blood loss, the patient's normal blood volume is inadequate to maintain perfusion of the cells.

NEUROGENIC SHOCK ONLY OCCURS IN THE PRESENCE OF A SPINAL CORD INJURY WITH COMPLETE PARALYSIS. NEUROGENIC SHOCK DOES NOT OCCUR WITH SPINAL FRACTURES ALONE.

Spinal shock is a RARE cause of shock in trauma victims, even those who have suffered spinal cord injuries. Trauma victims with shock are much more likely to be in hypovolemic shock caused by internal injuries. ALL INJURED PATIENTS FOUND IN SHOCK, REGARDLESS OF THE PRESENCE OF SPINAL INJURIES, MUST BE TREATED AS THOUGH THEIR SHOCK IS CAUSED BY ACUTE BLOOD LOSS.

Signs and Symptoms of Neurogenic Shock

* Paralysis and numbness of the lower extremities and variable portions of the trunk
* Possible impaired breathing as a consequence of paralysis of chest muscles (see Spinal Injuries, Part VI, Section D, page 147)
* The skin may feel warm and dry in the lower extremities
* There may not be a radial pulse

THE GENERAL PRINCIPLES OF MANAGEMENT OF SHOCK IN THE TRAUMA VICTIM

The evaluation and management of the injured worker in shock follows the Priority Action Approach outlined in Part III, page 20.

1. Begin with the primary survey.
2. Ensure an open airway with cervical spine control.
3. If a cervical injury is suspected with c-spine control, position the patient supine or in the lateral position (see Part VI, Section D, page 147). If there is no concern for cervical injury, the patient should be maintained in a horizontal position but may be positioned for comfort.
4. Expose the chest to assess for adequate breathing. AN OPEN AIRWAY DOES NOT ENSURE ADEQUATE VENTILATION. Look for open wounds or other signs of chest injury (e.g. inadequate and/or asymmetrical chest movements), bruising, abrasions or paradoxical movement. The chest injuries which most often compromise breathing are: a large flail chest with pulmonary contusion, tension pneumothorax and open pneumothorax.
5. Assess for respiratory distress or signs of oxygen deficiency (e.g. dyspnea, gasping, cyanosis or rapid breathing). If necessary, provide mouth-to-mouth respiration or assist ventilation with a bag-valve mask or pocket mask with supplemental oxygen. Time the assistance to the victim's breathing pattern.
6. Administer high-flow oxygen by mask (10 Lpm). Even patients with suspected chronic obstructive lung disease require high-flow oxygen if available in these cases.

7. Control life-threatening external bleeding.

8. ALL PATIENTS WITH SHOCK OR SUSPECTED OF DEVELOPING SHOCK FALL INTO THE RAPID TRANSPORT CATEGORY. Following the primary survey and initial management of life-threatening injuries, the patient must be transported rapidly to the nearest hospital.

9. **Avoid all unnecessary movement or rough handling because such action will aggravate the shock state.**

10. Protect patients from the elements and keep them comfortably warm. Do not apply external heat sources (i.e. heating pads or hot-water bottles), which will cause vasodilatation in the skin and worsen the shock state.

11. Give nothing by mouth.

12. Continually monitor the patient's vital signs every 10 minutes to determine if there is deterioration. If it does not distract the Attendant from performing necessary treatment, the vital signs should be recorded as they are taken.

In the past, certain treatments that have been emphasized must now be abandoned because they are unsound. They include:

- **The Head-Down Position**

  This position, with the patient's head down and the feet up at an angle of about 15°, makes breathing harder, because the abdominal contents fall against the diaphragm. The best position is horizontal (supine or lateral).

- **External Heat**

  As mentioned above, use of external heat from heating pads or hot-water bottles tends to cause the victim's skin blood vessels to dilate. With blood rerouted from the vital organs, this will aggravate the problem of a low circulating blood volume.

Part V, Section C
Bleeding and its Management

HEMORRHAGE CHARACTERISTICS

Bleeding (hemorrhage) is the escape of blood from arteries, veins or capillaries. Bleeding may be external or internal.

1. External — There is a break in the skin and blood escapes to the outside.
2. Internal — The skin is not broken, and bleeding may not be visible. Hidden bleeding into the thoracic or abdominal cavities or into muscle surrounding a fracture can account for a large amount of blood loss.

No matter whether bleeding is internal or external, it can be serious as it may cause shock.

Descriptions of bleeding are usually divided into arterial, venous and capillary, according to which vessel is involved. All wounds will include some capillary bleeding and most arterial bleeding will involve a corresponding vein.

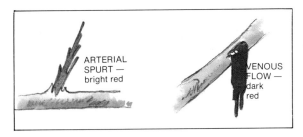

Hemorrhage characteristics

Arterial

Blood from an artery spurts or pulses out and is usually bright red. It may be very brisk if a large vessel is involved.

Venous

Blood from a vein generally comes in a steady flow and its colour is much darker than arterial blood. Venous bleeding may also be very brisk if a large vessel is involved.

Capillary

Bleeding from capillaries is a continuous, steady ooze.

The rate at which blood is lost is significant. The average adult may comfortably lose 500 ml (approximately one pint) of blood over 15 to 20 minutes (i.e. blood donor). During this 15-20 minutes, the body adapts to its loss quite well. If larger amounts are lost or this amount is lost more quickly, the patient may go into shock. If massive bleeding is not controlled and medically treated, the patient may die. Consequently, brisk hemorrhage should be identified and controlled in the primary survey. Rapid external blood loss is managed by direct pressure on the wound.

EXTERNAL BLEEDING

Bleeding from lacerations and nosebleeds are examples of external bleeding. Ordinarily, for most minor wounds, bleeding stops on its own within minutes, as the body has its own defense system against blood loss. When larger blood vessels are involved, however, it is often necessary for the Attendant to control bleeding.

The Body's Natural Response to Bleeding (Hemostasis)

- **Retraction of Blood Vessels**

  The elastic muscle fibres in the walls of the damaged blood vessels cause them to pull back into the tissue, thus constricting them at the cut ends. This will reduce bleeding.

- **Clotting**

  Special elements in the blood form a clot, which will seal the injured portion of the vessel and stop the bleeding.

In some cases, the injury is so severe that clots cannot form nor can damaged blood vessels constrict effectively. Blood loss may sometimes be so fast that if the Attendant waits for the body's natural response, the patient may go into shock or may bleed to death. In order for clotting to take place, the flow of blood from the wound must be slowed or stopped for at least a few minutes.

THE ATTENDANT MUST FOLLOW THE PRIORITY ACTION APPROACH.

A — Ensure a clear Airway, maintaining C-spine control.

B — Ensure adequate Breathing.

C — Assess Circulation and control bleeding.

THREE P'S HEMORRHAGE CONTROL

The control of external hemorrhage is simple. The Attendant must remember three principles:

1. **Pressure**

   There are two types of pressure, and in some cases the Attendant must use both:
   - direct (pressure directly on the wound)
   - pressure point (indirect)

2. **Patient Position — Lying Down**

   The patient should be at rest, lying down. Putting the patient at rest will lessen anxiety, and help the bleeding to slow down.

3. **Part Position — Elevation**

   Simply elevating a bleeding part will help to slow down the flow of blood. Elevation of the limb need not be more than 30 centimetres (1foot) above the trunk to be effective. Pressure in the veins of the upper and lower extremities is such that most venous bleeding can be reduced considerably by elevation. Elevation may also slow arterial bleeding. If moving the extremity causes extreme pain or aggravates the injury, do not elevate the limb until it is immobilized.

PRESSURE

1. **Direct Pressure**

   Pressure applied directly over the wound will control nearly all types of bleeding. At first, pressure may be applied with the fingers or a hand placed over any readily available material (i.e. shirt or handkerchief). In this situation, obviously a sterile pressure dressing or gauze pads are preferred. Formerly, it was recommended that initial direct pressure could be applied with the fingers or a hand directly over the bleeding site. Owing to the risk to the Attendant of blood-born infection (i.e. hepatitis, AIDS), this practice must be discouraged. Once the sterile pressure dressing is in place, pressure on the wound is maintained by a loop tie or elastic wrap that secures the dressing. To minimize further damage, the injured limb should be supported while the dressings are being applied. The entire sterile dressing should be covered above and below the wound by the bandage, tightly secured. If the dressing becomes blood-soaked, the Attendant should apply additional dressings over the initial one and direct pressure over it.

   On occasion, with persistent bleeding through the dressing, the Attendant may feel it necessary to

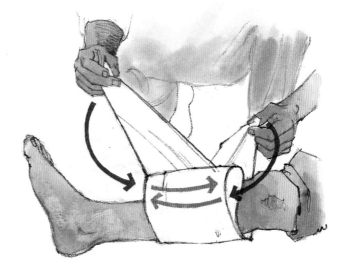

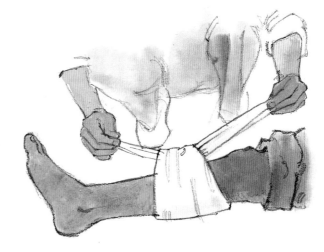

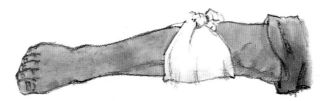

Tying a loop tie bandage

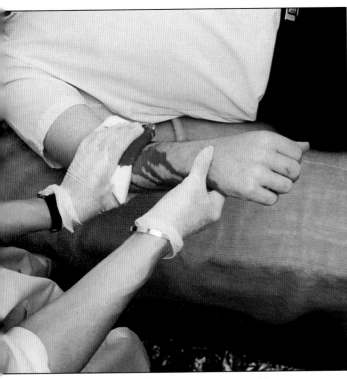

1. Pressure applied; Patient position; Part position

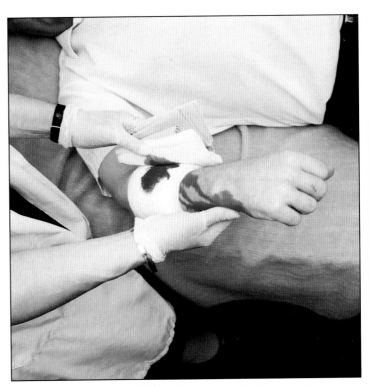

2. Additional pressure applied

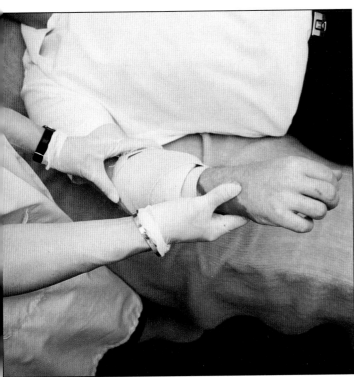

3. Pressure dressing used for pressure

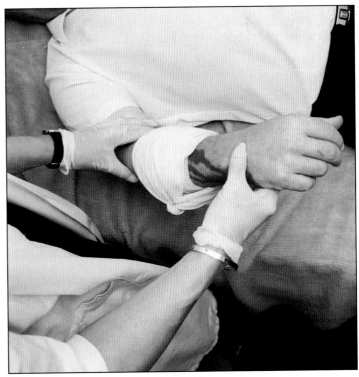

4. Loop tie used for pressure

remove the dressing once, in order to ensure that pressure is being applied directly on the wound. If bleeding persists despite additional dressings, the Attendant should apply firm pressure with a hand for five minutes or, alternatively, use a pressure point.

Scalp wounds are notorious for persistent bleeding owing to the difficulty of applying direct pressure with dressings, and also due to the fact that the scalp vessels do not vasoconstrict as readily as vessels in other locations.

2. **Pressure Points**

IF A PATIENT IS BLEEDING SEVERELY ENOUGH TO REQUIRE THE USE OF A PRESSURE POINT, THE PATIENT FALLS INTO THE RAPID TRANSPORT CATEGORY.

When dressing material is not immediately available and the patient is hemorrhaging from a major artery, the Attendant should apply pressure to a pressure point.

A pressure point may also be used when there is arterial bleeding from a wound that has a protruding bone or embedded foreign body.

A pressure point is any location at which pressure on the artery slows or stops bleeding at a distal injury. This generally means that the artery is close to the skin's surface and lies over a bone.

Some major arterial pressure points are listed on page 111, together with their location and the areas of bleeding they control.

Bleeding from a wound that has been controlled by a proximal pressure point may not entirely stop, but will significantly slow so that dressings and bandages can be applied. Once the wound has local, direct pressure and is elevated if possible, the proximal pressure point should be maintained for five minutes, then released slowly. The pressure point is held for five minutes to allow adequate time for clots to form. If there is further bleeding, the pressure point must be reapplied and the pressure bandages tightened. THESE PROCEDURES MAY BE PERFORMED AS THE PATIENT IS BEING PREPARED FOR TRANSPORT AND CONTINUED EN ROUTE IF NECESSARY.

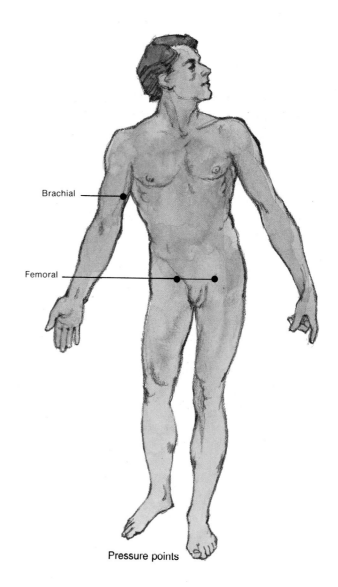

Pressure points

Do not use clamps or hemostats to stop bleeders; it may damage nerves or other structures that lie near arteries.

TOURNIQUETS

TOURNIQUETS ARE RARELY NEEDED. IF A PATIENT IS BLEEDING SEVERELY ENOUGH TO REQUIRE A TOURNIQUET, THE PATIENT IS IN THE RAPID TRANSPORT CATEGORY. A tourniquet can be used to control hemorrhage in the following circumstances:

• if all other methods fail;

- if another life-threatening priority demands the Attendant's attention;
- an amputation.

The tourniquet is applied proximal to the wound and on the upper arm or the thigh where the artery can be compressed against a single long bone. If there has been an amputation, it must be as close to the end of the stump as possible.

A tourniquet is best applied with an Esmarch bandage. This is a rubber bandage, approximately 10 cm wide by 90 cm long. Apply the bandage with even pressure on each wrap and each succeeding wrap providing a greater degree of pressure. The bandage should be applied so that there is 2 mm to 5 mm margin of the preceding wrap visible.

Tourniquets may be made from any suitable material but, if possible, avoid the use of belts, wire or rope, which are too narrow and seriously damage underlying structures. If an Esmarch bandage is not available, the best substitute is a 10 cm tensor bandage.

There are certain precautions that must be observed when using tourniquets:

1. **Do not use unless other means are ineffective.**
2. If at all possible, avoid using material such as belts, rope or wire that can cut into tissue.
3. Ensure that it is applied with sufficient pressure. A loose application will increase venous blood flow from wounds beyond the tourniquet.
4. If there is an extremity distal to the tourniquet, the tourniquet must be released for 1 minute every 45 minutes. This will provide some blood flow to the distal limb and prevent tissue death. When the tourniquet is released, try to prevent additional bleeding distally by applying direct pressure to the wound. If there is a complete amputation and the tourniquet is close to the severed end, then it should not be released.
5. TOURNIQUETS MUST NEVER BE COVERED BY BANDAGES.
6. THE PATIENT MUST BE CLEARLY MARKED AS HAVING A TOURNIQUET AND THE TIME IT WAS APPLIED. FIX A LARGE TAG TO THE PATIENT'S BODY, PREFERABLY NOT TO THE CLOTHES, BUT TO A LIMB. AN ALTERNATIVE METHOD WOULD BE TO WRITE IN INK ON THE PATIENT'S SKIN IN LARGE LETTERS

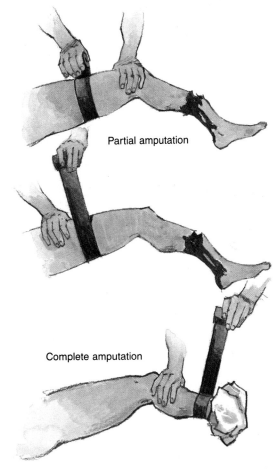

Partial amputation

Complete amputation

Application of an Esmarch bandage

"TOURNIQUET" AND THE TIME IT WAS APPLIED.

7. Patients requiring tourniquets fall into the Rapid Transport Category. The Attendant should not waste time applying local splinting techniques, unless they can be applied safely en route.

IMMOBILIZATION FOR HEMORRHAGE CONTROL

Bleeding from an injured extremity is often caused because muscles are lacerated by sharp ends of broken bones or because vessels lying in the fractured bone continue to bleed.

When there is a break in the tissue, whether it is soft tissue or bone, some of its ability to support itself is lost. Until the injured part is effectively immobilized, damage and bleeding can continue. For this reason, the application of splints to a fractured or lacerated extremity will help control the hemorrhage.

INTERNAL BLEEDING

The Attendant must rely on the mechanism of injury and the primary survey to suspect and diagnose internal bleeding.

Internal bleeding is usually associated with injury to the internal organs resulting in hemorrhage into one of the body cavities (i.e. thorax or abdomen). It can also occur with fractures of the pelvis or a femur. Because the bleeding is not directly visible, the Attendant must rely on the mechanism of injury and the primary survey to suspect and diagnose internal bleeding. These patients are in the Rapid Transport Category. In some cases, the onset signs and symptoms of internal bleeding may be delayed. The Attendant must therefore make a secondary survey and continual re-evaluations, watching for signs and symptoms of shock to diagnose internal bleeding. Although internal bleeding is not initially visible, it may become visible at one of the body's orifices, which may indicate the source of bleeding.

Internal bleeding must be suspected when a patient's condition deteriorates following an injury. Internal bleeding may produce shock. Some of the signs and symptoms are:
- skin becomes cool or cold, pale and clammy
- pulse becomes weak and rapid
- air hunger or shortness of breath
- the patient may faint or become dizzy
- the patient may be thirsty, anxious and restless
- the patient may be nauseated and may vomit

Please review the section on Shock, page 95.

SPECIAL HEMORRHAGE PROBLEMS

Neck

Bleeding from the neck presents several problems for the Attendant. If the bleeding is severe, the Attendant must provide immediate and continued direct pressure on the region until medical aid is reached. Swelling associated with this type of injury may also compress the airway. The Attendant must monitor the patient for signs of airway problems and treat accordingly (see Airway Management, Part IV, Section B, page 39).

ANY PENETRATING WOUND TO THE NECK THAT HAS PROGRESSIVE LOCAL SWELLING OR SEEMS TO HAVE PENETRATED THE MUSCLES FALL INTO THE RAPID TRANSPORT CATEGORY. This is because of the possibility of airway compression from hidden bleeding or damage to important underlying structures.

Severed Carotid Artery and Jugular Vein

Bleeding from the carotid artery or jugular vein is most effectively controlled by placing the fingers of both hands behind the patient's neck, with thumbs on either side of the wound. Put firm, direct pressure on the severed ends of the vessels against the vertebrae of the neck. Because of the rich collateral circulation in the head and neck, bleeding may come from both ends of the severed artery. Only apply pressure to the carotid artery on the affected side. Try to avoid putting any pressure on the airways.

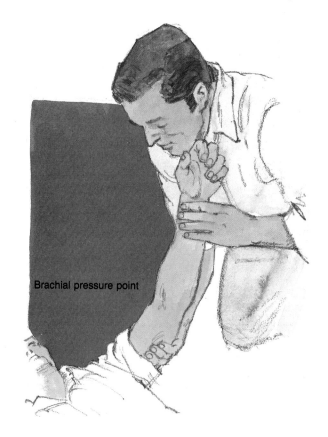

Brachial pressure point

Nosebleeds (Epistaxis)

Nosebleeds are common emergencies and, on occasion, can cause shock and even death. There may be only a small amount of blood visible, as it often goes down the throat and is swallowed. If blood is swallowed, vomiting may ensue.

Most nosebleeds can be treated at the accident scene or first aid room.

Management

- Apply constant pressure by pinching the nostrils for 15 to 20 minutes. Apply cold packs to the bridge of the nose and the forehead.
- Keep the patient sitting, if possible, with the head forward. The traditional practice of tilting the patient's head back is not recommended because blood may trickle down the throat. The person may swallow the blood or possibly choke on it. The patient should be encouraged to cough or spit out any blood but should not blow the nose.
- Keep the patient quiet. If the patient suffers from high blood pressure or is anxious, the agitation may increase blood pressure and the bleeding.

A person with a prolonged nosebleed (greater than 30 minutes) should be taken to medical aid. Nasopharyngeal packing should be done only by a physician.

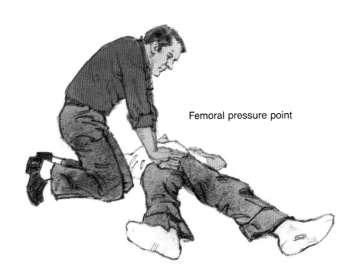

Femoral pressure point

MAJOR ARTERIAL PRESSURE POINTS

NAME	LOCATION	PURPOSE	METHOD
BRACHIAL	MIDWAY BETWEEN THE ELBOW AND ARMPIT ON THE INNER SIDE	TO CONTROL ARTERIAL BLOOD FLOW DISTAL TO THE MID ARM AREA	PLACE FOUR FINGERS ON THE MEDIAL SIDE OF THE ARM APPROACHING FROM UNDERNEATH. PUSH THE BICEPS MUSCLE TOWARDS THE FRONT OF THE ARM AND PRESS THE ARTERY AGAINST THE HUMERUS.
FEMORAL	IN THE CREASE OF THE GROIN APPROXIMATELY WHERE A TROUSER CREASE WOULD CROSS THE GROIN LINE	TO CONTROL ARTERIAL BLOOD FLOW TO THE LOWER LIMB	PLACE THE HAND DIRECTLY OVER ARTERY WHERE IT CROSSES THE INGUINAL AREA (THE PULSE IS EASILY FELT AT THIS POINT) AND PRESS DIRECTLY DOWNWARD.

Part V, Section D
Traumatic Cardiovascular Emergencies

CONTUSION TO THE HEART

The most common blunt traumatic injury to the heart is caused by impact with steering wheels, although contact sports and crushing accidents can also cause cardiac injury. Cardiac contusion may be caused either by compression of the heart between the sternum and the vertebral column or by sudden deceleration of the body, causing the heart to be thrust against the chest wall. All injured workers with blunt anterior chest trauma should be presumed to have a myocardial contusion.

Injury to the heart can vary from small areas of bruising to full thickness contusion of the cardiac wall; the latter may result in immediate or subsequent cardiac rupture.

The most common symptom of myocardial contusion is anterior pain, usually identical to that of a heart attack (myocardial infarction, see Section E, page 116). The chest pain starts immediately or within a few hours of the trauma. The patient may complain of palpitations, may be dyspneic or in shock. Myocardial contusion may co-exist with a hemopericardium, and present with the signs of cardiac tamponade (see below). Lethal cardiac rhythms are the major complication of myocardial contusion.

Management of Cardiac Contusion

Management of the patient with suspected cardiac contusion should follow the Priority Action Approach to the injured patient outlined in Part III, page 20. All patients with suspected cardiac contusion fall into the Rapid Transport Category. In managing such patients, the Attendant should follow the general principles of management of chest injuries as previously outlined (see Part IV, Section C, page 57).

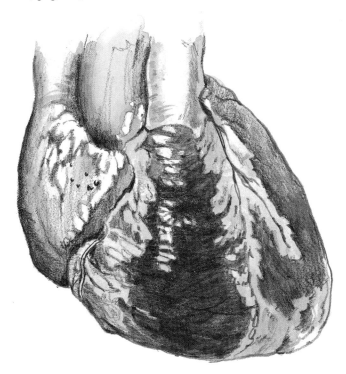

Multiple contusions of Heart

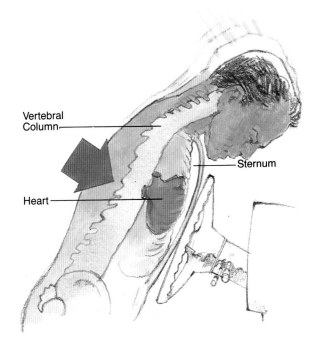

Vertebral Column

Sternum

Heart

Mechanism of injury
for Myocardial Contusion

PERICARDIAL TAMPONADE

Pericardial tamponade is a condition in which the pumping action of the heart is impaired by the entry of blood or other fluid into the pericardial sac. The pericardial sac is a very tough, fibrous membrane surrounding the heart. When the heart is perforated, blood leaks out and fills this sac, compressing the heart. The heart's chambers can no longer accommodate blood normally returned to them through the veins. The pressure of accumulated blood must be relieved or the patient will soon die.

Recognition of Pericardial Tamponade

In addition to the general signs of chest injury as outlined in Part IV, Section C, page 56, the patient may demonstrate any or all of the following:
- restlessness
- air hunger
- rapid and weak or absent pulse with other signs of shock
- cyanosis
- distended neck veins

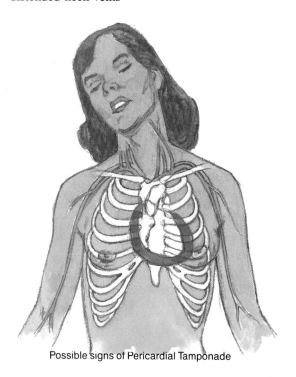

Possible signs of Pericardial Tamponade

Management of Pericardial Tamponade

This condition is a life-threatening emergency and requires urgent medical attention at a hospital. They should be managed according to the Priority Action Approach to the injured patient outlined in Part III, page 20. All patients with suspected pericardial tamponade fall into the Rapid Transport Category. In managing such patients, the Attendant should follow the general principles of management of chest injuries in Part IV, Section C, page 57.

INJURY OF THE MAJOR VESSELS

There are several large blood vessels in the chest. Injuries to any of these vessels may cause massive, rapidly fatal hemorrhage. Any patient who is in shock and who has a chest injury may have an injury to a large blood vessel. The bleeding may not be apparent, as it remains inside the chest cavity.

The major vessels may be damaged by either blunt or penetrating injuries to the chest, upper abdomen or lower neck. Other injuries may mask the signs of major vessel damage. Chest pain, dyspnea, back pain or inability to move the lower extremities may indicate injury to the major vessels. The patient may be in shock. Even without shock, an absent pulse in any limb may indicate major vessel injury — in the absence of any other obvious cause (fracture).

Management of Patients with Major Vessel Injury

Patients with major vessel injury may experience life-threatening exsanguination (excessive hemorrhage). Such patients fall into the Rapid Transport Category. Management should follow the Priority Action Approach to the injured patient, Part III, page 20. In addition, the Attendant should follow the general principles of management of chest injuries in Part IV, Section C, page 57.

Part V, Section E
Non-Traumatic Cardiac Emergencies

CORONARY ARTERY DISEASE

Introduction

The heart has its own system of blood vessels to supply its tissues with oxygen and nutrients and remove wastes. The two major arteries that carry blood to the heart muscle (myocardium) are the left and right coronary arteries. A heart attack is primarily caused by a sudden obstruction of the coronary arteries or their branches, with loss of blood supply and oxygen to the heart muscle beyond the obstruction. The result is hypoxia of the heart cells and subsequent death of a portion of the heart tissue (myocardial infarction or heart attack).

Coronary artery disease is the leading cause of death in the western world, killing 75,000 Canadians each year. One-quarter of the victims are under 65 years of age.

A majority of deaths from coronary artery disease occur before the person reaches hospital.

Of those people who reach hospital, the average time between the onset of symptoms and their arrival is four hours!

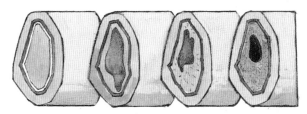

Progressive narrowing of coronary arteries with atherosclerosis

Atherosclerosis is a process by which the coronary arteries become narrowed. The process may take place in other areas of the systemic circulation, most particularly the brain, the kidneys and the large vessels of the lower aorta and the arteries of the lower extremities. Atherosclerosis is a build-up of fatty deposits in the inner walls of the artery. Fats and other particles combine to form a deposit known as plaque. With time, calcium can be deposited at the site of the plaque, causing the area to harden. The inner diameter of the artery is narrowed, restricting the flow of arterial blood. The hardening of the artery causes the vessel to lose its elasticity, which affects blood flow and increases blood pressure. Cholesterol is one of the major fatty deposits that participate in the formation of plaque. The plaque causes a roughened surface of the internal lining of the artery, which may lead to blood clots being formed, subsequently obstructing the vessel. At times, the clot may break off and form an embolus, which will cause a blockage of the vessel further along its course. It is the process of atherosclerosis with obstruction of the coronary artery that causes heart attacks.

There is an increased incidence of atherosclerosis and heart attack when one or more of the following risk factors are present:
1. smoking;
2. high blood pressure (hypertension);
3. high level of cholesterol or other fatty substances in the blood;
4. poor level of physical fitness;
5. obesity;
6. diabetes;
7. a family history of heart attacks in middle age;
8. prolonged stress.

A combination of two or more risk factors will increase the incidence of coronary artery disease and subsequent heart attack.

ANGINA PECTORIS

The heart muscle works with greater effort when the body is subjected to physical or emotional stress. Healthy coronary arteries will dilate to supply the heart muscle with more oxygen to meet its increased demands. In the presence of advanced coronary artery disease, the narrowed vessels cannot provide the increased requirements of the heart muscle and it becomes starved for oxygen. That lack of oxygen may precipitate chest pain, which is called angina pectoris. The pain is experienced differently by each individual. For some, it is very severe; for others, it is a discomfort or tightness.

The pain of angina pectoris usually will ease and disappear if the patient rests and the physical or emotional stress ceases. As the heart rate and strength of contraction return toward normal, the narrowed coronary arteries can once again meet the increased demands for oxygen and the chest pain recedes. Usually, angina attacks seldom last more than 15 minutes. If they do, the Attendant must presume the patient is having a heart attack.

Signs and Symptoms of Angina Pectoris

The signs and symptoms of an angina attack may vary from person to person but, for each individual, the pain is of constant intensity, duration and location. If any noticeable changes occur in the pattern, the patient must be managed as if suffering from a heart attack.

Pain

- The pain may occur suddenly or build up gradually.
- The pain is usually located beneath the sternum in the anterior chest, and may radiate across the anterior chest. It may be felt in the left or right arm, sometimes as far down as the wrist. It may also radiate up into the neck or jaw or through to the back. It sometimes is only felt in the upper mid-abdomen and assumed to be indigestion.
- The pain usually will last less than 15 minutes.
- The most common descriptions of the pain are mild to moderate heavy pressure, squeezing or vise-like tightness. Pain is relieved almost immediately by nitroglycerin tablets taken sublingually (under the tongue) and with the administration of oxygen.
- The pain is not influenced by deep respiration, cough or movement.

NITROGLYCERIN SHOULD NEVER BE GIVEN TO A PATIENT WITH CHEST PAIN UNLESS IT HAS BEEN PRESCRIBED FOR THE PATIENT. IT MAY CAUSE SERIOUS COMPLICATIONS IN SOME PATIENTS WHO ARE HAVING A HEART ATTACK.

Associated Signs and Symptoms

- Nausea
- Belching
- Apprehension or uneasiness
- Pallor
- Shortness of breath

Management of Angina Pectoris

Individuals suffering from angina are able to carry on reasonably normal lives by taking medications that dilate the coronary arterial blood vessels. Angina sufferers usually carry nitroglycerin tablets, which they take at the onset of anginal pain. The tablets are issued under prescription and are not to be swallowed, but placed under

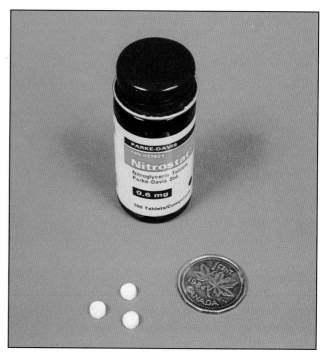

Nitroglycerin tablets are small white pills

the tongue to dissolve. Alternate preparations of nitroglycerin involve nitroglycerin spray and nitroglycerin skin patches. The patient should only take nitroglycerin as instructed by a physician. The Attendant can assist the patient in taking the medication and finding a comfortable position. Oxygen should be administered at 10 Lpm. Patients with anginal pain not relieved by nitroglycerin fall into the Rapid Transport Category. They should be transported in a recumbent position with continuing supplemental oxygen. Patients who have taken repeated doses of nitroglycerin may have a weak pulse as a result of generalized blood vessel dilatation. On occasion, such patients may have a brief fainting episode. They should be transported in the horizontal position with supplemental oxygen at 10 Lpm. The patient's pulse and respirations should be assessed frequently en route to hospital.

HEART ATTACK (MYOCARDIAL INFARCTION)

When part of the heart is deprived of oxygen and if the condition continues for long enough, the heart muscle cells in that area will die. This is called a heart attack or myocardial infarction.

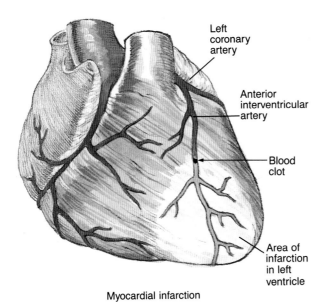

Myocardial infarction

Myocardial infarction is usually caused by a progressive narrowing of the coronary arteries. This is due to the result of atherosclerotic plaques which develop over the years within the lining of the coronary arteries. Actual occlusion (blockage) of the artery usually occurs suddenly. It is a result of either a thrombus (blood clot) forming on the rough surface of a plaque, or from an embolus.

Signs and Symptoms of Heart Attack

Chest pain is the classic symptom of most heart attacks.

Pain

- The pain may occur suddenly and may come on when the victim is at rest.
- It is usually substernal (anterior chest, beneath the sternum) and often radiates across the chest.
- Some patients may not experience chest pain but may have epigastric discomfort usually associated with belching, gas and indigestion.
- The pain may radiate to one or both arms (usually the left) sometimes as far as the wrist. It may also radiate up to the neck, jaw or through to the back.
- Pain is described as choking, squeezing, vise-like, burning or intense. Patients often experience a feeling of pressure.
- The pain usually lasts longer than 30 minutes and is constant.

- Pain is not affected by cough, movement or deep respiration; relief does not come with nitroglycerin or rest.

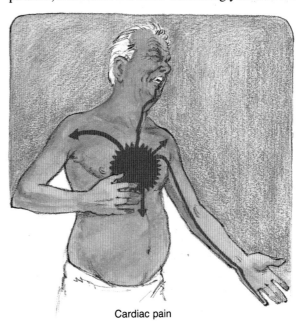

Cardiac pain

Associated Signs and Symptoms

- Apprehension (the patient may feel he or she is going to die)
- Marked weakness, especially in the arms
- Shortness of breath or difficulty breathing
- Sweating, sometimes profuse
- Pallor
- Nausea or vomiting
- Desire to defecate
- Weak and rapid pulse, although in some cases the pulse rate decreases

Three major complications which most often cause death are:

1. Arrhythmia — a disturbance in the heart's rate or rhythm;
2. Congestive heart failure;
3. Cardiogenic shock (see Section B, page 101).

Sudden Cardiac Death

Almost half of all patients with acute myocardial infarction die before reaching a hospital. This is most often due to an arrhythmia, which is an irregular rhythm of the heart preventing effective pumping of blood. The most common lethal arrhythmia is ventricular fibrillation. This arrhythmia occurs when the ventricles cease to beat with an organized forceful contraction and all the heart muscle cells contract randomly and independently. Another less common lethal arrhythmia associated with acute myocardial infarction is asystole, which means cardiac standstill. An irregular heart rhythm occurs most frequently within the first hour after the heart attack and its incidence is considerably reduced after three to five days of medical treatment.

Sudden cardiac death may also occur as a result of congestive heart failure or cardiogenic shock.

Management of the Heart Attack Victim

The presence of chest pain in a conscious patient must be considered as an urgent priority.
1. Perform a primary survey.
2. Keep the patient quiet and calm. Do not allow the patient to move unassisted onto the stretcher. The patient should be recumbent or in the position of comfort.
3. Administer high flow oxygen at 10 Lpm.
4. Keep the patient comfortably warm.
5. Monitor the vital signs and be prepared to assist ventilation if needed.
6. Patients with chest pain, suspected of having a heart attack, fall into the Rapid Transport Category.
7. The vital signs should be carefully monitored during transportation.

CONGESTIVE HEART FAILURE

The strength of contraction of the left ventricle is often decreased by myocardial infarction so that the heart fails to pump effectively.

The left ventricle cannot pump effectively when it is damaged. Because the ventricle cannot empty completely, blood backs up into the left atrium and the pulmonary veins. Pulmonary congestion develops because vessels in the lungs become swollen with blood. Pulmonary edema will develop if excessive back-pressure occurs in the capillaries of the lungs, causing plasma to leak into the alveoli and bronchial walls. Pulmonary edema interferes with normal oxygen and carbon dioxide exchange. The pulmonary congestion and pulmonary edema associated with heart-related causes is called congestive heart failure.

Other cardiogenic causes of congestive heart failure, aside from myocardial infarction, include:
• hypertension;
• valve disease in the left ventricle;
• failure to take cardiac medications;
• arrhythmia;
• too much salt in the diet;
• too much exercise or stress in an individual with heart damage, etc.

For further details on pulmonary edema, see the section on pulmonary edema (Part IV, Section D, page 74).

RECOGNITION OF CONGESTIVE HEART FAILURE

History

1. If caused by left heart failure, there may be:
   • chest pain associated with heart attack;
   • increased blood pressure;
   • history of previous attacks;
   • history of rheumatic fever and valve disease;
   • excess exercise or stress.
2. Dyspnea, often severe, with inability to lie down.

Physical Findings that May Be Present

• Increasing respiratory distress and the patient may become agitated, apprehensive, restless or confused. They may exhibit panic and air hunger.
• Chest pain may be present but it is not a reliable symptom.
• Pallor and cold clammy skin.
• Cyanosis is possible.
• Tachycardia with pulse greater than 100.
• Cough with frothy white or pink sputum.
• Wheezing respirations are possible.
• Patient will insist on sitting upright and the dyspnea worsens as the patient lies down.
• Neck veins may be distended.

Management of Congestive Heart Failure

1. Calm and reassure the patient.
2. Position the patient sitting upright in the position of comfort with the legs dangling, if possible.
3. High-flow oxygen (10 Lpm) is essential.
4. Periodic rapid suctioning of the airway may be necessary for accumulated secretions, if the patient cannot clear it.
5. If the patient becomes drowsy or is extremely dyspneic, assisted ventilation timed to the patient's breathing, with a bag-valve mask and high-flow oxygen, should be instituted.
6. The comatose patient with acute pulmonary edema will require suctioning and assisted ventilation with high-flow oxygen with a bag-valve mask.
7. PATIENTS WITH PULMONARY EDEMA FALL INTO THE RAPID TRANSPORT CATEGORY.

SUMMARY OF CHEST PAIN MANAGEMENT

Chest pain in the conscious patient should be regarded as a top priority.

Assessing the Patient

If the patient is comatose, not breathing and has no pulse, the need is for CPR, rather than examination and assessment. Remember to make sure the ABCs are present before proceeding with anything else.

A   Airways open.
B   Breathing is present and adequate.
C   Circulation is present.

History

- What is the patient's skin colour and condition?
- What are the vital signs?
- Are there any signs of distended neck veins or lower extremity edema?
- Is the patient coughing frothy sputum which may be blood-stained?
- When did the pain start?
- How does the patient describe the pain?
- How severe is the pain?
- Where is the pain?
- Does the pain radiate and where?
- What was the patient doing at the onset?
- Is the pain aggravated or lessened with respiration, exercise or rest?
- Has this happened before?
- Is the patient taking medication?
- Has the patient taken anything for pain?
- Is the patient nauseated?

These questions are designed to be a summary of all the important facts about the problem. Answers should be recorded and accompany the patient to the medical facility, if possible.

Part V, Section F
Cardiopulmonary Resuscitation (CPR)

Tissues, especially the brain, require an adequate supply of oxygenated blood to maintain vital functions. Organ functions will deteriorate rapidly if this supply is interrupted.

Cardiopulmonary Resuscitation (CPR) is the recognition and treatment of the following life-threatening conditions:

- airway obstruction
- respiratory arrest
- cardiac arrest

Basic Cardiac Life Support (BCLS) refers to the first aid techniques used to treat the above conditions. Advanced Cardiac Life Support (ACLS) includes all the methods of BCLS with the addition of advanced medical procedures (e.g. intubation, defibrillation and drug therapy).

Priority Action Approach outlined in this manual follows the BCLS guidelines recommended by the Canadian and American Heart Associations, except for the treatment of airway emergency in trauma patients.

WHENEVER A FIRST AID ATTENDANT APPROACHES A PATIENT, THE PRIORITY ACTION APPROACH MUST BE FOLLOWED.

Cardiopulmonary resuscitation consists of:

1. opening and maintaining the patient's airway;
2. artificial ventilation for the patient, if necessary;
3. artificial circulation for the patient, if necessary.

The sequence and method of CPR follows the Priority Action Approach (ABCs):

A — Airways Open (cervical spine control if trauma suspected)

B — Breathing checked and restored, if necessary

C — Circulation checked and restored, if necessary

CPR can be performed quickly and with minimal equipment or help from another person. CPR must be practised frequently to maintain a high standard.

CPR methods are frequently updated as new medical information becomes available. Therefore, the step-by-step procedures of CPR will not be covered in this manual. The student should refer to the current guidelines for basic CPR as recommended by the Canadian and American Heart Associations. An overview follows.

The first priority for successful resuscitation is opening the *airway*. See Student Syllabus or Canadian Heart Foundation Guidelines. The tongue is the most common cause

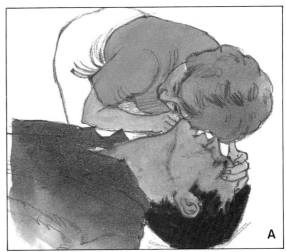

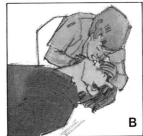 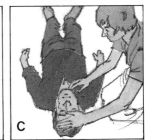

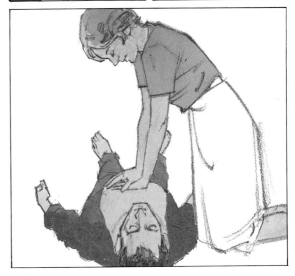

A. Airway open
B. Breathing restored
C. Circulation checked

of airway obstruction in the patient with a decreased level of consciousness. Often, opening the airway is all that is needed. If the patient resumes breathing, the airway must be maintained.

If the patient is *not* breathing or not breathing adequately, the Attendant must institute the breathing by artificial ventilation or assisted ventilation. Artificial ventilation is accomplished by mouth-to-mouth or pocket mask.

The next priority is *circulation*. The Attendant must check pulse. The carotid pulse at the neck is usually strong, readily accessible and easily palpable. Therefore, it is used to assess the circulation.

If the pulse is absent, the patient is in cardiac arrest. The Attendant must start external chest compression in an effort to artificially circulate the patient's blood. If the heart is beating, a pulse is usually detected. AS LONG AS THE PULSE IS PALPABLE, REGARDLESS OF THE STRENGTH OR CHARACTER, CHEST COMPRESSIONS MUST NOT BE PERFORMED.

Artificial ventilation may be all that is needed if a patient has a pulse. Mouth-to-mouth or pocket mask ventilation should be continued at one breath every five seconds and the pulse checked frequently to make sure that the heart has not stopped.

External chest compressions, when efficiently performed according to current guidelines, will provide approximately 25% of normal blood flow to the brain. If the blood is properly oxygenated by efficient artificial ventilation, this amount of circulation is usually sufficient to preserve life until cardiac function resumes or advanced life support becomes available. External chest compression must always be accompanied by artificial ventilation.

CPR is most effective when started immediately after cardiac arrest has occurred. However, this does not mean CPR should not be initiated if there is doubt as to when the cardiac arrest occurred. CPR must be started on all patients in cardiac arrest and continued until one of the following occurs:

- Spontaneous circulation and breathing are restored;
- Another person takes over resuscitation efforts;
- A physician assumes responsibility;
- The patient is transferred to a medical facility or ambulance personnel.

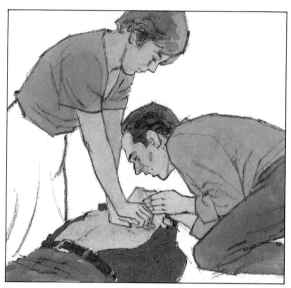

Two-operator CPR

FOREIGN BODY OBSTRUCTION OF THE AIRWAY ("CAFE CORONARY")

Foreign body obstruction of the airway occurs most often during eating. A variety of foods and foreign bodies cause choking in children and adults.

The victim with this emergency has often been mistaken for a heart attack victim, giving rise to the name "cafe coronary".

Early recognition of airway obstruction is the key to successful management. For a complete discussion of assessment of the airway and its management, see Part IV, Section B, page 39. Any patient with airway obstruction, cardiac or respiratory arrest fall into the Rapid Transport Category.

Part VI, Section A
Head and Nervous System Anatomy and Function

The nervous system is responsible for maintaining the individual's state of consciousness as well as controlling most body functions. Since ancient times, men have known that normal conscious behaviour depends on intact brain function. Hippocrates, the famous Greek scholar, wrote: ". . . and men should know that from nothing else but from the brain come joys, delights, laughter and jests, and sorrow, grief, despondency and lamentation." Consciousness means the awareness of self and of the surrounding environment. Because the hallmark of brain function is consciousness, any alteration or loss of consciousness (other than sleep) automatically indicates abnormal brain function.

The nervous system is composed of the brain acting as control centre and the nerves, which act as cables or wires connecting the brain to the various parts of the body. By learning the anatomy of the nervous system, the Attendant will be better equipped to understand neurological emergencies such as head injury, spinal cord injury, strokes, seizures, etc.

ANATOMY

BRAIN

The brain, as mentioned earlier, is the body's control centre. It is responsible for monitoring the state of normal consciousness, enabling us to respond to our environment. All sensory and motor functions are controlled by the brain. The brain receives input from all the sensory organs of the body and analyzes the information in specific areas of the brain. The brain responds to the sensory input as required and, through its motor functions, enables us to walk, talk, smile, etc. (i.e. respond to our environment). The brain is divided into three major structures: the cerebrum, the cerebellum and the brain stem.

1. The cerebrum is the largest part of the brain. It is responsible for all voluntary functions. Thinking, memory, pain, emotions — all the higher functions that make us human — are centred within the various parts of the cerebrum. Anatomically, the cerebrum is physically divided into two halves, or hemispheres, with many interconnections. The left hemisphere controls the right side of the body and the right hemisphere controls the left side of the body. This unique anatomical fact must be remembered by the Attendant

when assessing patients with neurological emergencies. For example, motor paralysis of the left side of the body usually indicates damage to the right side of the cerebrum.

Each half of the cerebrum is further subdivided into four lobes.

- The frontal lobe: All voluntary muscle activity is controlled by a small strip of tissue located in the frontal lobe. Swinging a baseball bat or sewing a button — each is controlled by the frontal lobe. The sense of smell is also located in this region.

- The parietal lobe: Sensations such as touch, pain and temperature are interpreted in this area. In most individuals, the speech centre is also located in the left parietal lobe with connections to the left frontal lobe.

- The temporal lobe: The brain's memory banks are located in these areas. As well, the sense of hearing is controlled and interpreted in this region.

- The occipital lobe, located at the back of the brain, contains the visual centre where our sense of vision is interpreted.

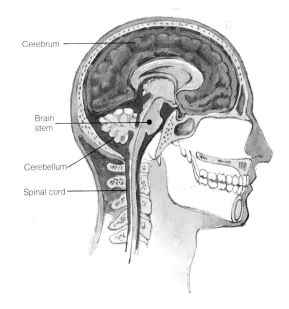

Figure VI-1 Anatomy of the Brain

2. The cerebellum is a smaller area of the brain located posteriorly and inferiorly to the cerebrum (see Figure VI-1). The cerebellum is primarily responsible for the coordination of motor activity. For example, the act of walking, which we often take for granted, requires the complex interplay of many different muscles of the body. The ability to walk steadily is coordinated by the cerebellum, but the actual movement of the limbs is controlled by the frontal lobe of the cerebrum.

3. The brain stem is located at the base of the brain. In this region are the centres that control most of our subconscious vital functions such as breathing (the respiratory centre), blood pressure, heart rate, etc. The autonomic nervous system alluded to in the section on shock is centred in the brain stem (see Part V, Section B, page 97). Furthermore, all the nerves that control the actions of the face and the special senses (e.g. the tongue, swallowing, eye movements, hearing, facial movements and sensations) connect to specific centres in the brain stem. Finally, all the nerves connecting other parts of the body to the cerebrum or the cerebellum pass through the brain stem. It should be apparent to the Attendant that major injuries to the brain stem quickly result in loss of vital functions, severe neurological disability and often death.

Blood Supply of the Brain

The carotid arteries in the neck and the vertebral arteries (two arteries running up through the cervical spine) provide the blood supply to the brain. Injuries to these vessels may reduce perfusion to the brain and restrict the supply of oxygen, glucose and other essential nutrients. That will result in injury and sometimes permanent damage of the affected areas of the brain. Branches of the carotid arteries supply the cerebrum, while branches of the vertebral arteries supply the cerebellum and brain stem. Occlusions (i.e. clots) within the branches of the carotid arteries are the most common causes of strokes. (See Part XIV, Section A, page 331.)

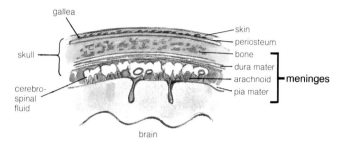

Brain coverings

Skull and Protective Coverings

The tissue of the brain is very soft and delicate. The brain is partially supported by three layers of specialized tissues called meninges. The pia mater lines the surface of the brain. The arachnoid membrane forms the middle layer. The dura mater forms the outermost layer and lines the inner aspect of the skull. These three layers of meninges protect the brain. Meningitis, a term familiar to many people, is a serious infection involving the meninges of the brain — hence the term meningitis.

Between the arachnoid membrane and the pia mater is the subarachnoid space. This space is filled with a clear watery fluid called cerebrospinal fluid, which completely surrounds the brain. The brain, in essence, is suspended in the cerebrospinal fluid.

The brain, with its protective coverings, is completely encased within the skull. The skull is composed of a series of bony plates fused together to protect the brain and give the head its characteristic shape. The forehead, top, side and back components of the skull are collectively referred to as the vault. The bony plates also extend underneath the brain to form the base of the skull, which separates the brain from the facial structures.

The spinal cord is really an extension of the brain stem and exits through the only major opening in the skull — the foramen magnum located at the base of the skull. Because of the unique anatomical relationship between the brain and the skull, any increase in the size of the brain (e.g. swelling from injury) is limited by the bony skull. The increasing pressure within the skull (intracranial pressure), which may result from injury, will, if it exceeds a certain level, compress the brain stem (the controller of the body's vital functions). Compression of the brain stem will often result in death.

SPINAL CORD

The spinal cord extends from the brain stem down to the lumbar spine. It is the main cable carrying all the individual circuits that connect the brain to all the other parts of the body. The spinal cord is contained and protected by the vertebral column which is composed of the individual bony vertebrae. Sensory and motor pathways are carried in separate parts of the spinal cord.

The spinal cord and the vertebral column are divided into cervical, thoracic, lumbar, sacral and coccygeal portions. There are openings between each vertebra for the spinal nerves. The spinal nerves connect the brain and the spinal cord to their respective body tissues, i.e. muscle or sensory receptors. At each vertebral level, two spinal nerves branch off, one for the left side and one for the right side. There are 31 pairs of spinal nerves. Each spinal nerve contains both sensory and motor fibres.

The spinal nerves are precisely organized anatomically. Branching off the cervical portion of the spinal cord are eight pairs of cervical spinal nerves that supply all the muscles, skin, etc. of the arms. Similarly, the 12 pairs of thoracic spinal nerves leave the spinal cord in the thoracic region and supply the muscles and organs contained within the thorax and the abdomen. Finally, the muscles and other tissues of the lower extremities are supplied by spinal nerves arising from the lumbar and sacral portion of the spinal cord. There are five pairs of lumbar spinal nerves, five pairs of sacral and one pair of coccygeal spinal nerves. The sacral portion of the spinal cord supplies the perineum and genitalia.

CRANIAL NERVES

The skin, muscles and special sensory organs of the head and neck region are supplied by 12 pairs of special nerves that do not branch off the spinal cord. These are called the cranial nerves. They travel through special holes or foramina in the skull to connect directly with the brain stem. The cranial nerves connect to those centres of the brain stem that control the special senses (e.g. sight, hearing, taste and smell). They also control facial movements and sensation, swallowing, eye movements and pupillary reaction.

Together, the brain and the spinal cord comprise the *CENTRAL NERVOUS SYSTEM*. The cranial nerves and spinal nerves, with all their branches, comprise the *PERIPHERAL NERVOUS SYSTEM*.

FUNCTION OF THE NERVOUS SYSTEM

In order to understand how to diagnose and treat neurological emergencies, the Attendant must have a basic understanding of how the nervous system works. The following examples illustrate how the nervous system is organized and functions. When an individual wants to wiggle the big toe of the left foot, an electrical signal is generated in the toe section of the right frontal lobe of the cerebrum. This electrical signal is carried down a nerve fibre through the brain stem and crosses over to the left side of the spinal cord. The electrical signal continues down the same nerve fibre through the cervical and thoracic portions of the spinal cord until it reaches the lumbar section. There, it makes a connection with the spinal nerve that controls the muscle that moves the left toe. When the electrical signal reaches that muscle located in the left leg, it causes the muscle to contract, thereby moving the left toe. If we consider an individual who is six feet tall, it is incredible to think that a small electrical signal generated in the top of the head travels almost six feet down to the left big toe in just a few microseconds.

What happens when an individual pricks the index finger of the right hand with a needle? Pain fibres in the tip of the right index finger are stimulated by the injury and they generate a small electrical signal which is carried by the sensory nerve fibres located in the index finger. The electrical signal is carried along this particular branch of the appropriate spinal nerve serving the right arm, ultimately connecting to the spinal cord in the cervical region.

Nature has created a unique mechanism for reacting to pain. When the pain signal connects to the spinal cord, two things occur. Firstly, the electrical signal triggers stimulation of the appropriate motor nerve fibres in the same cervical section of the spinal cord. A new electrical signal is then carried from the spinal cord along the spinal nerve serving the muscles of the hand and forehand that cause withdrawal of the injured index finger. Ultimately, the individual, by reflex, withdraws the finger from the offending needle prick. Secondly, another electrical signal is also transmitted up the spinal cord towards the brain. These fibres soon cross over to the left side of the spinal cord and pass up through the brain stem and into the left parietal lobe of the cerebrum, where the pain centre is located. The brain then triggers its own response: for example, a yell. The important points to remember are that the body responds to pain with a reflex withdrawal controlled by the spinal cord before the brain has had the opportunity to receive the pain signal and initiate its own response. That constitutes one of the fundamental aspects of the human preservation instinct.

The tissues of the brain are highly dependent on adequate supplies of oxygen and blood sugar (glucose) in order to function properly. Approximately 15% of the heart's output is required to maintain normal cerebral function. If brain cells are deprived of oxygen for more than 10 minutes, they will die. Even if the brain is deprived of oxygen for more than four minutes, permanent damage is possible. That is why the Priority Action Approach ranks airway and breathing first.

If the heart cannot pump enough blood to the brain, serious brain dysfunction will also occur. Therefore, shock associated with low blood pressure (i.e. hypotension) can cause brain dysfunction. Even though the body responds by trying to maintain perfusion of the vital organs, as discussed in the section on shock, a point is reached where cardiac output may be insufficient to supply adequate perfusion of the brain's tissues. As a result, brain dysfunction ensues. It often begins with lethargy and weakness and progresses to a diminished level of consciousness. Therefore, in the setting of major trauma with hypovolemic shock, it can be extremely difficult to determine whether the patient's coma is due to head injury or due to the presence of shock, or a combination of both. That is why perfusion of the brain's tissues is extremely important in order to maintain proper cerebral function. It also explains why the Priority Action Approach ranks "C" for circulation third on the list and why a cardiac arrest causes rapid loss of consciousness. Even if the heart beat is rapidly restored, the patient often suffers permanent neurological damage because the brain was deprived of oxygen for more than a few minutes.

Part VI, Section B
The Comatose Patient

The IFA Attendant may be called upon to treat a comatose patient. In this section, the Attendant will learn how to assess and treat the comatose patient, using a logical, systematic Priority Action Approach.

DEFINITION OF COMA

As previously mentioned, consciousness refers to the awareness of self and of the surrounding environment. Obviously, there are different degrees of consciousness varying from fully alert to unresponsive. Rather than relying on subjective terms like "sleepy" or "semi-conscious", the Attendant should refer to the Glasgow Coma Score (GCS) to determine the patient's level of consciousness. It provides an objective scale by which the Attendant can determine the level of consciousness. The truly comatose patient generally is unable to open the eyes to any stimulus, unable to speak coherently and unable to move voluntarily. This corresponds to a Glasgow Coma Score of "8" or less. Other patients with a higher Glasgow Coma Score are described best as having a "decreased level of consciousness".

There are groups of patients who may have a normal Glasgow Coma Score but obviously are not functioning normally. They may be confused (i.e. disoriented with regard to time, place or person), agitated, drowsy or hallucinating. A simple example is the patient who is quite intoxicated with alcohol. The patient's Glasgow Coma Score may be normal ("15/15") but he is obviously impaired, i.e. may be disoriented, may be agitated, may be drowsy, etc.

Finally, the duration of unconsciousness is important. The patient with a brief episode of unconsciousness, with full recovery, is said to have had syncope (e.g. fainting). There are many different causes of syncope (e.g. fear, pain, heart disease, strokes). The approach to the patient with syncope is exactly the same as treating the comatose patient.

COMMON CAUSES OF COMA

By understanding the common causes of coma, the Attendant is better prepared to focus on patient assessment. The Attendant must remember that patients can have more than one cause of coma. Patients intoxicated with alcohol may also have a serious head injury. THE ATTENDANT MUST NEVER ATTRIBUTE THE PATIENT'S COMA TO ALCOHOL OR DRUGS WHEN THERE IS ANY EVIDENCE OF HEAD INJURY OR OTHER MEDICAL CONDITIONS (E.G. DIABETES).

The following mnemonic is extremely useful to remind the Attendant to search out all possible causes of coma.

A — Alcohol	Is there alcohol on the patient's breath? Are there bottles lying around? Do any friends or bystanders know that the patient has been drinking?
E — Epilepsy (Seizure Disorder)	Does the patient have a history of epilepsy or seizure disorder? Is the patient carrying a medic alert bracelet? Does the patient take medication for seizures? Ask the bystanders if they witnessed any seizure-like activity. Is the patient seizing at the time the Attendant arrives?
I — Insulin (Diabetes)	Does the patient have diabetes? Is he or she taking insulin (injections) or other medications (pills) for diabetes? Both can cause low blood sugar and, in severe cases, seizures or coma.
O — Overdose	What medication is the patient taking? Has the patient taken an overdose of medication? Is there evidence of pills missing? Is there evidence of a suicide attempt? Does the patient abuse drugs intravenously? Are there syringes or needles about or on the patient's person? Does the patient have recent needle puncture wounds (track marks)?
U — Uremia (Kidney Failure)	Patients with severe kidney failure can deteriorate into coma from the accumulation of waste products that the kidneys are unable to excrete. The IFA Attendant will rarely encounter such patients in the workplace because of their chronic disability.

T — Trauma | Is there evidence of major trauma? Has the patient suffered a head injury?

R — Respiratory | Does the patient have an airway obstruction? Is the patient in cardiac arrest? Was the patient drowning? Does the patient have evidence of respiratory failure?

I — Infection | Does the patient have a fever? Has he or she had a recent infection?

P — Poisoning | Has the patient been exposed to any toxic gases or materials (e.g. carbon monoxide)?

S — Stroke | Intracerebral hemorrhage? Did the patient have a history of high blood pressure? Did the patient complain of a severe headache prior to the onset of coma? Is there evidence of paralysis involving one side of the body?

Using the above mnemonic (AEIOU TRIPS), the Attendant will be able to record all the information needed to identify the precise cause of the patient's unconscious state. The most common causes encountered in the workplace are trauma, seizures and diabetic hypoglycemic reaction. Because a patient is comatose and unable to provide any history, information must be obtained from friends and witnesses. A careful search must be made of the patient's clothes and valuables (i.e. wallet) for pill bottles, syringes, medic alert bracelets, etc.

PRIORITY ACTION APPROACH FOR THE COMATOSE PATIENT

Despite the many causes of coma and syncope, assessment and treatment of the comatose patient follows the Priority Action Approach, focusing on the ABCs.

1. ALL COMATOSE PATIENTS (GCS "8" OR LESS) FALL INTO THE RAPID TRANSPORT CATEGORY.

2. A — Assess and secure the airway (see Part III, page 16). Stabilize the neck if trauma is suspected.

3. B — Breathing. All comatose patients require supplemental oxygen. Assisted ventilation may be required (see Part III, page 17).

4. C — Circulation. Patients with hypotension and shock from any cause may be comatose. The Attendant must check the patient's pulses, looking for evidence of hypotension (absent radial pulses or arrhythmia [irregular, extremely slow or fast pulses]). CPR must be initiated if the patient is in cardiac arrest.

5. The Attendant must determine the level of consciousness using the Glasgow Coma Score (see Part III, page 26).

6. The Attendant checks the pupillary response to light. The presence of a dilated unresponsive pupil with coma is usually indicative of a life-threatening structural damage to the brain. (See Part III, page 28).

7. The Attendant must conduct a neurological assessment. In the comatose patient, sensory function is impossible to evaluate accurately. The Attendant must focus on the presence of any asymmetry in motor response between the left and right sides of the body including the facial muscles. The presence of any asymmetry in motor activity (e.g. paralysis of one arm) is another clue suggestive of a life-threatening structural damage to the brain.

Part VI, Section C
Injuries to the Head and Brain

Brain injury accounts for approximately 25% of all trauma deaths and 50-60% of all MVA deaths. Treating the trauma patient with a decreased level of consciousness presents a great challenge to the IFA Attendant. Careful attention to neurological assessment and the Priority Action Approach will optimize the outcome for these patients.

Head injuries vary from superficial soft tissue injuries of the scalp to severe disruption of brain tissue.

SOFT TISSUE INJURIES OF THE SCALP

The scalp is composed of the skin and soft tissues that cover the skull. Underlying muscles enable us to wrinkle our forehead and chew our food. The muscles that support the cervical vertebrae extend up over the back of the head. Because the scalp and the muscles have a rich blood supply, open wounds may result in extensive bleeding. Similarly, closed wounds may swell rapidly from bleeding underneath the scalp.

A profusely bleeding scalp wound does not mean that the blood supply to the brain is impaired. The brain obtains its blood supply from the carotid and vertebral arteries in the neck, not from the scalp.

Bleeding usually responds to direct pressure. Lacerations at the back of the head usually respond to the pressure of the head lying supine on a large dressing. Occasionally, a pressure or tensor bandage may be required to control the bleeding. If these dressings are required in patients with suspected cervical injury, appropriate C-spine control must be used. Treatment principles follow those outlined in the section on soft tissue injuries (see Part IX, Section D, page 210). Swelling associated with closed wounds responds best to ice packs if they are available.

ALL PATIENTS WITH A SOFT TISSUE INJURY TO THE SCALP MUST BE ASSESSED FOR POSSIBLE CERVICAL SPINE INJURY AND IMMOBILIZED ACCORDINGLY.

SKULL FRACTURES

If sufficient energy is transmitted to the head, a skull fracture may result. Skull fractures can occur without damage to the brain. Similarly, brain injury (even severe brain injury) can occur in the absence of a skull fracture. By itself, skull fracture is not an important cause of death or disability. Skull fractures may be classified as linear or depressed. Linear fractures are single fracture lines caused by trauma to the skull. On x-ray they resemble straight lines and are therefore called linear fractures. Characteristically, linear fractures are never displaced.

Depressed fractures are usually caused by the application of a localized force (e.g. hammer, crowbar). A segment of bony skull may be buckled inwards. The likelihood of associated brain injury and the need to surgically elevate the bony fragments means rapid transport to hospital is required for patients with these injuries. It is extremely difficult to diagnose a skull fracture except by x-ray. With a soft tissue injury, swelling is similar to that in patients without skull fractures. Unless the skull deformity is severe and obvious on examination, skull fractures are difficult to diagnose.

Skull fractures are further categorized into fractures of the vault and fractures of the base (basilar). As previously described, the bony plates of the skull extend beneath the brain to separate it from the facial structures. Therefore, basilar skull fractures cannot be directly detected and may not even be evident on x-rays. The diagnosis of basilar skull fractures is made indirectly by looking for specific signs.

Signs of Basilar Skull Fracture

- Bruising around both eyes — Raccoon Eyes
- Bruising and swelling behind the ear — Battle's sign
- Bleeding from either ear canal (not the ear lobe)
- Clear fluid (cerebrospinal fluid) leaking from the nose or ear canal

Skull fractures may also be classified as open or closed. An open skull fracture is associated with a scalp laceration. Penetrating injuries to the head from sharp objects or gunshot wounds represent a special subgroup of open skull fractures.

BRAIN INJURY

Brain tissue is semi-gelatinous in its normal healthy state. As previously described, it is suspended in a bath of cerebrospinal fluid (C.S.F.) and protected by the meninges. When the head is struck with sufficient energy, the brain in essence is "bounced around" within the skull. Characteristically, the brain tissue may be injured in a number of ways.

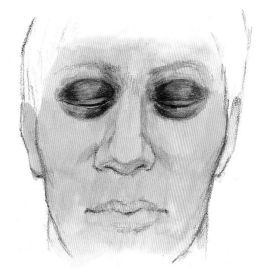

Raccoon eyes

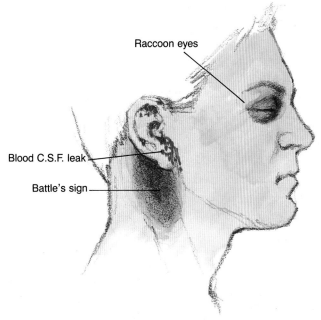

Raccoon eyes

Blood C.S.F. leak

Battle's sign

Signs of basilar skull fracture

- Concussion
- Damage to brain tissue
- Injuries to blood vessels — arteries or veins
- Inadequate oxygenation (hypoxia)
- Inadequate perfusion (ischemia)
- Combination of any or all of the above

Concussion

A concussion is a mild head injury that causes a brief "short circuit" of the brain. In actual fact, there is no damage or injury to brain tissue. This is the mildest form of brain injury. The head injury may cause a loss of consciousness for a variable period of time ranging from a few seconds to minutes. However, some patients may only be dazed and not actually lose consciousness. This is followed by a period of confusion where the patient may be disoriented, agitated or acting inappropriately. There may also be amnesia or loss of memory. The patient often cannot recall the injury or events leading up to the injury. Associated symptoms usually include headache, dizziness and nausea. All patients with a head injury severe enough to cause loss of consciousness (no matter how brief), confusion or other signs of concussion must be referred for medical assessment. Patients with concussion must also be assessed for an associated cervical spine injury (see page 132). If a cervical spine injury has been ruled out, the conscious patient may be transported to hospital in the position of comfort (e.g. lying, semi-sitting, or sitting).

Damage to brain tissue

Because brain tissue is rather fragile, a direct blow may result in bruising or tearing of the brain's tissues. Depending on the extent and location of the damage, the degree and nature of the neurological deficit will vary.

Classically, with a blow to the head, the area of the brain directly beneath the location of the blow may be injured. Because of the movement of the fragile tissue within the bony skull, characteristically, the region of the brain directly opposite the site of injury is also damaged from the force of the blow. The bruising of brain tissue is called a cerebral contusion. If bleeding is significant, an intracerebral (within the brain tissue) hematoma may develop.

Injuries to blood vessels

The arteries and veins supplying the meninges of the brain may also be injured directly or indirectly from the force of the blow. As with injuries to any other blood vessels, bleeding ensues and a hematoma develops. *Subdural hematomas* are caused by venous bleeding occurring below the dura mater layer. Because venous blood is under lower pressure than arterial blood, the hematoma accumulates gradually. *Epidural hematomas* are usually caused by arterial bleeding above the dura (between the skull and the duramater). Epidural hematomas may develop rapidly after injury. Some of these patients may exhibit a lucid interval between the initial head injury and the subsequent rapid deterioration. Both subdural and epidural hematomas are life-threatening neurosurgical emergencies and usually require emergency surgery. These hematomas may not necessarily be associated with any damage to brain tissue.

As with other tissues of the body, swelling is a natural response to injury such as bruising. Similarly, subdural, epidural and intracerebral hematomas will expand. Unfortunately, within the tight confines of the skull, there is no room to accommodate swelling from bruising, bleeding or an expanding hematoma. As swelling increases, the supply of blood and oxygen is reduced to brain tissue that has already been injured. This increases the extent of the initial injury. If the swelling or bleeding increases further, the pressure within the skull (intracranial pressure) increases dramatically, causing decreased blood flow to the uninjured parts of the brain. This worsens the patient's condition. Ultimately, the intracranial pressure may exceed a critical point, resulting in compression of the brain stem. This will cause the patient's death!

Depending on the extent of injury and the tissues involved, the bleeding or swelling may be minimal or severe. Similarly, the onset of significant bleeding or swelling will vary. The onset may be rapid or may be delayed for hours after injury.

THEREFORE, THE MOST IMPORTANT ASPECT OF THE NEUROLOGICAL EXAMINATION IS WHETHER OR NOT THE PATIENT'S CONDITION IS CHANGING AND IN WHAT DIRECTION IT IS CHANGING. The patient with a head injury whose level of consciousness is improving (GCS increasing) is less likely to have a severe head injury. On the other hand, the patient with a decreasing level of consciousness (GCS falling) may indicate the development of significant intracerebral swelling or bleeding. The Attendant must frequently reassess the patient for changes in the neurological status.

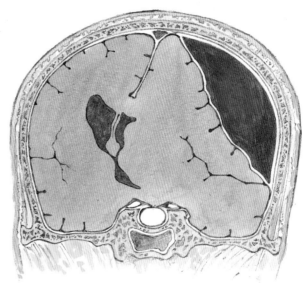

Subdural hematoma

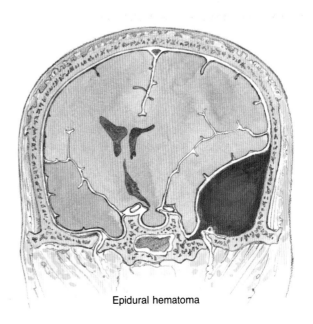

Epidural hematoma

Inadequate oxygenation (hypoxia)

As discussed in the section on brain function, cerebral tissue is highly dependent on an adequate supply of oxygen. If brain cells are deprived of oxygen for more than four or five minutes, permanent brain damage develops. This illustrates why airway and breathing are ranked as the major priorities in first aid.

Certain types of accidents or illnesses cause hypoxic brain injury without direct head trauma. Examples include drowning, choking and severe carbon monoxide poisoning. The primary treatment in these cases is to restore breathing and circulation as quickly as possible.

ALL TRAUMATIC INJURIES THAT RESULT IN AIRWAY PROBLEMS OR RESPIRATORY EMERGENCIES HAVE THE POTENTIAL FOR CAUSING HYPOXIC BRAIN INJURY. FURTHERMORE, IN THOSE PATIENTS WITH BRAIN INJURY, FAILURE TO CORRECT AIRWAY OBSTRUCTION OR HYPOXIA WILL WORSEN THE EXTENT OF THAT INJURY.

Inadequate perfusion (ischemia)

The circulatory system is responsible for maintaining the brain's essential oxygen supply. Obviously, failure of the circulatory system (i.e. shock or cardiac arrest) will seriously interfere with the supply of oxygen, resulting in brain injury. An occlusion (i.e. blood clot) in any of the major arteries supplying the brain may also result in brain injury. This is the major cause of strokes. A stroke illustrates the potentially devastating effect of an ischemic brain injury (see Part XIV, Section A, page 331).

In the setting of major trauma with hemorrhagic shock, the body attempts to preserve blood flow to the brain, but a critical point is reached, below which the cardiac output fails to maintain adequate cerebral blood flow. In this way, shock has the potential for causing ischemic brain injury or worsening an existing traumatic head injury. This illustrates why circulation is ranked third, after airway and breathing, in the Priority Action Approach.

ASSESSMENT AND MANAGEMENT OF THE PATIENT WITH HEAD INJURY

As with all trauma patients, the assessment follows the Priority Action Approach, beginning with the primary survey:

1. Clear the patient's airway while carefully controlling the cervical spine.

   ALL PATIENTS WITH HEAD INJURY HAVE A CERVICAL SPINE FRACTURE UNTIL PROVEN OTHERWISE.

   Patients with a decreased level of consciousness usually require the insertion of an oral airway to maintain patency of the airway.

2. Assess breathing. All patients with suspected brain injury require supplemental high-flow oxygen. (See Part IV, Section B, page 52).

   Those patients with a significant decrease in their level of consciousness (GCS "10" or less) have a high probability of severe head injury. Furthermore, these patients are at increased risk for the development of significant swelling or bleeding of brain tissue. As previously discussed, the swelling can progress and worsen the patient's condition.

   However, the Attendant can and must initiate treatment at the scene for those patients with severe head injury. Swelling of the brain is increased by elevated levels of carbon dioxide in the blood. Conversely, if the carbon dioxide level is decreased, swelling may be temporarily reduced. Hyperventilating the patient (increasing the respiratory rate) causes the level of carbon dioxide in the blood to fall.

   THEREFORE, THE ATTENDANT MUST PROVIDE ASSISTED VENTILATION TO ALL HEAD INJURY PATIENTS WITH A PERSISTENT GLASGOW COMA SCORE LESS THAN "10".

   In summary, assisted ventilation at a rate of 16-20 per minute will reduce the carbon dioxide level in the blood and reduce (but not stop) the degree of swelling and bleeding within the brain.

3. Assess the circulation. Head injury patients with evidence of shock and hypotension (decreased or absent radial pulses) are particularly difficult to assess. However, the Attendant must remember the following crucial points. IN ADULTS, SHOCK AND

HYPOTENSION ARE ALMOST NEVER CAUSED BY BRAIN INJURY. SHOCK AND HYPOTENSION ARE INVARIABLY CAUSED BY HEMORRHAGE IN OTHER PARTS OF THE BODY.

The Attendant must look diligently for other sources of bleeding (external or internal). The most common causes are intra-abdominal bleeding, thoracic injuries or pelvic fractures.

External sources of bleeding must be controlled with direct pressure. Scalp lacerations, even when bleeding profusely, are not usually the cause of shock and hypotension. The Attendant must look elsewhere.

4. Using the Priority Action Approach, the Attendant may have already determined from the mechanism of injury and the primary survey that the patient is in the Rapid Transport Category. If this is the case, the patient should be rolled onto a long spine board while stability of the neck is maintained. The critical interventions are performed and the patient is transported rapidly to hospital. The secondary survey is begun en route. If the patient has not yet met the criteria for rapid transport, the secondary survey is begun at the scene.

5. Neurological examination. For head injury patients, the secondary survey focuses on examination of the head, the patient's level of consciousness, the patient's pupillary response and the neurological assessment.

EXAMINATION OF THE HEAD INJURY PATIENT

The Attendant examines the head for evidence of trauma. Furthermore, the Attendant must look for the signs of a basilar skull fracture (see page 130). The scalp should be palpated and inspected for evidence of a depressed skull fracture.

LEVEL OF CONSCIOUSNESS (LOC)

The hallmark of brain injury is loss of consciousness. All patients with head injury who are alert must be asked if they incurred a loss of consciousness or were dazed by the event. Patients may not remember exactly what happened so bystanders should be asked. A head injury must be suspected in those patients who, as a result of the accident, are confused or have a decreased level of consciousness at the time of the initial assessment. All these

patients must be referred to a hospital for medical evaluation.

The level of consciousness is best assessed by the Glasgow Coma Score (GCS). Patients with coma usually have a GCS of "8" or less. Patients with severe head injury are those with a GCS of "10" or less.

Brain injury is a dynamic process and the patient's level of consciousness will reflect those changes. If the level of consciousness is improving (GCS increasing), the likelihood of a severe head injury is less. Similarly, if the level of consciousness is deteriorating (GCS decreasing), the likelihood of a severe head injury is very high. THEREFORE, THE MOST IMPORTANT ASPECT OF THE NEUROLOGICAL ASSESSMENT IS NOT ONLY THE INITIAL LEVEL OF CONSCIOUSNESS BUT WHETHER IT IS CHANGING AND THE DIRECTION OF THAT CHANGE.

Unfortunately, the patient's clinical condition may not change for hours or even days after injury. Therefore, it is impossible for the IFA Attendant to accurately determine which patients are at risk. ALL HEAD INJURY PATIENTS WHO ARE DAZED, CONFUSED OR HAVE EXPERIENCED A DECREASED LEVEL OF CONSCIOUSNESS REQUIRE REFERRAL FOR MEDICAL EVALUATION.

As previously discussed, patients with hypoxia or shock and hypotension may also have brain injury in the absence of head trauma. This usually manifests itself as a change in the level of consciousness. Therefore, it is almost impossible for the IFA Attendant to determine whether the patient's decreased level of consciousness is due to head injury, hypoxia, shock or a combination of all three. Nevertheless, the treatment does not change. The Attendant focuses on the ABCs and rapidly transports the patient to hospital.

Unfortunately, in our society, drug and alcohol abuse are becoming an increasing problem. Drugs and alcohol can also cause a decreased level of consciousness. Victims under the influence of drugs and alcohol have an increased risk of injury, especially head injury.

Patients with any head injury (even mild bruises, abrasions or lacerations) who appear intoxicated or impaired from alcohol or drugs must be referred for medical evaluation. THE ATTENDANT MUST NOT ATTRIBUTE

THE MILD HEAD INJURY PATIENT'S ALTERED MENTAL STATUS, CONFUSION, ETC. TO DRUGS OR ALCOHOL.

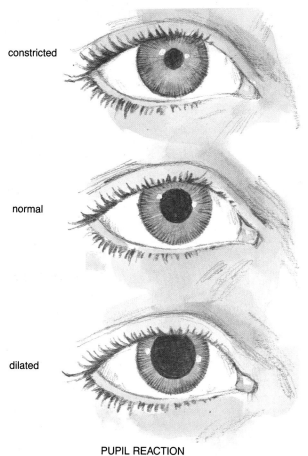

constricted

normal

dilated

PUPIL REACTION

PUPILLARY RESPONSE

The pupil size and response to bright light is an important aspect of assessing the severity of head injury. The nerve pathways that control the pupillary response travel a long distance from the eyes down to the brain stem. Therefore, any serious brain injury is likely to affect these pathways at some point. Furthermore, these nerve pathways are sensitive to changes in the intracranial pressure. This is manifested by a dilated pupil that responds sluggishly to light or not at all.

As discussed previously, swelling or bleeding within the brain causes the intracranial pressure to rise dramatically. If the intracranial pressure exceeds a critical point,

the brain stem becomes compressed and the patient will die. As the intracranial pressure approaches this critical point, the nerve pathways controlling pupillary size are usually affected, and one or both pupils will dilate.

Therefore, the presence of a dilated and sluggishly reactive or fixed pupil in the comatose patient, at the time of initial assessment, is an indication of severe head injury, with probable increased intracranial pressure.

Occasionally, direct trauma to the eye will also result in a dilated, sluggishly reacting or fixed pupil. These patients may easily be distinguished from those with severe head injury because they are usually alert and have a normal level of consciousness. Patients with a fixed dilated pupil from head injury usually have a significant decrease in their level of consciousness.

The swelling and bleeding of brain tissue from head injury that causes the rise in intracranial pressure may be delayed in onset. Therefore, as part of the neurological reassessment, the Attendant must re-examine the pupillary response. If the patient with an altered level of consciousness develops a dilated pupil while under the Attendant's observation, this indicates a medical emergency and the patient must be upgraded into the Rapid Transport Category.

NEUROLOGICAL ASSESSMENT

The brain controls sensory and motor function of the extremities. The assessment of sensory and motor function has already been discussed in detail. See Part III, page 32.

If the patient is able to cooperate, motor and sensory function is relatively easy to assess. The Attendant attempts to determine whether or not there is asymmetry between the left and right sides of the body. If the patient has a decreased level of consciousness, asymmetry of movement may be observed with or without a painful stimulus. The presence of asymmetry of movement or sensation between the left and right sides of the body indicates a severe head injury. There may not be a significant change in the level of consciousness as determined by the GCS.

Because of swelling or bleeding, the onset of the asymmetry may also be delayed. Once again, frequent reassessments of the neurological examination are mandatory.

COMPLICATIONS OF HEAD INJURY

1. **Convulsions (seizures).** Severe head injury may cause generalized or focal seizures (see Part XIV, Section B, page 335). Usually, they do not last more than ten minutes. There is no particular treatment except to maintain the ABCs. These patients must be upgraded into the Rapid Transport Category.

2. **Vomiting.** Patients with head injury are prone to vomiting, especially during transport. The Attendant must remain alert to this complication to prevent aspiration. Therefore, patients with a decreased level of consciousness must never be left unattended in the supine position.

   If the patient retches or vomits, the Attendant must log-roll the patient into the lateral position, maintaining immobilization of the cervical spine. The airway is cleared and the patient is repositioned (see Part IV, Section B, page 44).

SUMMARY

Assessment of patients with head injuries focuses on the ABCs and the neurological examination. The severity of brain injury can be established from the neurological examination in less than one minute by evaluating:

- The level of consciousness using the GCS
- Pupillary size and response to bright light
- Presence of extremity weakness or paralysis

From the foregoing discussion, patients with the following criteria must be considered to have severe head injury. All patients who meet these criteria for severe head injury fall into the Rapid Transport Category.

Criteria for Severe Head Injury

- Glasgow Coma Score less than or equal to "13"
- Decreasing GCS by "2" or more
- Pupillary inequality greater than 1 mm and sluggish response to light in the presence of an altered level of consciousness
- Extremity weakness or paralysis regardless of the GCS
- Depressed skull fracture
- Open penetrating head injuries

All patients with any decreased level of consciousness, confusion or who have been dazed from the force of injury must be referred for medical evaluation.

All open wounds should be covered. External bleeding should be controlled with direct pressure. Penetrating wounds to the brain with exposed brain tissue or leakage of cerebrospinal fluid should be covered lightly with a sterile dressing.

All patients with head injury must be frequently reassessed, focusing on the ABCs, level of consciousness, pupillary function, and extremity motor and sensory function.

Conscious patients with suspected cervical injury and all patients with a decreased level of consciousness must be transported fully immobilized on a long spine board (see Part XVI, Section A, page 355).

Head injuries are common and have the potential for causing death or permanent disability. The ultimate outcome depends, in large part, on the role of the IFA Attendant. It is hoped that rapid identification, effective initial treatment and rapid transport of patients with severe head injuries will improve their chances of recovery.

Part VI, Section D
Spinal Injuries and Their Management

INTRODUCTION

Neck and back injuries are the most common cause of disability among workers. The majority of these injuries are minor and resolve with rest and conservative treatment. At the other end of the spectrum, however, fracture of the spine has the potential to cause permanent paralysis as the result of spinal cord injury. The primary role of first aid — "Do no harm" — is never more important than in the evaluation and treatment of patients with spinal injury. The correct treatment, stabilization and transportation of spinal injuries may prevent a spinal cord injury. A possible scenario is to render a patient permanently quadriplegic from improper care of a spinal injury. Apart from the physical and emotional disability, the lifetime cost of medical care for a quadriplegic is expensive.

The key to preventing spinal cord injury is to always think about the possibility of a spinal injury before moving any patient. In this section, the Attendant will learn how to evaluate, treat, immobilize and transport patients with spinal injury.

ANATOMY AND FUNCTION

The spine or vertebral column is made up of 33 bony segments or VERTEBRAE stacked one on top of the other. The spine extends from the base of the skull to the tip of the coccyx (tail bone).

The vertebrae are divided into five groups:
1. cervical
2. thoracic
3. lumbar
4. sacral
5. coccygeal

The first 7 vertebrae are the CERVICAL vertebrae and form the bony framework of the neck. The 12 pairs of ribs are attached to the 12 THORACIC vertebrae. There are 5 LUMBAR vertebrae, which form the small of the back. The 5 SACRAL and 4 COCCYGEAL vertebrae are fused together to form the posterior wall of the pelvis. Anterior and lateral views of the vertebral column are illustrated in Figure VI-2.

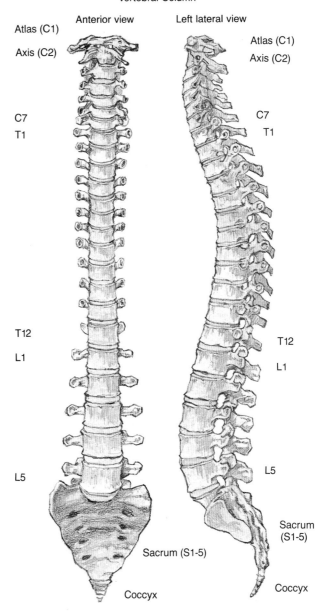

Vertebral Column

Anterior view — Atlas (C1), Axis (C2), C7, T1, T12, L1, L5, Sacrum (S1-5), Coccyx

Left lateral view — Atlas (C1), Axis (C2), C7, T1, T12, L1, L5, Sacrum (S1-5), Coccyx

Figure VI-2 Anatomy of the vertebral column

The vertebrae are identified by their grouping and position. For example, the 5th vertebra from the top is called C5 — the "C" refers to the cervical group and the number "5" implies the 5th vertebra down. The 11th vertebra from the top is called T4 — the "T" refers to the thoracic group and the number "4" identifies the vertebra as the 4th one down from the top of the thoracic group. Similarly, L3 refers to the 3rd lumbar vertebra.

Between each of the cervical, thoracic and lumbar vertebrae are the intervertebral discs. The discs are composed of a soft nucleus encased in a tough, fibrous shell. The discs act like shock absorbers between the vertebrae. They also permit the spine to bend in various directions without kinking the spinal cord inside.

Each intervertebral disc is identified by its adjacent vertebrae. For example, the disc between the 4th and 5th cervical vertebrae is called the C4-C5 disc. Similarly, the L5-S1 disc is the one between the 5th lumbar and 1st sacral vertebrae.

Each individual vertebra is made up of a bony ring attached to a bony core (the body). The spinal cord passes through the bony ring. The vertebral column is held together by specialized joints and ligaments which prevent shifting of any one vertebra on the other. A series of strong muscles run up and down the spine attaching to each vertebra. Together, these muscles, ligaments and joints not only provide support but also give the spine its mobility and flexibility. Figure VI-3 illustrates a top view of a typical vertebra. Figure VI-4 provides a side view showing how the vertebrae are joined together with the intervertebral discs interspaced between them.

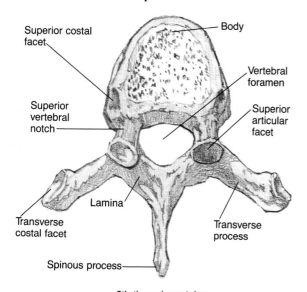

Superior costal facet

Body

Vertebral foramen

Superior vertebral notch

Superior articular facet

Lamina

Transverse costal facet

Transverse process

Spinous process

6th thoracic vertebra

Figure VI-3 Top view of a thoracic vertebra

The Attendant must note the special anatomical relationship between the spinal cord, the spinal nerves and the bony vertebrae. The bony rings of each vertebra, when stacked one on top of the other, form a long bony canal called the spinal canal which contains and protects the spinal cord.

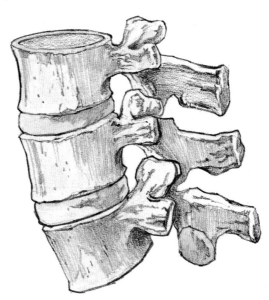

Figure VI-4 Side view of multiple lumbar vertebrae

The Attendant should recall, from the section on the nervous system, that there are 31 pairs of spinal nerves. Spinal nerves branch off from the spinal cord and connect the brain to the muscles and sensory receptors. At each vertebral level, a pair of spinal nerves branch off the spinal cord — one to the left and one to the right. The spinal nerves leave the vertebral column through bony passages between adjacent vertebrae. The anatomical relationship between the spinal cord, spinal nerves and the bony vertebrae is also illustrated in Figure VI-5 and VI-6.

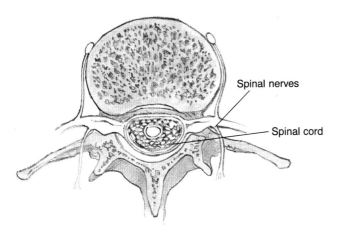

Figure VI-5 Top view of a thoracic vertebra
showing spinal nerves and cord

Lumbosacral Spine and Ligaments

Lateral view

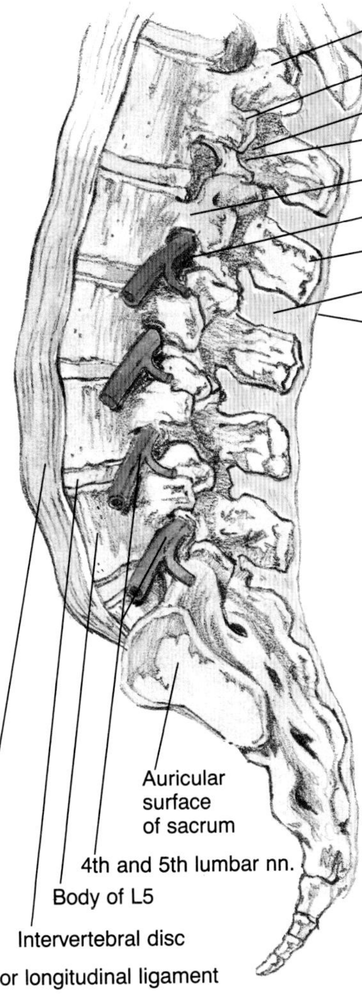

Superior articular process

Transverse process

Lamina

Inferior articular process

Pedicle

Intervertebral foramen

Spinous process

Interspinal ligament

Supraspinal ligament

Auricular
surface
of sacrum

4th and 5th lumbar nn.

Body of L5

Intervertebral disc

Anterior longitudinal ligament

Figure VI-6 Lumbosacral spine
showing ligaments and spinal nerves

The spinal nerves are numbered according to the level of the spinal column in which they emerge. The 1st cervical spinal nerve, C1, exits *above* the 1st cervical vertebra below the base of the skull. By consensus, the spinal nerve that exits above T1 (the 1st thoracic vertebra) and below C7 is called C8. The T1 spinal nerve exits *below* the 1st thoracic vertebra, T1. As a result, there are 8 pairs of cervical spinal nerves. There are 12 thoracic, 5 lumbar, 5 sacral but only 1 pair of coccygeal spinal nerves.

Because of the tight fit within the spinal canal, any fracture or ligament tear that allows slight displacement of one vertebra on the next will pinch or shear the spinal cord. This causes a spinal cord injury.

Similarly, significant narrowing of the bony passageways through which the spinal nerves pass, as a result of fracture, arthritis or protrusion of the intervertebral disc, may cause spinal nerve injury.

TYPES OF SPINAL INJURIES

Injuries to the spine may be classified as follows:
- muscle and/or ligament strain
- injuries to the intervertebral discs
- vertebral fractures and/or dislocations
- combination of the above

It is important that the Attendant recognize that spinal injury and spinal cord injury are different entities and may occur independently of each other.

Spinal injuries may be associated with spinal nerve or spinal cord injury but not necessarily so. To further complicate the issue, even unstable spinal fractures may not cause spinal cord or spinal nerve injury immediately. Inappropriate movement of the patient at any time may then cause sufficient displacement of the unstable fracture, resulting in permanent spinal cord or spinal nerve injury. Furthermore, spinal cord injuries may occur in the absence of spinal fractures. In this case, the spinal cord is injured by tearing, bruising or swelling.

SPINAL INJURIES

Muscle and/or Ligament Strains

The vast majority of spinal injuries are muscle/ligament strains or tears. Typically, muscle or ligament strains occur when the muscles are overloaded or overused —

i.e. when the patient lifts a heavy object or twists suddenly. The risk factors for muscle or ligament strains of the back are as follows:

- previous back injury
- overloaded muscles
- overuse
- poor muscle tone/poor physical conditioning
- poor posture

The key to the treatment of muscle/ligament strains is prevention.

Signs and Symptoms of Muscle/Ligament Strains

It is often difficult to differentiate muscle/ligament strains from more serious injuries such as fractures because the signs and symptoms overlap. The best indication is usually the mechanism of injury. Patients who report that they injured their back while lifting or twisting are more likely to have a strain. Spinal fractures are unlikely in the absence of a sufficient force to cause a fracture (e.g. fall down the stairs, direct blow, motor vehicle accident). Similarly, patients who cannot identify a specific injury that precipitated their back or neck pain, or who only develop the pain hours after the injury (rather than immediately), are also more likely to have a strain.

The major symptoms are pain and muscle spasm. The pain is usually limited to the site of injury and is worsened by movement. The pain may radiate away from the injury site into an extremity. This is suggestive of peripheral nerve irritation or injury. (See below.) Muscle spasm limits the range of motion of the vertebral column. The muscle spasm may be severe enough to cause the patient to assume a stooped, angled or rotated position and be unable to straighten out without increasing the pain.

Management

Patients with muscle or ligament strains of the spine should be referred to a physician for assessment. These injuries are not medical emergencies. The Attendant should document the presence of any previous neck or back problems as it may complicate the patient's acute injury. The patient should be transported in the position of maximum comfort. The Attendant should avoid heat lamps, liniments or massage therapy unless specifically directed by a physician. Ice packs are usually helpful for acute injuries. They should be applied for 10 minutes at a time. These injuries usually heal well without any complications, although the worker may be temporarily disabled.

Injuries to the Intervertebral Discs

The intervertebral discs may be injured acutely or slowly wear out with time. Certain types of work (e.g. heavy lifting, driving truck) increase the risk of intervertebral disc injury. As mentioned previously, the intervertebral disc consists of a soft nucleus surrounded by a tough, fibrous shell. The shell may be weakened acutely by injury or slowly wear out over time. If the shell is sufficiently damaged, it may bulge out under certain conditions. Sometimes, the soft material of the nucleus bulges out through a break in the shell, similar to a bubble in a bicycle tire. This bulging of the disc or its nucleus may cause pinching of the spinal nerve as it passes through the bony passageway out of the spinal cord. This is what happens with a "slipped disc". In many instances, the disc heals with rest and physiotherapy. In more severe cases, surgery may be required.

In other cases, the disc may pinch the spinal cord itself. This depends on the level of the intervertebral disc and may be associated with severe arthritis of the spine. These more serious cases often require surgery.

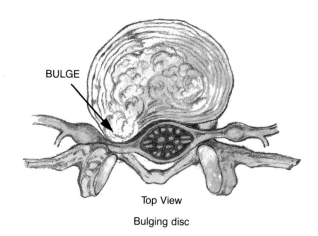

Top View

Bulging disc

Vertebral Fractures and/or Dislocations

As with fractures of the extremities, fractures of the spine may be stable or unstable. Stable spinal fractures are not at risk for any displacement. Therefore, they have little risk of causing spinal cord or spinal nerve injuries.

The unstable and/or dislocated spinal fractures have the greatest risk of spinal cord or spinal nerve injury. They do not necessarily cause spinal cord or spinal nerve injury immediately. Inadvertent movement of the patient at any time can cause displacement of the fracture and result in spinal cord injury. There are many examples of patients with unstable spinal fractures who have been walking around the accident scene with little apparent pain. The Attendant must realize that, at the scene of an accident, it is impossible to differentiate between simple muscle or ligament strains of the spine and unstable fractures or dislocations. They can be correctly diagnosed only with the help of x-rays at the hospital. Therefore, the IFA Attendant must treat all spinal injuries as if they were the worst case (i.e. an unstable fracture) and immobilize all these patients. Furthermore, the IFA Attendant must always suspect spinal injury and look for the mechanism of injury that commonly causes spinal injury.

SPINAL CORD INJURY

Approximately 10% of multiple trauma victims have spinal cord injury; 15-20% of all serious head injuries are associated with spinal cord injury.

The spinal cord is similar to a large telephone cable with thousands of individual circuits. Spinal cord injury is exactly like someone breaking the telephone cable. The break usually occurs at one point along the cable. Similarly, the spinal cord is usually injured in one specific area rather than along its entire length. As with the broken telephone cable, service is interrupted only to those households that are connected further down the line. Circuits that branch off before the break are unaffected. Similarly, spinal cord injury affects only those areas of the body below but not above the site of the injury.

There are two general types of spinal cord injuries — complete or incomplete. Complete spinal cord injuries result in *total* loss of motor and sensory functions on both sides of the body below the level of the injury. Incomplete spinal cord injuries result in *partial* loss. The degree of motor and sensory function that is lost depends on the exact extent and location of the injury. However, as with complete spinal cord injury, incomplete injuries only affect those areas below but not above the level of the injury. For example, a complete spinal cord injury at T12 characteristically causes complete paralysis and loss of sen-

sation from the waist down. An unstable fracture of C7 with complete spinal cord injury results in partial loss of motor and sensory functions in both arms and complete loss of sensation and total paralysis from the collar bones down. An incomplete spinal cord injury at C5 will produce partial loss of motor and sensory function in the arms and the legs.

It is important to remember that incomplete injuries may worsen with time (because of swelling or bleeding) or with rough handling of the patient, ultimately resulting in a complete injury.

One of the other physical findings that may be associated with spinal cord injury in male patients is persistent erection of the penis (priapism). The Attendant should not be embarrassed by this finding. It is beyond the patient's voluntary control and the patient cannot feel or notice its development. The Attendant should just reassure the patient and consider his dignity by covering with a blanket.

SPINAL NERVE INJURY

The spinal nerves are most commonly damaged by conditions that cause narrowing of the bony passageways through which they pass. Fractures, arthritis or intervertebral disc protrusions (slipped disc) may pinch or kink the spinal nerves. Usually only one spinal nerve (the left or right) at one particular level is affected. As a result, the most common findings with spinal nerve injury are pain and partial loss of sensation and motor strength in one extremity. Therefore, those patients with pain, tingling and/or weakness in one extremity may have a spinal nerve injury.

It is extremely difficult for the Attendant to differentiate spinal nerve from spinal cord or even brain injury. THEREFORE, ALL PATIENTS WITH ANY COMPLAINTS OF NUMBNESS, TINGLING OR WEAKNESS IN ONE OR MORE EXTREMITY MUST BE TREATED AS A POSSIBLE SPINAL CORD INJURY AND BE FULLY IMMOBILIZED.

MECHANISMS OF SPINAL INJURIES

Certain types of accidents must alert the Attendant to the possibility of spinal injury. By always thinking about the possibility of spinal injury, the Attendant will not miss this diagnosis. In all patients with the following mechanisms of injury, the Attendant must assume the presence of a spinal injury until proved otherwise.

- Motor vehicle accidents are the most common causes of spinal fractures and spinal cord injury. Even when seatbelts are worn, the force of the impact can cause spinal (especially cervical) fractures. The frequency of whiplash injuries attests to the high-risk nature of motor vehicle accidents. Whiplash injury is a muscle and ligament strain of the neck associated with flexion and extension of the neck, which occurs on impact. If the force of injury is high enough, cervical fracture results. Accidents involving bicycles, motorcycles, all-terrain vehicles (ATV's), skidders or tractors have an increased likelihood of causing spinal fracture, especially if seatbelts are not worn.

- Falls are another frequent cause of spinal fracture. The height of the fall and the manner in which the body strikes the ground often determine the type and location of the spinal injury. Jumping down from a wall and landing on the feet often result in fracture of the lower thoracic or upper lumbar vertebrae. This is especially true if the force of impact is sufficiently strong to fracture the heel bone. The patient who falls down a flight of stairs is also at risk of spinal injury, especially the cervical spine.

- Direct blows. Any direct blow to the spine has the potential to cause a spinal fracture. Assaults, crush injuries, blunt injuries from falling or swinging objects are some examples of accidents that may result in fractures of the spine.

- Diving into shallow water such as a lake or pool is another common cause of cervical spine fracture. The Attendant must consider the possibility of cervical spine injury when called to rescue a drowning victim, especially in shallow water. The management of near-drowning victims with suspected cervical spine injury is discussed in Part XI, Section F, page 302.

- Sports injuries are also associated with spinal fractures. Football, rugby, surfing and gymnastics are some examples of high-risk sports.

- Gunshots, deep knife wounds or other penetrating injuries may directly injure the vertebral column or the spinal cord.

- Severe electrical shock can cause direct spinal cord injury or cause spinal fracture from the violent muscle spasms that often accompany these injuries. Comatose victims of electrical injury must be assumed to have a spinal injury and immobilized accordingly.

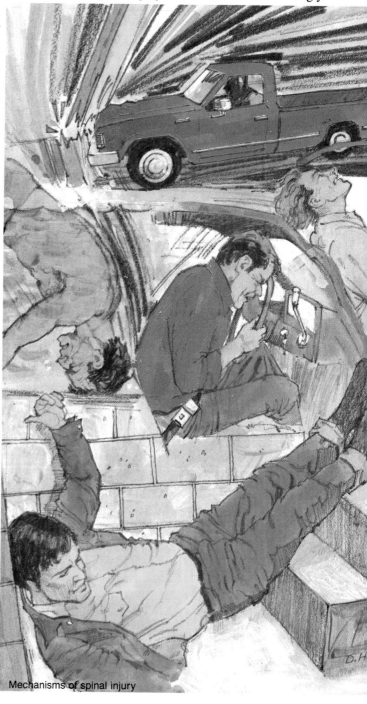

Mechanisms of spinal injury

• Facial and head injuries are also associated with cervical spine fracture. The same mechanism of injury that causes structural damage to the face or head (lacerations, contusions or fractures) can also result in cervical spine fracture.

In summary, the Attendant must suspect spinal injury in all the conditions listed above and treat the patient accordingly. The first step in the treatment of these patients is to "think spinal injury".

The Attendant is often called to evaluate patients with severe neck or back pain as a result of seemingly minor injuries such as twists or heavy lifting. Although the pain associated with such injuries can be severe, a spinal fracture is unlikely. These patients invariably have ligament and muscle strains or disc injuries. In the absence of any of the previous mechanisms of injury, spinal fracture is unlikely.

SIGNS AND SYMPTOMS OF SPINAL INJURY

PAIN: Conscious patients invariably complain of pain or stiffness in the affected area of the spine. These patients are usually able to indicate the region of the neck or back that is injured. It is impossible to differentiate the pain associated with a mild strain from a disc injury or an unstable spinal fracture.

• ALL CONSCIOUS PATIENTS WITH ANY OF THE ABOVE MECHANISMS OF INJURY WHO COMPLAIN OF PAIN OR TENDERNESS IN THE SPINAL REGION MUST BE ASSUMED TO HAVE AN UNSTABLE SPINAL FRACTURE AND BE FULLY IMMOBILIZED.

• ALL TRAUMA PATIENTS WITH A DECREASED LEVEL OF CONSCIOUSNESS MUST BE ASSUMED TO HAVE A SPINAL FRACTURE AND BE FULLY IMMOBILIZED.

• ALL PATIENTS WITH SEVERE HEAD OR FACIAL INJURY MUST ALSO BE ASSUMED TO HAVE A SPINAL FRACTURE AND BE FULLY IMMOBILIZED.

Patients with other serious injuries or those who are intoxicated with alcohol or under the influence of drugs may not notice pain in the spine. Therefore, the Attendant must rely on the mechanism of injury and treat these patients accordingly. It is always better to err on the side of caution and immobilize these patients rather than risk a spinal cord injury.

NUMBNESS, TINGLING OR WEAKNESS: If the conscious patient complains of any tingling, numbness or weakness in one or more extremities, a spinal cord or spinal nerve injury may exist. It is extremely difficult for the Attendant to differentiate brain injury from spinal cord or spinal nerve injury.

PAIN ON MOVEMENT: The patient may voluntarily indicate that movement of the spine causes or increases the pain. The Attendant should never attempt to test for this by moving the patient or asking the patient to move unassisted.

TENDERNESS: The Attendant may discover tenderness over the bony projections (processes) of the spine or in the muscles alongside the spine. The presence of tenderness is a strong indication that a spinal fracture exists.

DEFORMITY: The presence of any noticeable deformity of the spine is extremely rare and is only found with severe injuries. Absence of a deformity does not rule out the possibility of a spinal fracture.

SWELLING: Fractures or other injuries of extremities are usually associated with soft tissue swelling. However, swelling associated with a spinal injury is very unusual. The absence of swelling also does not rule out a spinal fracture.

ALL PATIENTS WITH ANY COMPLAINTS OF NUMBNESS, TINGLING OR WEAKNESS IN ONE OR MORE EXTREMITIES MUST BE TREATED AS A SPINAL FRACTURE WITH POSSIBLE SPINAL CORD OR SPINAL NERVE INJURY.

PRIORITY ACTION APPROACH FOR THE PATIENT WITH SUSPECTED SPINAL INJURY

The initial assessment of these patients focuses on the ABCs — Airway, Breathing and Circulation. However, the Attendant has the opportunity to prevent paralysis by "thinking about spinal injury" while approaching the patient.

1. Consider the mechanisms of injury that are known to cause spinal injury. If any are present, any movement of the patient must include careful control of the entire spine.

2. Assess and clear the airway. The airway is best assessed without moving the patient. If an airway obstruction is suspected, the Attendant must open the airway with careful C-spine control. The Attendant MUST use a jaw thrust manoeuvre coupled with careful realignment of the neck to the neutral position to open the airway. Care must be taken never to extend the neck of a trauma patient with a suspected cervical spine fracture. In the patient with a decreased level of consciousness, an oral airway is often required. In the presence of blood, vomitus or foreign debris in the airway, suctioning equipment is recommended to clear it. A finger sweep may be used but care must be taken not to move the neck.

In the presence of active bleeding or vomiting, the ¾ prone position is not usually recommended because the cervical spine is excessively rotated. The lateral position is preferred because it maintains the spine in the neutral position and still allows drainage by gravity. See Figure VI-7. These patients must be rapidly moved to the lateral position with C-spine control to clear the airway. Patients with airway problems are in the Rapid Transport Category.

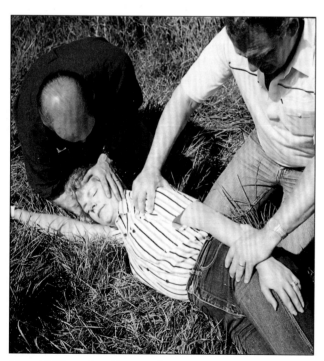

Figure VI-7 Lateral position with C-spine control

3. The Attendant must ensure adequate breathing. Patients with cervical or thoracic spinal cord injuries will have paralysis of the chest wall muscles. Therefore, these patients will have shallow respirations. The Attendant must provide supplemental oxygen at 10 Lpm to all patients with spinal cord injury and assist ventilations if required. Patients with respiratory difficulties are in the Rapid Transport Category.

4. The Attendant then assesses the circulation and controls any severe external hemorrhage with direct pressure. Patients with spinal cord injury may develop a shock-like state with decreased pulses as a result of the damage to the pathways of the autonomic nervous system contained in the spinal cord. This is called neurogenic shock. Neurogenic shock occurs only in the presence of a spinal cord injury with complete paralysis. Neurogenic shock does not occur with spinal fractures alone.

It is very difficult to differentiate neurogenic shock from hemorrhagic shock due to internal bleeding. Therefore, the Attendant must treat all trauma patients with shock as if they had hemorrhagic shock from internal bleeding. These patients are in the Rapid Transport Category.

Upon completion of the primary survey, the Attendant will have determined whether or not the patient has a mechanism of injury capable of producing a spinal injury. Any life-threatening emergency will have been identified and treatment initiated. The Attendant then follows these steps to determine whether or not a spinal injury exists:

1. The Attendant asks the conscious patient if there is any pain or stiffness in the neck or back. If the patient answers yes, the Attendant must treat the patient as if an unstable spinal fracture exists. Remember, it is impossible to differentiate at the accident scene simple strains of the neck or back from unstable spinal fractures.

2. If the patient is comatose, or too confused to indicate whether a spinal injury exists or not, the Attendant must assume that a spinal injury is present. For example, the intoxicated patient who falls down the stairs has a mechanism of injury capable of producing a cervical spine injury. The patient may be too drunk to notice any pain in the neck or may be unable to respond appropriately to the Attendant's questions. In these situations, the Attendant must assume the presence of a spinal injury and immobilize the patient accordingly. Similarly, patients with a head injury who are comatose or too confused to respond appropriately must be treated as if a spinal injury exists.

3. Patients with multiple injuries may be distracted by the pain associated with those other injuries and not "notice" or "feel" the pain in their spine. Therefore, all patients with multiple trauma must also be treated as if a spinal injury exists.

4. The Attendant asks the patient if there is any numbness, tingling or weakness in any of the extremities. The presence of any of those findings, in the absence of any obvious extremity injury, indicates the presence of a possible spinal cord or spinal nerve injury. These patients must be treated as if an unstable spinal fracture is present.

5. The Attendant gently palpates the spine and the paraspinal (alongside the spine) muscles for tenderness, bleeding or wounds. If there is tenderness to palpation, the Attendant must suspect the presence of a spinal injury and treat accordingly.

   Ideally, the Attendant should look for evidence of swelling or deformity involving the spine. However, the patient may have to be rolled to expose the area and properly examine the spine. IF A SPINAL INJURY HAS ALREADY BEEN DIAGNOSED, THIS STEP SHOULD NOT BE DONE. Patients with spinal injury should not be moved unnecessarily because of the risk of aggravating the injury. Further-

more, the patient's spine can usually be palpated in the position found without necessarily moving the patient.

If a wound or bleeding is discovered, the patient will have to be log-rolled with careful spine control to examine and treat the injury.

6. THE ATTENDANT CONDUCTS A NEUROLOGICAL EXAMINATION AS PART OF THE SECONDARY SURVEY. Weakness or paralysis may be checked in the upper extremity by asking the patient to lift the arms and squeeze fingers (hand grip). To check the lower extremities, the Attendant should ask the patient to wiggle the toes and test ankle flexion and extension. The Attendant should always compare the left and right sides and record the observations. The Attendant must carefully assess each extremity. Sensation may be tested by lightly touching the arms, legs and trunk for evidence of numbness or tingling. The Attendant must remember to carefully assess each extremity in its entirety.

   If any abnormality is detected, the patient must be treated for possible spinal cord injury. Remember, it is extremely difficult to differentiate brain injury from spinal cord or spinal nerve injury. Furthermore, many head injury patients also have an associated spinal cord injury. Therefore, all patients with any neurological abnormality detected on examination must be treated as a possible spinal cord injury.

7. If all the above steps have been performed and no spinal injury has been found, the patient may be asked to gently move the neck or back. If any pain or stiffness is found, the Attendant must tell the patient to stop and return to the original position. The Attendant must then treat the patient as a potential spinal injury. Only if the patient can complete a full range of motion without pain can the Attendant safely rule out the possibility of a spinal injury.

The following table summarizes the Priority Action Approach to patients with suspected spinal injury.

TABLE VI-a

PRIORITY ACTION APPROACH TO PATIENTS WITH SUSPECTED SPINAL INJURIES

1. Recognize the mechanisms of injury that are capable of producing spinal injury:
    - motor vehicle accidents including motorcycles, bicycles, ATVs, tractors and skidders
    - falls
    - direct blows to the neck or back
    - head and facial injuries
    - diving into shallow water
    - sports injuries
    - penetrating injuries that may involve the spine
    - high voltage electrical injuries

2. Complete the primary survey focusing on the ABCs. In the presence of a life-threatening emergency, the patient may have to be moved but care must be taken to control the spine.

3. All comatose or confused patients must be treated as if they have an unstable spinal fracture.

4. Ask the patient if there is pain or stiffness in the neck or back.
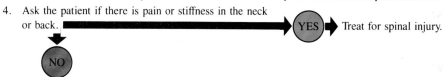
    YES → Treat for spinal injury.
    NO ↓

5. Is the patient too confused or drowsy to respond accurately to your questions?
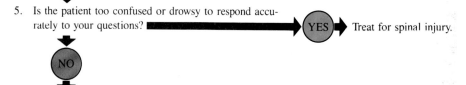
    YES → Treat for spinal injury.
    NO ↓

6. Does the patient have multiple injuries or another painful injury that may impair ability to feel pain in the spine?
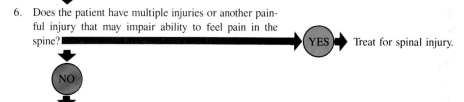
    YES → Treat for spinal injury.
    NO ↓

7. Ask the patient if there is numbness, tingling or weakness in any of the extremities.
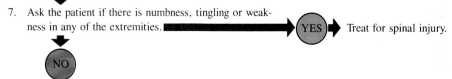
    YES → Treat for spinal injury.
    NO ↓

8. Gently palpate the spine and paraspinal muscles for tenderness.
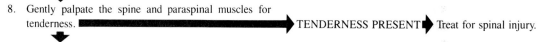
    TENDERNESS PRESENT → Treat for spinal injury.
    NO TENDERNESS TO PALPATION ↓

9. On palpation or observation, is there evidence of a wound or bleeding close to the spine?
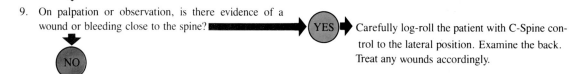
    YES → Carefully log-roll the patient with C-Spine control to the lateral position. Examine the back. Treat any wounds accordingly.
    NO ↓

10. Perform a careful neurological examination.
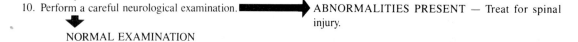
    ABNORMALITIES PRESENT — Treat for spinal injury.
    NORMAL EXAMINATION ↓

11. Ask the patient to gently move the neck and back. If any pain or stiffness is found, tell the patient to stop and return to the original position. The Attendant must then treat the patient as a potential spinal injury.

    NOTE: This step must not be performed if a spinal injury has already been diagnosed from any of the preceding steps. This step must also *not* be performed if, on the basis of other injuries, there are contraindications to having the patient move the neck or back.

SPECIAL PRECAUTIONS FOR PATIENTS WITH SPINAL CORD INJURY

Patients with spinal cord injury are at very high risk for developing two specific problems:
- respiratory difficulties
- pressure sores

Respiratory Difficulties

In the presence of cervical or thoracic spinal cord injury, the respiratory muscles of the chest wall are paralyzed. The patient is able to breathe only by movement of the diaphragm, which has a unique nerve supply. Therefore, the Attendant will only observe the abdomen moving in and out with each respiration and little movement of the chest wall. As a result, the patient with spinal cord injury will have respiratory difficulties and supplemental oxygen must be provided. The Attendant must prevent aspiration in these patients.

Pressure Sores

When the body is lying down, its prominences are subject to pressure (e.g. shoulder blades and sacrum when lying down supine). The pressure may reduce the blood supply to the skin. The normal healthy person shifts position slightly or applies padding to prevent the problem. The patient with spinal cord injury who has lost sensation and motor strength is unable to do so. Over a long period of time, the blood supply to the skin over these bony prominences may be reduced to the point that the skin and underlying soft tissue are injured or die. This is called a pressure sore. The sore may begin as a reddened mark but may progress to a large infected ulcer that extends down to the bone. It may vary in size from a few millimetres in diameter to as large as several centimetres across. Pressure sores may become infected and often require surgery with skin grafts in order to heal.

Pressure sores are preventable. The Attendant must take extra precautions to prevent their development in patients with spinal cord injury. Hard objects such as keys, wallets and belts must be removed from under the patient. The stretcher or spine board must be padded. The patient must be rotated slightly every two hours. (The technique is described in a later section.)

In summary, the Attendant must be aware of the specific complications of patients with spinal cord injury and take extra precautions to prevent them.

SPECIFIC TREATMENT OF SPINAL INJURIES

Once a spinal injury has been diagnosed or strongly suspected, the Attendant must initiate specific treatment to stabilize the injury. There are no essential differences between those patients with and those without spinal cord injury. Patients with spinal cord injury must be carefully stabilized to prevent further injury to the spinal cord. Patients with a suspected spinal fracture without spinal cord or spinal nerve injury must be carefully stabilized to *prevent* spinal cord injury.

These general principles of spinal stabilization are similar to the treatment of injuries to the extremities:
- Prevent further injury.
- Realign and gently rotate to the anatomical position.
- Immobilize.
- Maximize patient comfort.
- Provide supplemental oxygen by mask if necessary. All patients with spinal cord injury should be provided with supplemental oxygen by mask.
- Keep the patient warm with blankets. Prevent hypothermia.
- Do not give the patient anything by mouth.

1. Further injury can be prevented by carefully moving the patient as a unit at all times. Even in the presence of life-threatening airway or respiratory emergencies, the patient still can be moved rapidly yet with stability of the spine maintained.

2. Realignment of the spine. The anatomical position of the spine is a straight line from head to toe without flexion, extension or rotation. The head is positioned with the eyes forward and the chin in the midline. For proper spine alignment the head must be put in the neutral position. The neutral position is obtained when the head is on a flat surface and gently tilted so the corner of the mouth is in approximate alignment with the earlobe (see Figure VI-8). The neutral position of the head is obtained as the head and neck are being anatomically aligned. The anatomical position can be achieved effectively only with the patient supine (see Figure VI-9) or in the lateral position with the head

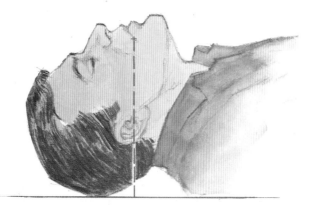

Figure VI-8 Neutral position of the head

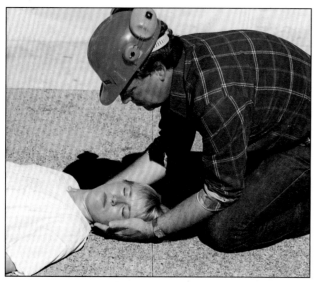

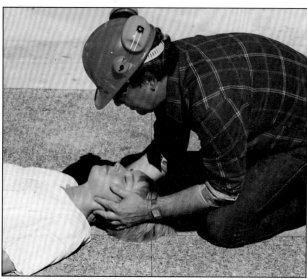

Figure VI-9 Top: placing the hands
Bottom: head realigned to the anatomical position

supported (see Figure VI-10). In the ¾ prone position, the spine is not in the anatomical position because there is excessive rotation of the neck.

The patient with suspected spinal injury must therefore be carefully realigned to the supine or lateral position. The supine position is preferred because patient assessment and monitoring is easier. Immobilization of the head and neck is also simpler in the supine position. However, there are specific situations and factors that make the lateral position preferred. Patients with suspected spinal injuries and the following conditions must be maintained in the lateral position:

- facial injuries with active bleeding in the nasal or oral airway;
- active vomiting;
- patients with a decreased level of consciousness who cannot be continuously monitored by the Attendant;
- stretcher limitations, i.e. inability to rotate the spine board or stretcher should the patient vomit;
- helicopter evacuations; if the stretcher is suspended below the helicopter during rescue operations, the patient cannot be monitored effectively so the lateral position is required.

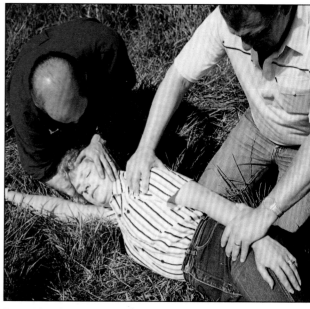

Figure VI-10 Maintaining the cervical spine alignment in the lateral position

TECHNIQUES FOR REALIGNMENT OF THE SPINE

The basic principles for realignment of the spine involve moving the head, neck, trunk and extremities as a unit. In most cases, the Attendant will require the assistance of at least one co-worker. The Attendant must assume responsibility for the head and neck whenever the patient is moved.

If the patient is conscious, the Attendant should explain ahead of time what will happen, to ensure the patient's relaxation and cooperation. The following cases listed below illustrate the step-by-step procedures to be followed for realigning the spine, depending on the position in which the patient is found.

CASE A — PATIENT FOUND SUPINE (SEE FIGURE VI-11)

1. The Attendant manually stabilizes the head and neck by grabbing the muscles at the base of the neck (trapezius muscles) with one hand and the patient's head with the other hand (see Figure VI-11). Note that the patient's head is supported between the Attendant's hand and forearm.

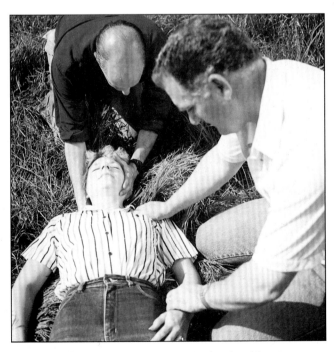

Figure VI-11 Support the head between the hand and forearm.

2. With gentle hand traction, the Attendant gently moves the head to the neutral position, and realigns the chin to midline (i.e. the anatomical position). If resistance is met, do not forcefully rotate the neck. The Attendant should manually stabilize and immobilize the neck in the anatomical position.

3. The Attendant manually stabilizes the head in the neutral position until the neck has been immobilized. By holding the trapezius muscles at the base of the neck, the Attendant is able to ensure that the head, neck and trunk move as a unit.

4. If the patient's trunk is twisted or rotated, the Attendant should direct an assistant to align the spine while the head and neck are maintained in the neutral position. This is best achieved by having the assistant grasp the patient's waist and gently slide, push or pull the trunk into the neutral position.

5. Continuous manual stabilization of the head and neck must be maintained until the patient can be properly immobilized. A hard cervical collar alone is not considered adequate spinal immobilization. Adequate spinal immobilization is only achieved when the patient is fully secured to a spine board or stretcher.

CASE B — PATIENT FOUND PRONE (SEE FIGURE VI-12)

1. a) If the patient is conscious, the Attendant should begin the primary survey, leaving the patient in the position found. If the airway is clear, the Attendant proceeds to log-roll the patient to the supine position and completes the primary survey.

   b) If the patient has a decreased level of consciousness or other critical conditions are found on the primary survey, the patient must be log-rolled to the lateral position immediately. In the absence of any contraindications (oral or nasal bleeding, vomiting), the log-roll may be continued until the patient is supine.

2. If a lifting device is readily available, the patient should be rolled directly onto the spine board or clamshell, to avoid moving the patient again at a later time.

3. The primary survey is completed and life-threatening conditions are treated in the lateral or supine position, taking into account the factors and conditions previously mentioned.

4. Continuous manual stabilization of the head and neck must be maintained until the patient can be properly immobilized. A hard cervical collar alone is not considered adequate spinal immobilization. Adequate spinal immobilization is only achieved when the patient is fully secured to a spine board or stretcher.

TECHNIQUES FOR LOG-ROLLING THE PRONE PATIENT

By following these steps, the Attendant will be able to safely move the patient. This technique requires at least one and preferably two assistants.

1. The Attendant is positioned at the head of the patient. The Attendant must kneel to achieve the necessary control of the patient's head and neck. The Attendant's leg on the direction to which the patient will be rolled may be extended for stabilization. The Attendant should grasp the patient's trapezius muscle at the base of the neck on the underside to control the patient's head and neck. The Attendant's thumb of this hand should rest on the patient's scapula (see Figure VI-13).

2. The Attendant positions the other hand on the patient's head and face, using the fingers to support the head and angle of the jaw.

3. The patient's head and neck are firmly controlled by the Attendant's forearm and hand. The Attendant may support the downside arm on the flexed knee.

4. The Attendant directs an assistant to firmly grasp the patient's shoulder and waist or belt.

5. If there is another assistant available, he/she should be directed to stabilize the patient's legs and hold them together at the knees.

6. The Attendant directs the assistant(s) to roll the patient as a unit to the lateral position. The Attendant's responsibility is to maintain alignment of the patient's head and neck with the torso and *follow* the movement of the assistant(s). The Attendant should *not* turn the patient's head and neck ahead of the assistants' roll. The patient must always be rolled in the direction that keeps the face up, unless there are extenuating circumstances (e.g. insufficient space) (see Figure VI-14).

7. Once the patient is in the lateral position, the alignment of the head, neck and back must be maintained.

8. At this point, with the patient in the lateral position, an assistant should be directed to grasp the cheek bones anteriorly with one hand. The assistant's hand is stabilized in this position by bracing the forearm and elbow against the patient's anterior chest. With the other hand, the assistant grasps the patient's neck posteriorly at the base of the skull. This hand is also stabilized by bracing the forearm firmly against the patient's back. In this position, the assistant is able to manually stabilize the patient's cervical spine. Then, and only then, the Attendant may release the patient's head (see Figure VI-15).

9. If the patient must remain in the lateral position, continuous manual stabilization of the head and neck must be maintained until the patient can be properly immobilized. Assistant(s) may have to support the patient in the lateral position to prevent any rolling, as placing blankets under the patient's head may not be sufficient.

10. If there are no contraindications, the patient may be rolled directly to the supine position from the lateral position as follows. The Attendant repositions as in Figure VI-16. The assistant then releases his/her grip and is repositioned at the patient's shoulder and waist. The roll is then completed to the supine position.

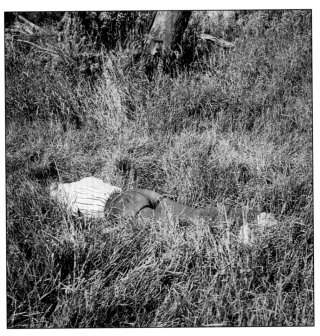

Figure VI-12 Patient found prone

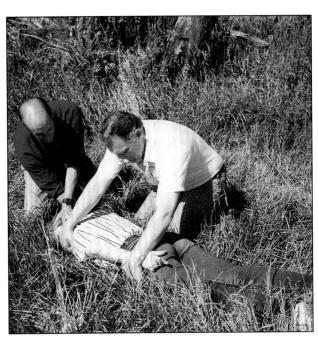

Figure VI-13 Preparing to roll patient

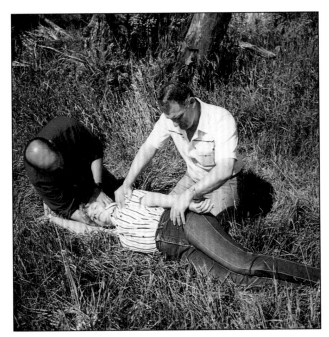

Figure VI-14 Patient in lateral position

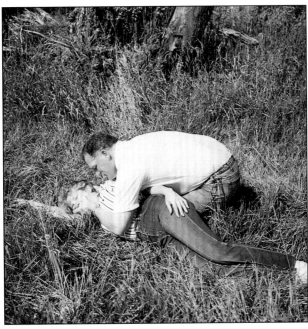

Figure VI-15 Assistant stabilizing the cervical spine

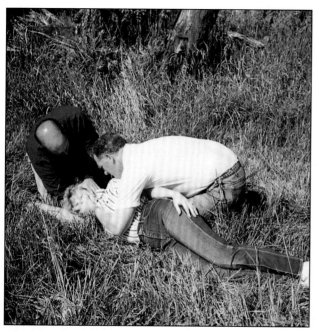

Figure VI-16 The attendant is repositioned

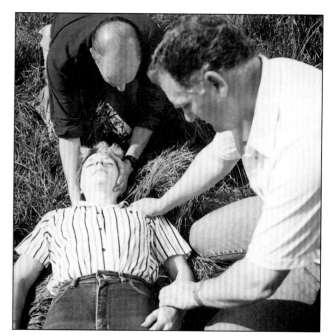

Roll completed to supine

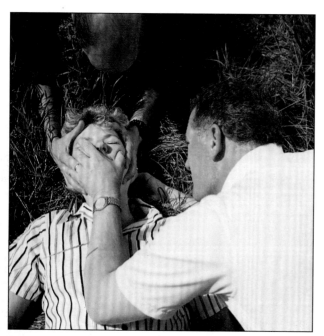

Assistant stabilizes head while attendant repositions hands

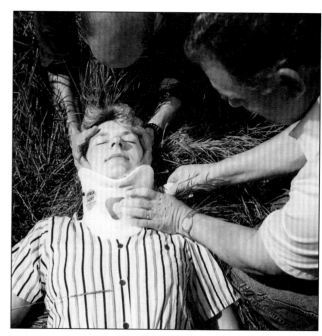

Collar applied to patient by a trained assistant

CASE C — PATIENT FOUND SITTING UP

1. The Attendant or assistant manually stabilizes the head and neck in the neutral position with the patient upright. The primary survey is begun.
2. a) If the patient is conscious, he or she should be told not to move the head while the Attendant completes the primary survey. Alternatively, the Attendant directs one of the co-workers to hold the head and neck in the neutral position. A hard cervical collar may be applied at this time.
    b) If the patient has a decreased level of consciousness or a life-threatening condition is identified, the patient must be immediately moved to the supine or lateral position to initiate treatment.
3. The Attendant retakes control of the head and neck by grasping the trapezius muscles with one hand and the patient's head and face with the other hand.
4. The Attendant directs an assistant to straighten and free up the legs.
5. The Attendant directs another assistant to grasp the patient's waist.
6. Together and as a unit, lift the patient slightly and turn to whatever position is necessary to allow the patient to be laid down.
7. The patient is then carefully lowered to the supine or to the lateral position. If a spine board is available, it may be faster to lower the patient onto the spine board.
8. Continuous manual stabilization of the head and neck must be maintained until the patient can be properly immobilized. A hard cervical collar alone is not considered adequate spinal immobilization.

CASE D — PATIENT FOUND ON UNEVEN GROUND OR IN AN AWKWARD POSITION

The same principles of realignment apply except that, in this case, the patient must be moved to a level surface. The procedure outlined below should not be used to carry a patient over a few metres. It should only be used to transfer patients found on uneven ground onto a spine board or stretcher.

The Attendant begins with the primary survey:

1. a) If the patient is conscious, the Attendant should ask the patient not to move and explain briefly what will happen next.
    b) If the patient has a decreased level of consciousness or a life-threatening condition is identified on the primary survey, the patient must be moved quickly to a level surface.
2. The Attendant selects a level surface as close to the patient as possible or preferably moves the patient directly onto a spine board or stretcher.
3. The Attendant will usually require at least three assistants. Two additional assistants may be required to hold and stabilize the stretcher.
4. The Attendant manually stabilizes the head and neck by grasping the trapezius muscle on one side with one hand and the head and face with the other hand. The head and neck are stabilized between the Attendant's hand and forearm.
5. The Attendant directs an assistant to hold the patient under the chest. Another assistant is directed to hold the patient's waist or belt.
6. The Attendant directs another assistant to straighten and free up the legs and then hold the patient's knees together.
7. Together, with the Attendant manually stabilizing the head and neck, the patient is gently lifted as a unit (multi-person lift) and moved to a level surface or directly onto the spine board or stretcher.
8. The Attendant completes the primary survey and initiates treatment for any life-threatening condition.
9. Continuous manual stabilization of the head and neck must be maintained until the patient can be properly immobilized. A hard cervical collar alone is not considered adequate spinal immobilization.

EXTRICATION FROM A VEHICLE FOR PATIENTS WITH SUSPECTED SPINAL INJURY

With the increasing frequency of vehicular accidents, the Attendant may be faced with the problem of extricating the patient from a vehicle. In certain instances, the scene assessment will reveal conditions that immediately endanger the patient and/or the Attendant (e.g. risk of explosion). Sometimes the Attendant identifies a life-threatening condition during the primary survey that cannot be treated adequately inside the vehicle (e.g. respiratory failure requiring assisted ventilation). In such cases, the Attendant must remove the patient from the vehicle and then initiate treatment. The following procedure outlines the steps to be followed to extricate a patient safely and rapidly from a vehicle:

1. The Attendant or assistant manually stabilizes the head and neck in the neutral position with the patient sitting upright. The primary survey is begun at the same time. A hard cervical collar may be applied at this point to minimize neck movement during the subsequent procedure.

2. If the scene assessment/primary survey reveals a life-threatening situation, the patient must be extricated quickly from the vehicle. It will require at least three and preferably four or five assistants for quick, safe action.

3. Slide the spine board onto the seat and slightly under the patient's buttocks and thighs. The patient may have to be lifted gently from the waist by another assistant working from the opposite side. The head and neck must be maintained in the neutral position at all times by one rescuer throughout the procedure.

4. With one rescuer lifting the knees and the waist from the opposite side, and another assistant holding the upper torso, the patient is lifted and rotated so that the patient's back is toward the spine board. The legs may have to be carefully manoeuvred to clear the gear shift.

5. One of the assistants keeps the head and neck in line with the body throughout this manoeuvre, then passes control to another assistant standing outside the door.

6. The patient is lowered to the spine board (supine or lateral position whichever is appropriate), then slid to the full length of the board as the legs are carefully straightened.

7. The patient is carried from the vehicle (to the ambulance if available) and treatment is continued.

8. In extremely dangerous situations (e.g. fire, rising water), the patient and Attendant may be exposed to very high risk. It may be necessary to extricate the patient as quickly as possible without following the above protocol.

Special Situation — Helmet Removal

Over the years, there has been a steady increase in the use of helmets for motorcycling and bicycling (in some cases, mandatory helmet laws apply). Furthermore, inju-ries from hockey or football may also result in spinal injury. The Attendant may be faced with a patient who is wearing a helmet. In order to perform a thorough assessment or provide airway stabilization and assisted ventilation, the helmet must be removed.

1. The patient's spine is realigned to the neutral position, and rotated to the anatomical position with the helmet on, following any of the procedures outlined above.

2. The head and neck should be maintained in the anatomical position by grasping the trapezius muscles on one side. The other hand is positioned on the patient's head, using the fingers to support the lower jaw.

3. The chin strap is undone or cut. It may be useful to remove the face shield. With football helmets, the face guard can be lifted out of the way by releasing the clips that hold it to the helmet.

4. The Attendant directs an assistant to place one hand on the lower jaw, the thumb on one side and the index and middle finger on the other side. The other hand is placed behind the patient's neck at the base of the skull. The Attendant directs the assistant to maintain the head and neck in the neutral position.

5. The Attendant then removes the helmet by remembering these tips:
    *   The helmet will have to be widened to clear the ears.
    *   If the patient is wearing glasses, they will have to be removed *before* the helmet.
    *   With full face helmets, the helmet must be tilted up to clear the face. Be careful not to hyperextend the neck.
    *   It is better to go slow and easy rather than force the helmet off.

6. Once the helmet has been removed, the Attendant completes the primary survey treating any life-threatening conditions while ensuring that continuous stabilization of the head and neck is maintained.

SPINAL IMMOBILIZATION

By now the Attendant should realize the difference between manual stabilization, spinal realignment and spinal immobilization. Once the spine has been realigned to the neutral position, it must be immobilized in that position. The principle is exactly the same as the treatment for a fracture dislocation of the extremity. Previously, the Attendant learned the basic procedures to realign the spine in patients with suspected spinal injuries. In this section, the technique of spinal immobilization will be reviewed.

The lumbar, sacral and coccygeal portions of the spine are adequately immobilized with the patient secured in the supine or lateral position on a firm surface such as stretcher or spine board. As long as these elements of the spine are maintained in a straight line and the patient is secured, no additional immobilization is required. The body's weight, together with the powerful muscles running up and down the spine, are sufficient to keep the vertebrae reasonably immobilized. Patients with only lower spine injuries do not require full immobilization of the neck unless the patient has signs or symptoms suggestive of cervical spine injury.

If the patient is unable to indicate whether an upper spinal injury exists, the Attendant must also immobilize the cervical spine. All patients with multiple injuries must also have their cervical spines immobilized.

The cervical and upper thoracic spine are much more mobile and therefore require additional immobilization. Even the patient resting quietly on the spine board may let the head fall to one side. This is sufficient to cause further injury in patients with unstable cervical or upper thoracic spinal fractures.

A number of devices have been developed to immobilize the neck. No one device, even the rigid hard collar, adequately immobilizes the spine. The traditional soft collar does not provide adequate support to prevent flexion, extension or rotation. Therefore, the soft collar is virtually useless if immobilization of the cervical spine is required. Even the hard collar *alone* is inadequate.

The only effective technique currently available for fully immobilizing the cervical spine is a hard collar applied to the neck, with the head immobilized to the spine board or stretcher with tape and supports (sand bags or blankets). The procedure is illustrated below. If proper first aid is to be applied to patients with suspected cervical or thoracic spine fractures, full immobilization is required in all cases. Half measures are totally inadequate, potentially dangerous and provide a false sense of security.

Examples of half measures include:

- patients with soft cervical collars applied and transported sitting in a chair;
- patients with hard cervical collars lying on a stretcher without tape or supports to prevent rotation;
- patients with suspected cervical spine fractures, wearing hard collars and asked to walk to the ambulance.

As discussed previously, it is impossible to differentiate at the scene between patients with simple strains of the neck and those with unstable fractures. Therefore, all cervical spine injuries must be treated as potential unstable fractures. By treating every suspected cervical spine injury as if the patient had a spinal cord injury, the Attendant will avoid any problems. There is no point in partially treating the patient. If a cervical or thoracic spine injury is suspected, the neck must be fully immobilized.

HARD COLLARS

A variety of rigid cervical collars are available for spinal immobilization. The hard collar is usually made of lightweight plastic or fibreglass and is fully padded. Unlike soft collars, they may come in a variety of adult sizes that vary by height. Therefore, the Attendant may have to carry all sizes in the first aid kit. Hard collars, when properly applied, do not cause airway obstruction and do not interfere with assisted ventilation.

There are a variety of commercially available hard cervical collars currently on the market. The Attendant should use the following general guidelines when selecting a particular brand for use at the work site:

- The collar must firmly support the weight of the head in the neutral position.
- It must independently provide and maintain adequate traction on the neck.
- It must independently limit lateral movement of the head and neck.
- It must limit rotational movement of the head and neck and limit flexion and extension of the neck (forward and backward motion).
- The collar must be relatively comfortable when applied.
- The collar must be translucent for x-ray examination.
- The cervical collar should fit readily into the first aid kit.

- The collar should be simple to apply, even for individuals who are not necessarily familiar with its use. It is not uncommon for Attendants to ask bystanders or co-workers to assist in the application of these collars.
- The cervical collar should be capable of easy cleaning, either in soap and hot water or with a disinfectant.
- The best choice is a cervical collar that fits as wide a range of neck sizes as possible, using the fewest collar sizes, in order to limit the quantity that would have to be carried in the first aid kit.
- The collar must be sufficiently flexible, even in the extremes of cold weather.
- The price should not be exorbitant, so that the Attendant could stock at least two in each major size category.

Sizing the Hard Collar for the Patient

Proper sizing of the hard collar is important for good first aid. Too short a collar does not provide enough support and may compromise the patient's airway. Too tall a collar may hyperextend the neck. The key dimension used for sizing is the distance between the top of the patient's shoulders and the bottom of the chin (see Figure VI-17).

- The Attendant uses the fingers to measure the shoulder-to-chin distance on the patient (see Figure VI-17).
- This distance is matched to the corresponding distance on the hard collar. In the example shown, this is the distance between the black fastener and the lower edge of the plastic portion of the collar (see Figure VI-18). The Attendant should choose the best match.

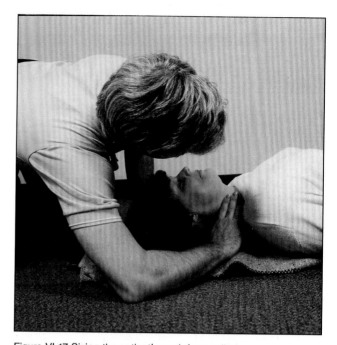

Figure VI-17 Sizing the patient's neck for a collar

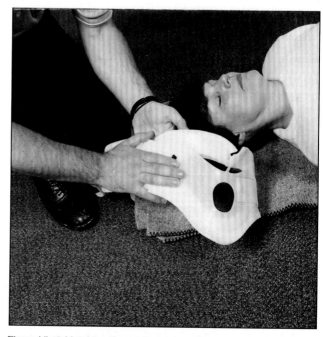

Figure VI-18 Matching the neck size to collar

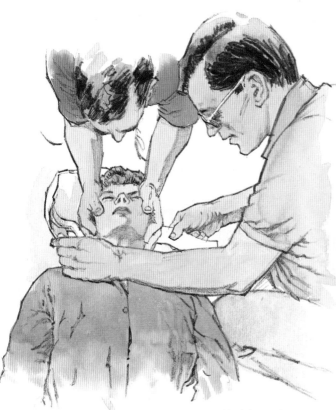

Figure VI-19 Slide the back portion behind the neck

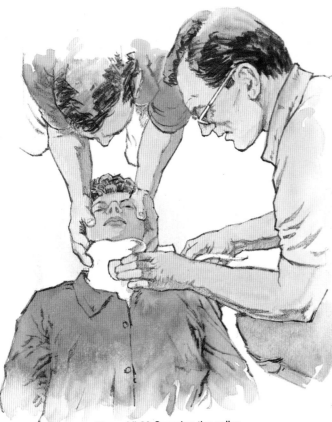

Figure VI-20 Securing the collar

Application of the Hard Cervical Collar

1. Once the correct collar size has been determined, the chin piece may have to be assembled. Hold the collar as shown. The chin piece is formed by sliding the black fastener up and into the small hole. Press firmly to snap it into place.
2. Hold the collar as shown. Flex inward to pre-form the collar to simplify its application.
3. Slide the back portion of the collar containing the Velcro® strap behind the patient's neck (see Figure VI-19).
4. Position the front of the collar underneath the patient's chin. Maintain the patient's head in the neutral position. The chin piece of the collar should rest snugly up against the patient's chin (see Figure VI-20). The lower portion of the collar should rest on the patient's breast bone.
5. Tighten the collar by gently pulling and attaching the Velcro® strap as shown in Figure VI-20.
6. The collar should be firmly tightened until adequate support is obtained. Care must be taken not to apply pressure anteriorly over the neck while tightening the collar.
7. To disassemble the collar, loosen the Velcro® strap and reverse the above procedures. The chin piece is disassembled by working the black fastener (not the white fastener) out of its hole.
8. *Once the patient has been immobilized, the collar should not be removed except by a physician.*
9. It may be difficult to apply the hard collar on a patient in the lateral position. If the patient cannot be rolled supine because of active bleeding in the mouth, the head and neck must be stabilized as best as possible using appropriate padding and secured to the spine board.

TECHNIQUES OF SPINAL IMMOBILIZATION

Once the patient's spine has been realigned to the neutral position and a hard cervical collar applied (if necessary), the patient's spine has to be immobilized. The following procedure outlines the steps to be followed to safely immobilize the spine:

1. The patient who is conscious and can cooperate should be instructed not to move the head, neck or back.

2. The legs should be tied together in extension with padding (e.g. blankets or jacket) inserted between them (only if the patient is not in the Rapid Transport Category).

3. The stretcher or spine board should be prepared. If transport to hospital is prolonged (more than one hour) or over very difficult terrain, extra care must be taken to ensure maximum patient comfort. The Attendant must remember that patients with spinal cord injury are especially prone to pressure sores.

   If a spine board is used for long transports, it must be padded with blankets or foam padding. Spine boards are extremely uncomfortable to lie on for any length of time. (The Attendant may wish to try lying on one.) By maximizing patient comfort, the patient is less likely to move or agitate, thereby reducing the risk of further injury.

   The Attendant should ensure that there are no hard objects such as keys, wallets, belts, etc. under the patient to cause discomfort or pressure sores. Therefore, the Attendant should "think ahead" when selecting the most appropriate spinal immobilization device.

4. The Attendant must decide whether the patient is to be immobilized supine or in the lateral position. Injured patients are more susceptible to motion sickness during transport, especially over difficult terrain. The patient who is strapped down to a spine board or stretcher that cannot be rapidly flipped, should the patient vomit, is at very high risk of aspiration. Once again, the Attendant must "think ahead" and consider the type of transportation that will be used to get the patient to hospital.

   Patients with a decreased level of consciousness who may vomit should be immobilized in the lateral position. (The Attendant must realize there is a difference between patient assessment, which is best performed supine, and transportation, where the lateral position is recommended.)

5. Use a "multi-person" lift or "clamshell" (Robertson scoop stretcher) to lift the patient onto the stretcher or long spine board.

6. The patient will have to be secured to the spine board or stretcher in order to prevent further movement. Velcro® straps, triangular bandages or long straps may be used. The advantage of the Velcro® straps or triangular bandages is that they may be applied and loosened rapidly. They also permit the spinal cord patient to be turned easily. The disadvantage of the long straps is that they can take a long time to apply and do not readily permit turning of the spinal cord injury patient. The ultimate choice is left to the judgment of the Attendant.

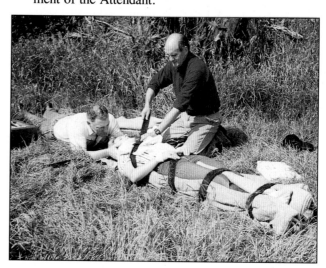

Securing the patient to the spine board

7. Once the patient has been secured on the stretcher or the spine board in the most appropriate position, the head and the neck are further immobilized by applying sand bags or rolled blankets on either side of the head (see Figure VI-21). A Velcro® strap (or strips of 2″ tape) is then applied across the patient's forehead and attached to the spine board. A dry gauze dressing may be used to prevent the tape from sticking to the patient's hair.

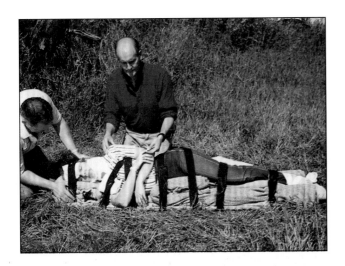

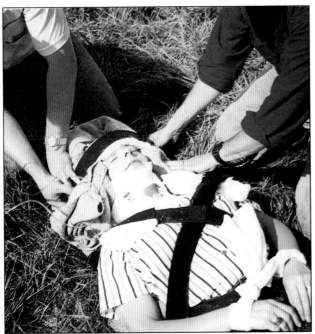

Figure VI-21 Top: head secured in the lateral position
Bottom: head secured in the supine position

8. Additional padding should be provided under all pressure points — the shoulder blades, sacrum and heels.

9. The arms may be kept free at the patient's side or, if the lateral position is used, one arm may be used to support the head.

10. The patient's vital signs and neurological status must be frequently reassessed (at least every ten minutes en route).

11. The patient must be kept warm. Cover the patient with blankets and keep the interior of the transport vehicle or ambulance warm. Spinal cord injury patients are at risk for hypothermia.

12. Patients with spinal cord injury must be turned slightly every two hours to prevent pressure sores. The patient is log-rolled slightly from the supine position to one side and supported with a few inches of padding. The next time the patient is rolled in the other direction to the opposite side and supported again with padding. The Attendant should massage the skin areas over the body's bony prominences after each rotation, such as shoulder blades, sacrum, heels and elbows.

SUMMARY

The best first aid for spinal injuries is to always think about spinal injury during patient assessment and treatment. By remembering the mechanisms of injury that are associated with spinal injury and then carefully looking for the signs and symptoms of spinal injury, the Attendant will minimize the risk of spinal cord injury. Once the Attendant has suspected or diagnosed a spinal injury, the correct techniques for spinal realignment and immobilization must be followed. The Attendant must take extra care to prevent the complications of spinal cord injury. By "thinking ahead", the Attendant will also avoid unnecessary movement of the patient and ensure maximum patient comfort and safety.

Part VII, Section A
Facial Injuries and Their Management

For a variety of reasons, the face is particularly prone to injury. Soft tissue injuries and fractures to the face are common. Facial injuries can be life threatening because of the possibility of precipitating airway obstruction. Furthermore, facial injuries can be very dramatic and may divert the Attendant's attention away from more serious injuries that are not as obvious.

ANATOMY AND FUNCTION

The key bones of the face are the mandible (lower jaw), the maxilla (upper jaw), the zygoma (cheek bone), the nasal bones and the bones of the orbits. The sinuses are small cavities contained within some of the facial bones. The sinuses drain into the nasal cavity. The most important organs of the face are the eyes, which are protected by the bones of the orbit. The skin and muscles of the face are richly supplied with blood vessels. This explains the profuse bleeding that usually occurs with open facial wounds.

ASSESSMENT AND TREATMENT OF FACIAL INJURIES
General Principles

The Attendant follows the Priority Action Approach beginning with the scene assessment and the primary survey. Several factors associated with facial injuries may cause airway obstruction:
- bleeding within the oral cavity or from the nose
- vomiting
- loose teeth or dentures
- fractures of the mandible and/or maxilla producing significant deformity of the airway
- swelling of the soft tissues, which encroaches on the airway
- direct injury to the anterior neck (i.e. voice box or trachea)
- brain injury causing coma

The Attendant's first priority is to clear the airway as described in Part IV, Section B, page 40.

Due to the mechanism of injury, facial injuries are often associated with cervical spine fractures. The Attendant must suspect a cervical spine injury in all patients with facial injuries. If the patient is conscious, a cervical spine injury may be ruled out if, and only if:
- the patient does not complain of any pain or stiffness of the neck; or

- there is no pain on palpation or movement of the neck. If the patient has a decreased level of consciousness, a cervical spine injury must be assumed and the patient's neck must be properly immobilized.

Facial injuries are also associated with brain injury. In conscious patients, the Attendant must determine if the patient suffered a loss of consciousness. ANY DECREASED LEVEL OF CONSCIOUSNESS OR "DAZING" FROM THE FORCE OF INJURY INDICATES A HEAD INJURY. THESE PATIENTS MUST BE REFERRED FOR MEDICAL EVALUATION. Obviously, any patient who is confused must also be referred.

After completion of the primary and secondary survey, the Attendant may have to initiate treatment. The following paragraphs outline the treatments required for specific facial injuries.

SOFT TISSUE FACIAL INJURIES

The treatment principles for soft tissue injuries of the face follow those outlined in First Aid Room Techniques (see Part IX, Section E, page 215). Bleeding is best controlled by direct pressure. Through-and-through lacerations involving the lip or cheek usually require pressure from both sides to control the bleeding. The Attendant must wear gloves before putting fingers into the patient's mouth.

Facial lacerations often require suture repair to ensure a good cosmetic result. The guidelines indicating which lacerations require physician referral are listed in First Aid Room Techniques (Part IX, Section E, page 215). Wounds that require suturing are not medical emergencies in themselves. As long as the patient is referred to a physician within six hours of injury, a good result is usually assured.

Avulsed skin should be retrieved from the accident site if possible. It should be cleansed and packaged exactly as an amputated part (see Part IX, Section D, page 210).

Flap-type soft tissue injuries should be repositioned, cleansed and bandaged in position. If the flap is left in its twisted or kinked position and then bandaged, the blood supply to the flap may be cut off. The flap may be permanently damaged and any subsequent attempt at repairing the laceration will fail, leaving the patient with a permanent disfigurement.

Dental injuries are discussed in Section D, page 175.

Laceration of the tongue may be difficult to control with pressure. The Attendant must ensure proper drainage to prevent the development of airway problems. Ice cubes or chips (if available) may be useful to control bleeding.

Nosebleeds usually result from blunt trauma and may be associated with nasal fractures. The patient should be maintained upright with the head forward or in the lateral position to prevent blood from draining into the back of the throat and compromising the airway. Patients with nosebleeds associated with suspected cervical spine injury must be treated with cervical spine immobilization in the lateral position. Bleeding is best controlled by direct pressure (i.e. pinching the nostrils together) and ice packs applied to the bridge of the nose. The Attendant should avoid placing any gauze or tissue into the nostrils.

FACIAL FRACTURES

Fractures of the facial bones usually involve the nose, the orbit, the cheek bone (zygoma), the maxilla (upper jaw) or the mandible (lower jaw). Clues to the presence of fracture are swelling, deformity and bleeding. Fractures of the maxilla or mandible may be suspected by irregularities of the patient's bite or the inability to open the mouth fully.

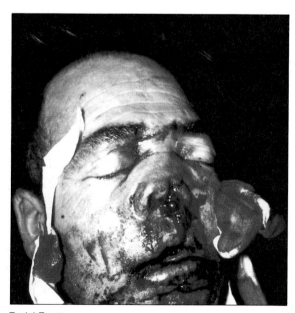

Facial Fractures

In all such injuries, especially those involving the maxilla and/or the mandible, the airway must be carefully assessed and cleared. These patients are at *continuous* risk of developing airway obstruction because of ongoing bleeding or swelling. All patients with suspected facial fractures must be assessed for the possibility of brain and/or cervical spine injury.

Fractures of the Nose

Nasal fractures by themselves are not medical emergencies. In the presence of significant swelling, it is often difficult to assess the degree of deformity. These fractures may not be "straightened" by the physician for four to seven days after injury, until the swelling has subsided. Unless there are other associated injuries or ongoing bleeding, these patients may be referred the following day to their physician.

Fractures of the Maxilla or Mandible

The Attendant must ensure that the airway remains patent. These patients are best managed in the lateral position. The Attendant should avoid supporting or wrapping the jaw with padding because the patient's airway may become blocked. The mouth must be kept open to ensure drainage of blood or vomitus.

Fractures of the Orbit or Cheek Bone (Zygoma)

These fractures are often associated with eye injuries as well as brain or cervical spine injuries. The treatment of eye injuries is discussed in Section C on page 167. Swelling is best controlled with ice packs. Bleeding is controlled with direct pressure, although the Attendant must be careful not to apply pressure to the eyeball. The Attendant should refer these patients for assessment by a physician.

INJURIES TO THE THROAT AND ANTERIOR NECK

Located in this region are the upper airway structures — the larynx (voice box) and trachea, as well as the carotid artery supplying the brain. Therefore, both open and blunt injuries to this region are potentially life threatening. Open wounds of the neck, no matter how innocent they appear, are in the Rapid Transport Category. Examples of blunt injuries are direct impact from steering wheels in MVA's, clothesline-type injuries sustained while riding a bicycle or running, and suicide attempts from hanging.

The immediate priority is stabilization of the airway. Clues to the existence of airway problems are the presence of swelling, hoarseness, stridor or subcutaneous emphysema. A cervical spine injury must be suspected in all these injuries and appropriately immobilized.

The patient should be managed in the position of maximum comfort. If a cervical spine injury is suspected, the patient is best managed supine or in the lateral position. Supplemental high-flow oxygen must be supplied to all of these patients.

Bleeding may be controlled with direct pressure although care must be taken not to compress the airway (located in the midline) and not to apply a circumferential dressing around the neck. Open wounds must not be probed as it may worsen the degree of injury. The remainder of the primary survey is completed and the patient is rapidly transported to hospital.

This is one of the few cases where a hard cervical collar should not be used to stabilize a suspected cervical spine injury. The collar will interfere with the continuous monitoring of the patient's injury and does not allow for swelling. The cervical spine must still be manually immobilized by the Attendant with the assistance of sandbags or padding. The patient must be firmly secured to the spine board.

SUMMARY

Facial injuries are very common and potentially life threatening. By following the basic principles of the Priority Action Approach and general treatment principles for soft tissue injuries, the Attendant will be able to provide optimal care to these patients. Early recognition and effective treatment of airway problems are life saving. Appropriate treatment of soft tissue injuries at the scene will minimize any permanent scarring or disfigurement.

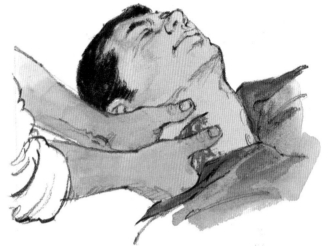

Direct pressure proximal and distal to the wound

Part VII, Section B
The Eye Anatomy and Function

The eye is an organ adapted for vision. It has many intricate parts, all of which are important for its proper function.

The eyeball is globe-shaped and about 2.5cm in diameter. The shape is maintained by the fluid contained in it. The fluid is a clear, jelly-like substance called the vitreous humor.

The anterior wall of the globe is a clear, transparent window through which light enters the eye. It is called the cornea. The sclera (white part of the eye) is a tough tissue making up the outer wall of the rest of the globe. The sclera is covered by a layer of clear membrane called conjunctiva. This membrane also covers the inside of the eyelids. When the eyelids move, the two smooth conjunctival surfaces slide over one another.

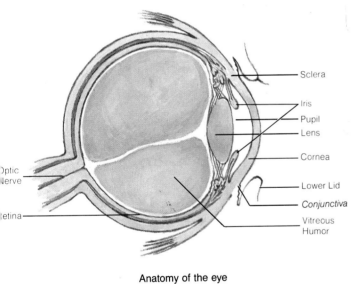

Anatomy of the eye

The coloured portion of the eye, the iris, is an adjustable circular muscle behind the cornea. It has an opening, like that of a camera, which regulates the amount of light entering the eye. The opening in the iris is the pupil. Behind the iris is a lens that focuses an image on the light-sensitive layer, the retina. The retina is a layer of cells at the back of the eye, which changes the light image into electrical impulses. These are carried by the optic nerve to the brain. The pressure of the vitreous humor supports the retina.

The lacrimal system is composed of lacrimal (tear) glands and ducts. Tears produced by the lacrimal glands protect, clean and lubricate the eye.

The tear glands are located beneath the upper eyelid. The tear ducts are on the inner side of the eye, along the lower lid.

Upper and lower eyelids protect the eyes. The smooth conjunctival lining of the eyelids is kept moistened by tears. The upper eyelids glide up and down over the eye to protect it from dust and other irritants. The eyelids are closed by the contraction of a circular muscle around the eye.

The pupil of the eye constricts or dilates as it adjusts to various degrees of light. The pupil also adjusts when viewing close or distant objects. Pupil adjustment is automatic and almost instantaneous.

Normally, when a light is directed into the eyes, the pupils constrict (become smaller). When in darkness, as the eye is shaded or the lids closed, the pupils dilate (become larger). The size of the pupils and any difference in size between the two pupils and their reaction to light are important signs which may help determine the nature and severity of a head injury.

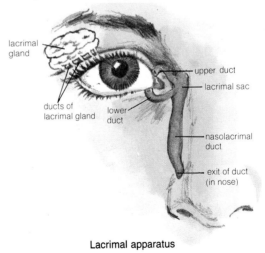

Lacrimal apparatus

Part VII, Section C
Eye Injuries and Their Management

A relatively minor eye injury can cause very serious, lasting consequences if it is not treated promptly and correctly. Proper initial care of an eye injury not only relieves pain but can also help prevent permanent loss of sight.

TYPES OF EYE INJURIES

Eye injuries include:

1. Foreign bodies
2. Blows from sharp or blunt objects
3. Burns (chemical, thermal or radiation)

GENERAL PRINCIPLES OF EYE EXAMINATION FOLLOWING INJURY

A. **Obtain Information Concerning the Accident**
   1. Time and location
   2. Details of injury — blow, foreign material, sharp object
   3. Nature of foreign material — acid, alkali, steel, glass, fume, etc.

B. **Measurement of Vision**
   1. Vision should be assessed prior to the initiation of treatment except in the case of:
      - chemical burns
      - penetrating injury
      IN THESE CASES, EMERGENCY TREATMENT TAKES PRIORITY.
   2. Techniques for assessing vision:
      - Can the patient see light?
      - Can the patient count fingers?
      - Ask the patient to read.

C. **Examination — General Approach**
   1. The Attendant's hands should be washed thoroughly.
   2. Attendant should be in front of and slightly above patient.
   3. The examining room should be as bright as possible. Patients with eye injuries are often very light-sensitive and a better examination may be obtained with room light rather than with a direct penlight beam.
   4. The patient should be comfortable, seated or lying down, with the head well back and firmly supported.
   5. Use great care and gentleness.

6. The hand holding any instrument used in treating the eye must rest steady on the patient's cheek or forehead.

D. **Procedure**
   1. Stabilize the hand on the patient's face.
   2. Gently place thumb on lower lid margin.
   3. Have patient look up to expose the lower conjunctiva of the eye and the inside of the lower lid.
   4. Shift thumb to upper lid margin.
   5. With the eyelids well separated, have the patient move the eyes slowly to the left and right, then up and down. The Attendant must carefully inspect the inner and outer canthus (corners) and the folds of the conjunctiva of the lower lid. This is where many foreign bodies will be carried by gravity. A foreign body may lodge itself under the upper lid and be missed quite easily unless the upper lid is everted.
   6. Look for any sign of scleral injury, inflammation, hemorrhage or congestion of conjunctival tissue and for any foreign body. The underside of the top lid must be everted for examination.

E. **Examination of Underside of Top Lid (Everting Lid)**
   NOTE: DO NOT EVERT LID IF PENETRATING INJURY IS SUSPECTED.
   Procedure
   1. Hold the top lashes firmly between the thumb and first finger.
   2. Instruct the patient to look down.
   3. Place a cotton-tipped applicator against the outside of lid, about halfway down (see Figure VII-1).
   4. Pull the lid out and up over the applicator.

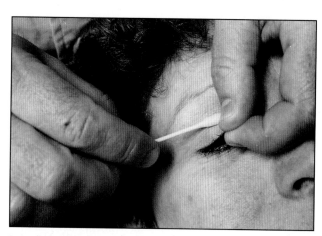

Figure VII-1 Everting the eyelid

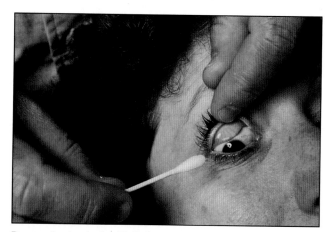

Remove foreign body with Q-tip

F. **Examination of Cornea**

1. Because of the extreme sensitivity of the cornea, the examination may be difficult without the use of a local anesthetic (see page 173).

2. With the patient looking straight ahead, shine the penlight at the cornea from an angle. The eye is examined best with the light source shining across it, so that a foreign body or lesion can be easily seen when it casts a shadow. The position of the foreign body can be described by the clock method (see Figure VII-2).

3. Move the penlight to the left and right and then up and down.

4. Look for any dark spots or irregularities on the clear corneal surface as the light moves. (Room lights may need to be dimmed.)

5. Look for any clouding of the cornea; normally it is clear.

G. **Examination of the Anterior Chamber**

The anterior chamber is the space immediately underlying the cornea but in front of the iris.

Using a penlight, examine the anterior chamber and iris.

1. Anterior chamber — look for any blood or foreign body. Blood may be seen best in the seated patient.

2. Iris — look for any irregularity or a tear in the iris.

H. **Examination of the Pupil**

1. Pupil size — are pupils equal in size? Check this in dim light.

2. Pupil shape — is it round (normal) or irregular?

3. Pupillary response to light (light reflex) — with penlight and in a dimly lit room, examine for inequality of pupil size and the pupils' response to bright light.

    •   Shine the light into each eye and watch for rapid pupillary constriction in the same eye.

    •   Repeat the procedure and watch for rapid constriction in the opposite eye. Slow or absent constriction is abnormal. These patients must be referred to a physician for further assessment.

I. **Examination of Eye Movements**

1. Have the patient watch an object or a light as the Attendant moves it in all directions of gaze, i.e. to the right, left, up and down, following an "H" pattern.

    The Attendant looks for:

    •   failure of either eye to follow the object or light

    •   any pain reported by the patient

    •   double vision

2. Eye position — is one eye more protruding or sunken than the other?

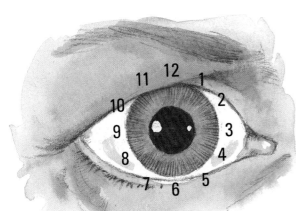

Figure VII-2 Clock method of reporting foreign body location

FOREIGN BODIES

Foreign bodies in the eye may be divided into two groups:

Superficial: These are objects such as eyelashes, welding slag and dirt particles. Some are easily removed and some may be stuck to the eye surface or the underside of the lids — most commonly the upper.

Penetrating: These are usually small high-velocity foreign bodies. They are sharp enough or have enough velocity to penetrate the outer eye. All are serious.

Management of Foreign Bodies

Most foreign bodies in the eye are easily removed without any complications.

- Tell the patient not to rub the eye.
- Obtain history. Suspect a penetrating injury with hammering, grinding, chiselling or explosions.
- Examine the eye as previously described.

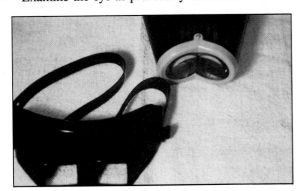

Sample magnification devices

Removal of Superficial Foreign Bodies

These techniques can be effective for foreign bodies that are non-adherent, or those that are adherent to the conjunctiva or to the underside of the upper lid.

1. Wipe away any loose foreign material from facial area.
2. If a foreign body is present but loose, use an eye cup filled with clean water or saline. The patient bends forward and makes a seal with the rim of the eye cup and the eye socket, then tips the head back and blinks several times. The head is then tipped forward with the eye open and the eye cup removed. This can be repeated several times. A clean cupped hand and clean tap water can be used in an emergency.
3. Some non-sharp foreign bodies can be dislodged by manipulating the eyelid; for example, a foreign body under the upper eyelid. The foreign body can be dislodged by holding the upper eyelashes and gently pulling the eyelid down over the lower lid. The eyelashes from the lower eyelid will brush the inside of the upper eyelid. Do not do this more than twice.
4. Conjunctival foreign bodies can be removed without anesthetic, if done gently.

If tolerated, more adherent conjunctival foreign bodies can be removed with a moist cotton-tip applicator. NEVER USE THIS TECHNIQUE FOR CORNEAL FOREIGN BODIES.

Only one attempt should be made to remove a conjunctival foreign body by this method.

Place the tip of the moistened applicator gently on the foreign body. Give the applicator a very gentle slight twist or short wipe to pick up the foreign body.

Removal of Corneal Foreign Bodies

The cornea is very sensitive. Removal of foreign bodies from the cornea can usually not be done without local anesthetic and must be referred to a physician.

A rust ring may develop on the cornea. This occurs when any foreign body containing iron has not been removed for several hours. Once the foreign body is removed, a small round ring remains. This should be removed by a physician.

If either a superficial foreign body or a corneal foreign body cannot be removed by the above methods, patch the eye and assist the patient to medical aid. Because depth perception is impaired with one eye patched, these patients should not be allowed to drive a motor vehicle.

After the successful removal of a foreign body, the patient may still complain of a foreign-body sensation. This usually indicates a corneal abrasion. Patch the eye and refer to a physician.

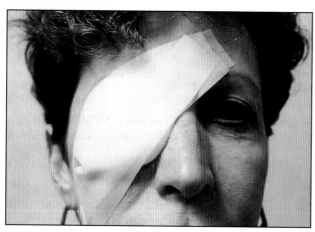

Example of eye patch

PENETRATING FOREIGN BODY

Penetrating wounds of the eye are very serious. A metallic projectile may penetrate the eyeball causing little or no pain. The wound may not be noticed on routine examination. IF THE HISTORY SUGGESTS A PENE-TRATING EYE INJURY, MEDICAL ATTENTION IS URGENTLY REQUIRED. NO ATTEMPT SHOULD BE MADE TO WASH OUT THE EYE OR TO APPLY LOCAL ANESTHETICS. Foreign bodies may impale or protrude from the eye or eyelid. They should be removed only by a physician.

Treatment for Penetrating Eye Injuries

- Both eyes must be covered with sterile dressings and the patient should be transported lying down with the head sandbagged.
- If the injury makes it impossible to close the eye, a moistened dressing should be used.
- It is important to patch both eyes so the eyes will not move about, which could cause further damage.
- Dress the area with sterile gauze to support the object.
- Use ring pads or a disposable drinking cup to cover the object and tape it firmly in place.
- The uninjured eye should be covered with a dressing.

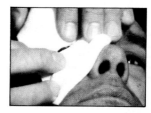
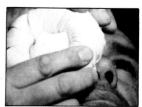
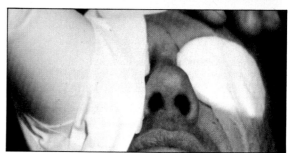

Paper cup or ring pad used for stabilization

- After initial stabilization, the patient is upgraded to the Rapid Transport Category.
- If the patient has a recognized life-threatening condition which places the patient in the Rapid Transport Category, minimal time should be spent securing the object prior to packaging.

LACERATIONS AND CONTUSIONS

Eyelid lacerations usually bleed profusely because the eyelids have a rich blood supply. If the eyeball itself is not involved, the bleeding can be controlled by direct pressure. If the eyeball is lacerated, do not apply pressure to the eye as this could force fluid out of the eyeball. The patient must be transported face up on a stretcher with the head and neck well secured to prevent movement. Dress the eyes loosely and apply ring pads or a disposable cup and then bandage lightly.

EYELID INJURY

If the eyeball itself is not lacerated, the torn eyelid may be flushed to remove dirt. Flushing solution should be restricted to saline or water. An attempt should then be made to re-align the eyelid tissue so as to achieve coverage of the eyeball, especially the cornea. This will prevent further injury to the cornea, either from drying out or from friction of the dressings.

Then apply a moist gauze dressing.

Be sure to send any avulsed (detached) tissue, also wrapped in moist gauze, to the hospital with the patient.

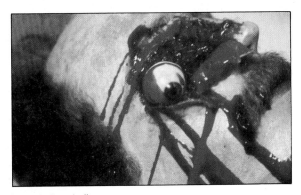

Extruded eyeball

EXTRUDED EYEBALL

An eye that has been torn from its socket must never be pushed back into place. These injuries should be treated as for penetrating foreign bodies except that the dressing should be moistened with sterile saline. The injured eye must be protected from any pressure by use of a ring pad or a paper cup and bandaged lightly (see Figure VII-3).

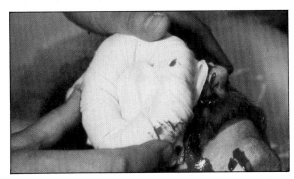

Figure VII-3 Application of ring pad

CONTUSIONS

Blunt trauma to the eye can result in:
1. superficial bleeding (conjunctival hemorrhage)
2. bleeding within the eyeball (hyphema)

1. Conjunctival Hemorrhage

This injury is actually a bruise of the transparent conjunctiva or underlying sclera. It is seen as a very obvious, bright red colour overlying the white part of the eye (sclera). These are commonly seen but are not serious unless associated with a laceration or penetrating injury to the eyeball. Conjunctival hemorrhage requires no treatment and generally resolves spontaneously within a few days.

2. Hyphema

Blood may be seen overlying the iris or pupil. During transport to the hospital, the patient must be:
- kept still with both eyes covered, and
- in the sitting position (other injuries permitting)

The patient should be in the sitting position to allow the blood to collect in the bottom of the eye.

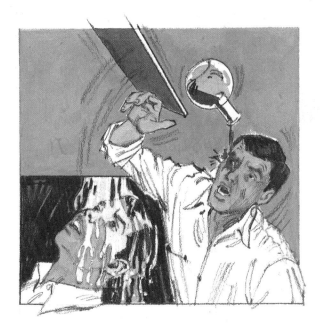

Chemical spill to eye

CHEMICAL INJURIES

Severity of damage varies with:
- properties of the chemical
- concentration of chemical
- the duration of exposure

Damage from Alkalis

Strong alkalis produce the worst injuries due to rapid penetration into tissue cells. Spreading cell death can be reduced by immediate dilution of alkali in the eye. An eye can look normal for several hours after a blinding alkali burn.

Common alkalis are: caustic soda (e.g. sodium hydroxide), lye, drain cleaners, cleaning agents, ammonia, cement and plaster.

Damage from Acids

Acids cause a more visible immediate damage, but penetrate less deeply. They are more easily washed out. If washed out immediately, serious injury can be reduced.

Common acids are: sulphuric (battery) acid, hydrochloric acid, nitric acid and acetic acid.

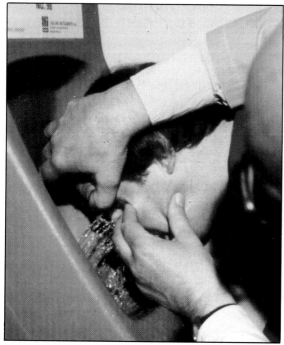

Flushing the eyes

Management of Chemical Burns

1. Where chemical burns are possible, an eye wash station should be immediately available. Personnel at risk should be taught the fastest method of washing a contaminated eye.
2. Effective irrigation should start immediately. Eyes should be irrigated for 30 minutes by the clock. Use running tap water or preferably normal saline to continually flush the eye. Remaining particles of cement or lime should be removed from behind the eyelids with a moist applicator.
3. Transport all patients to hospital with cold wet dressings on eyes and other affected areas for comfort.
4. Eyes burned by strong alkalis or acids should be flushed continually in transit if possible. If available, use sterile normal saline from an IV bottle or bag. The IV tubing can be held at the inner corner of the eye. Saline is allowed to run across the eye and out of the outer corner. If saline is not available, tap water will suffice.

Chemical neutralizing agents or solutions are not practical and may cause more damage. Water is readily available and is much more suitable for eye irrigation.

THERMAL BURNS

With exposure to heat, the eyelids rapidly close, usually protecting the eyes from damage. However, the eyelids are frequently burned. The treatment of burned eyelids requires specialized medical care. The patient should be treated as any burn victim, using the Priority Action Approach. (See Part III, page 20.) Injury management requires that the eyes be covered with sterile dressings. Do not examine the eye as this may injure the burned tissue. THE USE OF HOME REMEDIES OR BURN OINTMENTS IS CONTRAINDICATED.

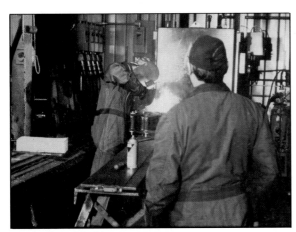
Mechanism of flashburn

ULTRAVIOLET INJURIES (FLASHBURNS)

Direct or reflected ultraviolet light from an electric arc or welding torch may cause a surface burn. Corneal burns become more painful after some hours. Although flashburns are very uncomfortable, they are not serious and usually heal in 12 to 24 hours.

Management

1. Examine the patient to rule out any foreign bodies.
2. Cold compresses and mild pain medications (ASA or acetaminophen) may help the patient to sleep at night.
3. A patient with severe ultraviolet burns may be unable to return to work for 1-2 days.
4. Dark glasses may be required for a couple of days due to photosensitivity (light sensitivity).

USE AND ABUSE OF LOCAL ANESTHETICS

The use of local anesthetic by the attendant in some circumstances will facilitate proper eye examination (e.g. simple corneal foreign bodies and ultraviolet flashburns). ANESTHETICS MAY BE ONLY USED ONCE, AND ARE NOT TO BE REPEATED UNLESS ADVISED BY A PHYSICIAN.

Anesthetics (e.g. amethacaine drops) are best supplied in droplet form from individual use dispensers. Do not use local anesthetic ointments.

CAUTION: THESE MEDICATIONS SHOULD NEVER BE GIVEN TO PATIENTS FOR SELF-ADMINISTRATION. They provide instant relief but can also cause problems.

- They delay healing.
- The anesthetized eye is subject to further injury due to the loss of normal protective reflexes; e.g. a foreign body would not be felt and could cause further damage without being noticed by the patient.
- The worker must not return to his job or drive a vehicle for at least one hour following the application of a local anesthetic. By this time, eye sensitivity will have returned.

EMERGENCY PROCEDURES FOR CONTACT LENS REMOVAL

Importance of Contact Lens Removal

A contact lens left on the eye for a long time may produce damage to the cornea. Contact lenses are to be removed from a patient's eyes if this will not cause further injury.

If a patient is known to be wearing contact lenses and they have not been removed, place adhesive tape marked "contact lenses" on the patient's forehead.

TYPES OF CONTACT LENSES

1. Hard — plastic discs 8-10 mm in diameter, non-flexible, may be coloured.
2. Soft — plastic discs 12-15 mm in diameter, flexible, rarely coloured.

REMOVAL OF CONTACT LENSES

1. Patient is Conscious
   - Ask if he/she is wearing contact lenses and, if so, what type.
   - Have the patient remove the lenses, if possible.
   - If patient cannot remove the lenses, the Attendant should remove them.

2. Patient is Comatose
   - Check for contact lens ID card, medic alert bracelet or necklace. Check for driver's license restrictions.
   - Check for contact lenses by gently separating the patient's eyelids. Shine a penlight onto the eye from the side. The front edge of the lens should reflect the beam and the far edge should cast a shadow.
   - If the lens is the same size or larger than the coloured part of the eye, it is probably a soft lens. If it is smaller than the coloured part, it is probably a hard lens.

Hard Lens Removal

1. With clean hands, gently separate the lids so they are clear of the bottom and top of the lens.
2. Move the lids together close to the edge of the contact lens, pressing slightly harder on the lower lid while sliding it upward.
3. When the lens pops over the lower lid, move the lids further together so that it slides out between the lids.

Soft Lens Removal

1. With clean hands, gently separate the lids. Pull the lower lid down with the second finger. Place the index finger on the lower edge of the lens. Slide the lens down onto the white part of the eye. If the lens does not move easily, flush the eye with normal saline and repeat the procedure. Do not remove the lens while it is over the coloured part of the eye (iris).
2. When the lens is pulled down, pinch it lightly between the thumb and index finger and remove it from the eye.
3. Store the lenses in water in separate containers, marked left and right.

Part VII, Section D
Dental Injuries

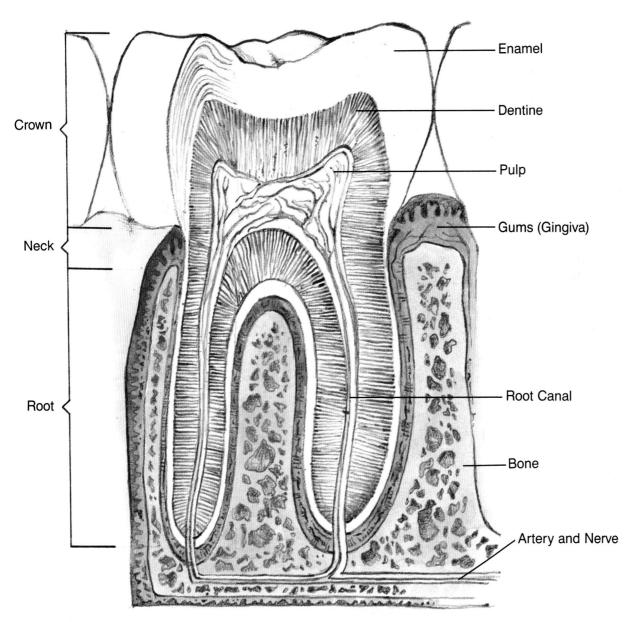

Cross section of tooth

Labels: Enamel, Dentine, Pulp, Gums (Gingiva), Root Canal, Bone, Artery and Nerve, Crown, Neck, Root

Dental injuries can occur in a variety of ways. Sometimes they are an isolated injury or they may occur in association with other injuries, such as a jaw fracture. Often, bleeding may obscure an underlying dental injury. Look or gently feel in the victim's mouth, when practical. Dental appliances may also be involved such as bridges, crowns or dentures. These may also be fractured, possibly adding to the soft tissue injury.

LOSS OF A TOOTH (AVULSION)

Stop bleeding from the gums with local pressure. When possible, locate the missing tooth at the accident scene. Wash the tooth gently in cold saline or water. Do not rub excessively. Place tooth in sterile cold saline, and place on ice or in refrigerator. Be sure to send the tooth with the patient when he/she is evacuated. Avulsed teeth can often be reimplanted. Ideally, this should be done within a half-hour. After 24 hours, the success rate is poor.

If the patient is conscious and considerable time may pass before a dentist is available, the Attendant may try to implant the tooth. After cleaning, gently but firmly reinsert the tooth into its socket. The patient may stabilize it with very light pressure on a piece of gauze placed between the jaws. Instruct the patient not to bite down hard on it until a dentist has been consulted.

LOOSE TOOTH

If a tooth is loose, but not actually displaced, refer the patient to a dentist.

If the tooth is loosened, and displaced more than 2 mm, gently push it back to its normal position. Refer the patient to a dentist.

CROWNS, BRIDGES, PLATES, ETC.

Where a fractured appliance remains in the mouth following injury, gently remove it to prevent further injury. Do not use force. Again, refer the patient to a dentist.

TOOTH FRACTURES

These may be very painful, and require early referral to a dentist for pain relief.

Part VII, Section E
Ear Injuries

THE EAR

The ear is a commonly injured sensory organ, often associated with serious head injuries. Correct management of ear injuries in the early stages can prevent both long-term hearing impairment and unacceptable cosmetic consequences.

ANATOMY OF THE EAR

The ear can be divided into three distinct anatomical parts:
1. the external ear
2. the middle ear
3. the inner ear

1. **The External Ear**
    The purpose of the external ear is to trap sound waves and direct them down the ear canal to the eardrum (tympanic membrane).
2. **The Middle Ear**
    The middle ear is a small air-filled cavity behind the eardrum, which connects the external ear to the nerve centre in the inner ear. It does so by the means of three tiny bones called ossicles.
3. **The Inner Ear**
    The inner ear is composed of two parts:
    *   the cochlea — responsible for interpretation of sound
    *   the vestibular apparatus — responsible for balance

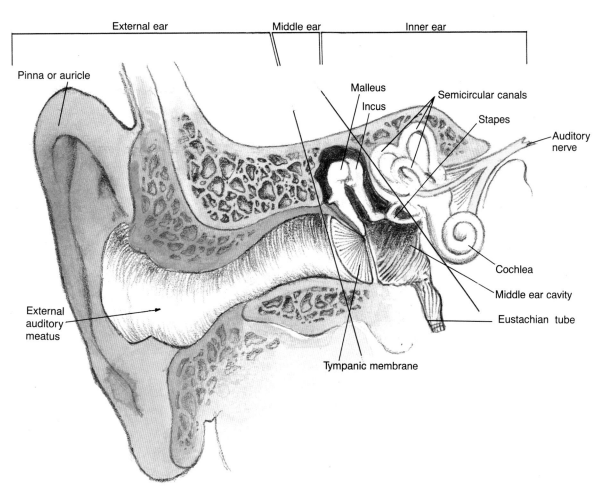

Anatomy of the Ear

EXTERNAL EAR

Foreign Bodies

It is imperative to have full cooperation from the patient with a foreign body in the ear. There is a high probability that the Attendant may cause significant injury to the eardrum and underlying structures if the patient is struggling.

Objects such as insects, dirt, sawdust and slag can usually be removed by flushing with warm water or mineral oil. Larger objects such as pebbles, etc. are best removed by a physician. If there is any bleeding or severe pain in association with a foreign body in the ear, the correct treatment involves only covering the ear with a sterile dressing and referring the patient to a physician.

Where there is an associated burn to the ear canal or to the eardrum (such as with hot slag), the patient must be referred to a physician.

Lacerations/Avulsions

Control bleeding by direct pressure. Position the ear as close as possible to its normal anatomical position, being careful to check for any tissue loss. Place sterile gauze bandage both behind and over the ear (see First Aid Room Techniques, Part IX, Section E, page 215). Retrieve any avulsed parts, gently clean (do not rub!), pack in moist gauze (not wet!) and send with patient to a physician as outlined in Part IX, Section D, page 210.

Hematoma

Significant bruising or hematoma formation of the external ear can produce permanent disfigurement (e.g. cauliflower ear). Use intermittent ice packs locally to minimize further swelling and bruising, and refer to a physician for further management.

Infection

If infection occurs following either blunt trauma or a laceration to the ear, the likelihood of permanent disfigurement is much greater! Again, the Attendant should refer to a physician.

Ear Injuries Associated with Skull Fractures

Fractures of the skull that extend into the ear canal (basilar skull fractures) are always potentially dangerous, because of the risk of introducing infection into the middle or inner ear, or even into the brain. Therefore, any handling or cleansing of this region should be restricted to removal of gross dirt or blood clots. Ensure that no fluid is allowed to enter the ear canal.

Any clear fluid seen dripping from the ear following blunt head injury represents cerebrospinal fluid (CSF leak). This is indicative of a serious basilar skull fracture — serious because of the risk of meningitis. In the absence of direct ear trauma, blood coming from the ear canal may also represent a basilar skull fracture. These patients should have a sterile dressing applied to the ear and be transported immediately to hospital. (See Head Injuries, Part VI, Section C, page 132.)

MIDDLE EAR
Middle Ear Injuries

Perforation of the eardrum often occurs with either blast, decompression or penetrating injuries to the ear, or in association with head injuries. Depending on the nature and severity of the injury, the deeper structures can also be damaged to varying degrees, sometimes resulting in permanent hearing impairment and/or dizziness.

Middle Ear Infections

Pain in the ear with hearing impairment at the time of an upper respiratory infection are the main symptoms of middle ear infection (otitis media). Refer to a physician.

INNER EAR

It is most commonly damaged by loud noises. Damage can occur with brief exposure to very loud sounds or with chronic exposure to lesser amounts. This is called "noise deafness". Blunt trauma to the head may result in disturbance of the balance mechanism, which will cause dizziness and sometimes vomiting. Injury suggesting middle or inner ear injury should also be referred to a physician.

Part VIII, Section A
Abdominal Organs Anatomy and Function

ABDOMINAL CAVITY

The two major cavities in the body are the thoracic cavity and the abdominal cavity. The abdomen is inferior to the thorax.

The abdominal cavity is bound above by the diaphragm and below by the pelvic region. The pelvic region is contained within the bones of the pelvis.

The abdominal cavity contains most of the digestive organs, the liver, spleen and the female reproductive organs. The pancreas, kidneys, bladder, parts of the large intestines and the major blood vessels are all located posterior to the abdominal cavity behind the peritoneum (see below). These organs are embedded in the soft tissue of the back, flank and pelvis, respectively. The liver, spleen and pancreas are considered solid organs, whereas the stomach, intestines, gallbladder, ureters and urinary bladder are hollow organs.

The abdominal cavity is lined by a smooth, glistening membrane called the peritoneum. The peritoneum has two layers, similar to the pleura that lines the thorax. One layer lines the wall of the cavity and another layer covers the organs.

DIGESTIVE SYSTEM

All food must be in a suitable form before it can pass through the wall of the bowel and actually "enter" the body. The different chemical changes by which food is made usable are the processes of digestion. Once the food is digested, it is transferred to the bloodstream by absorption. Digestion and absorption are the two main functions of the digestive system.

The digestive tract begins at the mouth. It is a long tube, coiled in the abdomen and terminating at the anus, where the solid waste products of digestion are expelled from the body. Beginning at the mouth, the tract consists of the pharynx, esophagus, stomach, small intestine and large intestine. The liver and pancreas are also involved in the process of digestion.

The breakdown of food begins in the mouth, where it is chewed by the combined action of the tongue and teeth. Salivary glands deliver their secretions (saliva) to the mouth, to help chewing and swallowing.

Swallowed food passes down the esophagus into the stomach. The stomach mixes and churns the food with the gastric juices. The food is moved into and through the small intestine by muscular contractions (peristalsis).

Absorption takes place in the small intestine. When the food enters the small intestine, additional digestive juices are supplied by the liver, pancreas and intestinal glands. These convert the food into basic sugars, fatty acids, proteins, water and salt.

The basic food products are transported in the blood to the liver where they are changed to substances that nourish individual tissues and cells. These substances are then transported in the blood through the circulatory system to all body cells.

Once the processes of digestion and absorption have been completed, the remaining substances are expelled. The large intestine contains layers of involuntary muscle, which move the solid waste products, called fecal matter, toward the rectum. Absorption of water also takes place through the walls of the large intestine.

SOLID ORGANS OF THE ABDOMEN AND THEIR FUNCTIONS

Liver

Liver functions include:
* Production of bile;
* Detoxification of poisons as well as the breakdown and elimination of many drugs;
* Storage of proteins, fats, minerals and vitamins;
* Storage and secretion of the simple sugar, glucose;
* Production of many body proteins and clotting factors.

Pancreas

Pancreatic functions include:
* Manufacture and release into the blood stream of insulin, which regulates the amount of sugar "burned" in the tissues;
* Production of pancreatic juice, which aids digestion.

Spleen

The spleen, although not associated with a digestive system, is in the abdominal cavity. It has functions related to the circulatory and lymphatic systems, including:
* Destruction of old red blood cells;
* Manufacture of some white cells;
* Removal of potentially infectious matter from the blood.

Kidneys

The three main functions of the kidneys are:
- To extract wastes from the blood;
- To aid in the maintenance of water balance;
- To aid in regulating the acid-base balance of the body.

HOLLOW ORGANS OF THE ABDOMEN AND THEIR FUNCTIONS

Stomach

The main function of the stomach is to convert food into a semi-solid mass by means of muscular movements and gastric juices.

Small Intestine

The main function is the absorption of nutrients.

Large Intestine

The main function is the absorption of water and excretion of waste products.

Gallbladder

The main function is to concentrate and store bile, which is used in the digestion of fats.

Ureters

Ureters are two tubes that pass urine from the kidneys to the urinary bladder.

Urinary Bladder

The bladder stores urine until voided.

Urethra

The urethra is a tube leading from the urinary bladder to the exterior of the body. Urine is passed through this tube to the exterior (voiding).

Esophagus

Stomach

Gall Bladder

Spleen

Liver

Pancreas

Large intestine

Small Intestine

Appendix

Rectum

Digestive System

Part VIII, Section B
Abdominal Injuries

INTRODUCTION

Often, intra-abdominal injury may not be evident when the patient is initially examined. If the victim obviously has signs of shock in association with abdominal trauma, internal bleeding must be suspected. Such cases fall into the Rapid Transport Category. For the most part, a HIGH DEGREE OF SUSPICION is required if abdominal injuries are to be diagnosed and receive proper treatment. Injuries to the abdominal contents should be suspected on the basis of:

- the mechanism of injury, i.e. a sudden deceleration as with a free-fall from a height or a motor vehicle accident;
- the anatomy of the injury, i.e. a blow to the abdomen or to the lower chest wall;
- the presence of abdominal pain;
- the presence of bruises or abrasions on the abdominal wall OR thorax;
- evidence of a penetrating wound on the abdominal wall OR thorax.

Initially, the Attendant must carefully examine the abdomen and then make periodic re-evaluations to detect any new findings or a deterioration in the patient's condition.

The most important factor in the first aid treatment of abdominal trauma is not the diagnosis of a specific injury but determining that an intra-abdominal injury exists, then rapidly transporting the patient to hospital.

All the solid abdominal organs are close to the diaphragm and protected by the ribs. The Attendant should be aware of possible trauma to these underlying organs when the lower ribs are injured.

Hollow organs may be ruptured or lacerated and spill their contents into the peritoneal cavity. This will cause peritonitis, an inflammation of the peritoneum.

The symptoms of advanced peritonitis are:
- Severe abdominal pain, aggravated by any movement
- Guarding of abdominal muscles, which become more tense upon palpation; this may be localized at first, then spread until the whole abdomen is rigid
- Fever and distension in some cases
- Dehydration, sepsis and ultimately septic shock in some cases

TYPES OF ABDOMINAL INJURIES

Abdominal wounds may be classified as either BLUNT or PENETRATING injuries, depending on whether the abdominal wall has been penetrated.

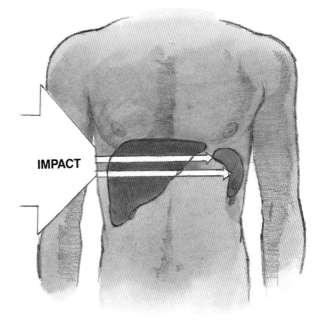

IMPACT

Blunt injury

Blunt Injuries

Blunt abdominal injury is caused by the direct transfer of energy to an organ, by compression of the abdominal organs against the spinal column, or by rapid deceleration, which may tear abdominal structures or their blood vessels. Seat belts may contribute to abdominal injuries while preventing lethal head injuries. It must be *emphasized* that blunt trauma to the lower chest can produce injuries within the abdomen, i.e. a fractured rib may rupture the spleen or pierce a kidney. Usually, the most significant immediate danger to patients with blunt abdominal trauma is serious hemorrhage. The patient with such injuries may reveal little on the initial examination. The Attendant must maintain a high degree of suspicion, regularly re-evaluate the patient and be prepared for the development of hypovolemic shock. Rupture or lacerations of abdominal organs may cause severe bleeding. Shock may be evident before peritoneal irritation becomes apparent. Victims with injuries to major blood vessels in the abdomen may bleed to death very quickly.

Penetrating Injuries

Penetrating injuries are more obvious, but serious damage to internal organs is possible with little or no evidence of external injury. Penetrating wounds of the abdomen are more commonly caused by knives or gunshot wounds but they can also be caused by shards of glass or sharp metal (e.g. an industrial accident). Penetrating abdominal injury usually results in:

- bleeding from damage to a solid organ or major blood vessel;
- perforation of the small or large bowel.

Severe bleeding will be evident early and presents with increasing abdominal distension, abdominal rigidity and varying degrees of shock. The onset of abdominal pain may be delayed especially in the case of bowel perforation. However, it may be equally life threatening.

If a person is impaled by a foreign object, it should not be removed, because the patient may bleed to death. INJURIES TO THE ABDOMINAL ORGANS MAY INCLUDE PENETRATING WOUNDS OF THE LOWER CHEST, BACK, FLANKS AND BUTTOCKS. All such cases should be evaluated by a physician.

A careful examination of the abdomen and the back is an important part of the secondary survey. The mechanism of injury should alert the Attendant of the possibility of an abdominal injury.

GENERAL SIGNS AND SYMPTOMS OF ABDOMINAL INJURY

- Abdominal Pain
  Ascertain its location, intensity, time of onset and duration, and whether it radiates or not (use the mnemonic PQRST — see Part III, page 30).
- Visible Soft Tissue Injury
  Redness, bruising, abrasions or an external wound will indicate the site of impact and will alert the Attendant to internal injury.
- Rigidity or Guarding of Abdominal Muscles
  Palpation may cause protective muscle tightening or guarding if the underlying peritoneum is irritated or inflamed.
- Nausea and Vomiting
  The patient may vomit. The Attendant must clear the

airway by positioning the patient according to the protocols outlined in Airway Management, Part IV, Section B, page 43. The Attendant should also note the contents of the vomit — whether it contains undigested food or blood. The presence of blood at any of the body openings must be noted.

- Shock
  Signs and symptoms of shock may be present. Distension, restlessness, air hunger and complaints of thirst may be the only indication that there is internal abdominal bleeding.
- Abdominal Distension
  Internal bleeding or bowel perforation may cause abdominal distension. In the patient with a decreased level of consciousness, who cannot complain of abdominal pain, abdominal distension may be the only sign of internal abdominal injury.
  NOTE: Non-penetrating or blunt injuries may leave little or no evidence of external injury.

EXTERNAL INJURIES AND MANAGEMENT

Any wound involving the abdominal wall must be considered as serious, regardless of the patient's condition at the time of injury. The Attendant should assume that major damage has been done even if there is no obvious sign of internal injury, i.e. the bowel may be perforated in several places. If these internal wounds are small, they may seal themselves and may not leak for several hours. The patient may feel fine during this time.

GENERAL PRINCIPLES OF MANAGEMENT OF ABDOMINAL INJURIES

The evaluation and management of the injured worker with abdominal injuries follows the Priority Action Approach outlined in Part III, page 20. ANY PATIENT WITH A PENETRATING INJURY TO THE ABDOMEN, OR WHO HAS EARLY SIGNS OF SHOCK, FALLS INTO THE RAPID TRANSPORT CATEGORY. The Attendant must limit management to the primary survey and treatment of life-threatening injuries. The patient must be rapidly transported to hospital.

Providing there is no contraindication, (e.g. C-spine injury or decreased level of consciousness,) the patient

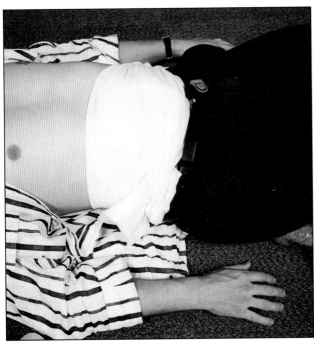

Abdominal dressing

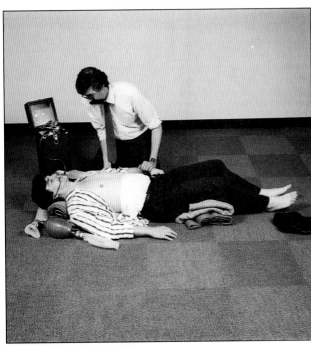

Positioning for abdominal injury

should be helped into a more comfortable position, usually the modified recumbent position — head and shoulders raised with the knees flexed and supported. A patient who is in shock should be transported in the horizontal position, usually supine, with the knees flexed over a pillow.

Once the Priority Action Approach has been completed and you are en route, the main points in caring for a protruding bowel are:

1. Gently cover the protruding bowel with several sterile gauze pads moistened with saline or water (sterile if available). If the intestine dries out, it may be permanently damaged.

2. If a coil of intestine or an organ is protruding from the abdomen, support it with drainage dressings or other bulky dressings placed over the moistened sterile gauze to avoid unnecessary traction on the blood vessels to the protruding part. Bandage the area securely enough to provide support and to keep the bowel clean, warm and moist. Protection from further injury is sometimes accomplished by "corralling" the abdominal contents that are protruding. The Attendant must use material that will not apply direct pressure to the bowel. Circumferential padding, which may be used, should be thick, soft and compressible. NOTE: If the treatment for protruding bowel contents is given in a cold environment, the application of fluid may not be feasible. The application of sterile dressings and bandaging may have to suffice.

3. Foreign bodies embedded in the abdominal wall must not be removed except at surgery. Do not remove any foreign body. It may cause a lethal hemorrhage. Use ring pads, bulky dressings or supportive bandages to maintain the protruding foreign body and protect the patient from further injury.

DO NOT GIVE THE PATIENT WITH ABDOMINAL INJURIES ANYTHING BY MOUTH.

DO NOT DELAY THE RAPID TRANSPORT OF PATIENTS WITH PROTRUDING BOWEL OR PENETRATING FOREIGN OBJECTS FOR THE PURPOSE OF COMPLETING COMPLICATED DRESSINGS THAT CAN BE DONE EN ROUTE TO HOSPITAL.

Part VIII, Section C
Non-traumatic Abdominal Emergencies The Acute Abdomen

The term "Acute Abdomen" refers to any severe problem involving the abdominal organs. The acute abdomen is recognized through the signs and symptoms of peritoneal irritation. Peritonitis is primarily indicated by severe pain, especially on movement or palpation. Other signs and symptoms include nausea and vomiting, fever in the presence of septic conditions, and abdominal wall rigidity. Peritonitis also causes an ileus of the bowel, which means a paralysis of the normal intestinal peristaltic movement. With the presence of ileus, the bowel may become distended and lead to abdominal distension, which will add to the pain and nausea and vomiting.

Peritonitis is commonly caused by acute appendicitis, perforation of a peptic ulcer, inflammation of the gallbladder and, in women, pelvic inflammatory disease and ectopic pregnancy. Any condition that allows pus, blood, urine, gastric juice, intestinal content or feces to come in contact with the lining of the abdominal cavity (peritoneum) can produce the signs of an acute abdomen.

EXAMINATION OF THE ACUTE ABDOMEN

The examination of the patient with acute abdomen should be brief and gentle, and should include the following:

- assess the patient's vital signs and observe any restlessness.
- observe the patient's position.
- check for abdominal distension.
- gently palpate the abdominal wall for rigidity and location of pain.
- reassess and record the patient's vital signs frequently.

MANAGEMENT OF THE PATIENT WITH THE ACUTE ABDOMEN

The Attendant should be aware that swollen or distended abdominal organs are very fragile and may be damaged by rough handling and excessive movement. As the degree of pain and tenderness usually indicates the degree of severity, the Attendant can assess the urgency of the abdominal situation through examination. If the Attendant suspects an acute abdominal condition, the patient falls into the Rapid Transport Category. Unless contraindicated, these patients should be placed in the position of comfort (usually semi-recumbent) and transported to hospital with urgency.

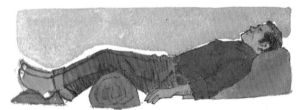

Semi-recumbent position

Part VIII, Section D
Genitourinary System Anatomy and Function

The urinary and genital systems share many structures.

The urinary system removes waste products from the blood and eliminates them from the body. The genital system is involved with reproduction.

The kidneys are solid urinary organs. The female reproductive system (uterus, ovaries and fallopian tubes) is situated in the lower abdomen, protected by the pelvis. The male reproductive system (testicles, vas deferens and penis) is mostly outside the abdomen.

URINARY SYSTEM

The main parts of the urinary system are:
1. two kidneys
2. two ureters
3. urinary bladder
4. urethra

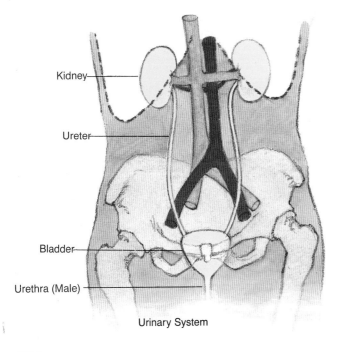

Urinary System

Kidneys

The kidneys lie against the muscles of the back in the upper abdomen, behind the peritoneum (the lining of the abdominal cavity). Posteriorly they are protected by the ribs of the lower chest wall.

The kidneys consist of a large number of microscopic filtering units that filter the blood, removing certain body wastes and excreting them as urine. These filters have the unique ability to conserve important body chemicals and fluids, and to get rid of only the unwanted material. The urine produced by the kidneys then passes down through small tubes called ureters leading to the bladder.

Ureters

The two ureters are long, slender, muscular tubes that extend from the kidney down and into the urinary bladder. The muscle of the ureter is capable of the same rhythmic contraction found in the digestive system, known as peristalsis. The peristaltic action moves the urine along from the kidneys to the bladder at frequent intervals.

Urinary Bladder

The bladder lies behind the pubic bone when empty. As it fills, it rises up into the abdominal cavity. The urinary bladder functions as a temporary reservoir for urine. When the bladder is full, sensory cells send messages to the brain that the bladder is ready to be emptied. When it is time to urinate (void), the bladder contracts, forcing urine through the urethra, and out of the body.

Urethra

The urethra is the tube that extends from the bladder to the outside, through which the bladder is emptied. The urethra is longer in men than in women and is also part of the male reproductive system.

GENITAL SYSTEM

In the higher life forms, reproduction occurs by sexual means. A specialized sex cell from the male (sperm) must unite with a specialized sex cell from the female (ovum) to produce a fetus. The function of the reproductive system is to produce the specialized sex cells, and to allow for their union and growth.

MALE REPRODUCTIVE SYSTEM

The male reproductive system consists of the testicles, seminal ducts and vas deferens, seminal vesicles, prostate gland, urethra and penis.

Testicles

There are two testes (testicles), which are found outside the abdominal cavity in a sac called the scrotum, suspended between the thighs. Each is oval in shape and

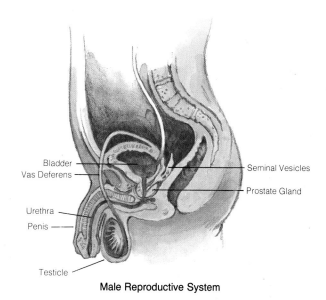

Male Reproductive System

Penis

The external genital organ, through which the urethra passes, is composed of erectile tissue. This tissue, when distended with blood during sexual activity, allow the penis to erect. The foreskin (prepuce) is a fold of skin which covers the end of the penis (the glans).

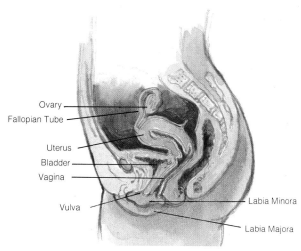

Female Reproductive System

consists of specialized cell types. Here are produced the male sex hormones (testosterone) and also the sex cells (spermatozoa).

Seminiferous Tubules and Vas Deferens

As the sperm-collecting seminiferous tubules leave each testis, they combine to form the vas deferens. This long tube travels up and out of the scrotum, under the skin of the abdominal wall for a short distance. It then passes through an opening in the abdominal wall (the inguinal canal) and into the abdominal cavity. From there, it extends down to the prostate gland where it joins the urethra.

Seminal Vesicles

The seminal vesicles are two storage pouches situated posterior to the urinary bladder. They receive and store the spermatozoa. The vesicles empty into the urethra at the prostate.

Prostate Gland

The prostate gland, about the size of a walnut, surrounds the urethra where it exits from the urinary bladder. The prostate adds its secretions to the spermatozoa from the seminal vesicles, and the resulting fluid is called semen. The semen is expelled from the urethra by rhythmic contractions of the vas deferens and prostate (ejaculation).

FEMALE REPRODUCTIVE SYSTEM

Ovaries

Two small, oval-shaped glands below the brim of the pelvis produce female hormones and the female sex cells (ova). A mature ovum is released by an ovary (ovulation) about every 28 days (the menstrual cycle) from puberty to menopause.

Fallopian Tubes

The fallopian tubes are two tubes leading from beside each ovary to the uterus, which is near the centre of the pelvic cavity. The fringe-like end of each tube near the ovary is open and the ovum is drawn into the tubes. It is carried to the uterus by peristalsis.

Uterus

The uterus is a hollow, muscular, pear-shaped organ in the centre of the pelvic cavity. The bottom, narrow part is firmly attached between the urinary bladder and the rectum. The upper, larger portion is movable and held in place by ligaments. The narrow, lower part of the uterus which enters the upper part of the vagina is called the cervix. There is an opening in the cervix which allows the passage of sperm into the uterus and of menstrual fluid from the uterine cavity into the vagina. When a baby is born, it passes from the uterus through the dilated cervix and vagina (birth canal).

Vagina

The vagina is a muscular, distensible tube connecting the uterus with the vulva (the external female genitalia). It is situated behind the urethra and in front of the rectum. During intercourse, the semen is deposited into the vagina.

Vulva

The external parts of the female reproductive system (vulva) consist of the labia (major and minor) and clitoris. The perineum is the area between the vaginal opening and the anus.

Part VIII, Section E
Genitourinary Injuries

INJURIES TO GENITOURINARY SYSTEM

About 10% of injuries requiring hospital care involve the genitourinary (G-U) system to some degree. Early recognition is desirable to prevent serious complications.

Assessment

The primary assessment is directed towards hemorrhage or shock, or any other associated life-threatening injury which may be present.

A detailed history of the mechanism of injury should be taken. Special concern for G-U system injury should arise with the following types of injuries:
- direct blows to the kidney or other G-U structures
- fractured pelvis
- sudden deceleration injury

Inspection — Look for evidence of bruising or swelling, which might suggest deeper injury. Where practical, check the urethral opening for evidence of bleeding.

Palpation — Feel the abdomen. Generalized tenderness may represent a perforated organ, internal bleeding, or leakage of urine. Localized tenderness over a kidney or lower posterior ribs should raise the level of suspicion for a kidney injury.

SIGNS OF GENITOURINARY INJURY

- blood in the urine;
- difficult or painful voiding following trauma;
- blood at the urethral opening;
- penetrating wound, bruising or tenderness over the kidney (flank);
- fracture of 10th, 11th or 12th ribs;
- tenderness or bruising in lower abdomen or groin.

Kidney Injuries

Most kidney trauma is minor but warrants close observation. Major bleeding from kidney trauma is rare. Blood in the urine is common following blunt kidney trauma.

Bladder Injury

The bladder is normally protected by an intact pelvis. Pelvic fractures can result in direct bladder injury. With pelvic fractures, blood loss can be significant. Transport quickly when suspected. Blunt trauma can rupture a full bladder. Generalized abdominal tenderness may be present. This is not a common injury.

Urethral Injuries

Urethral injuries occur most often in men, usually occurring following a straddle injury or a pelvic fracture. They are rare in women, and are not common generally. The most reliable finding is blood at the urethral opening and/or difficult or painful voiding.

Injury to External Genitalia

These injuries are often very painful due to the extensive nerves in the region. Anxiety may be high. Use care and be gentle.

These injuries should be dressed with sterile moistened bandages. Bleeding can usually be controlled with direct pressure. Ice may alleviate pain. The simplest dressing is a diaper-type bandage. Transport in position of most comfort. Retain any detached tissue (see Soft Tissue Injuries, Part IX, Section D, page 210). Pack in a saline dressing and transport with patient.

INJURIES DURING PREGNANCY

The Attendant must be aware that a seemingly minor mishap may have serious consequences in the pregnant patient. Any blunt trauma (e.g. MVA, fall, or blow to the abdomen), even minor, must be considered potentially serious.

These injuries can result in conditions that could threaten the life of the fetus or mother. Follow the Priority Action Approach. In the absence of any abnormalities of Airway, Breathing and Circulation, the Attendant should look for, and specifically ask about:
- abdominal pain;
- periodic pains of premature labour;
- vaginal bleeding;
- leakage of clear (amniotic) fluid that surrounds the fetus.

Any patient with abnormalities of the ABCs or any of the above findings are in the Rapid Transport Category.

Often, there may be hidden injury which could threaten the fetus or the mother. Therefore, all pregnant patients without any of the above abnormalities, even with normal vital signs, must be referred to hospital by routine transport.

Management

1. Stabilize the ABCs, if necessary.
2. Administer oxygen at a 10 Lpm flow.
3. Place the patient, ideally, on her left side. This improves perfusion of the fetus. If, as a consequence of injuries, the patient cannot be placed on her left side, the right hip should be elevated.
4. If there is a discharge or bleeding from the vagina, cover the vagina with a sanitary napkin or well-padded dressing. DO NOT PACK THE VAGINA.

MEDICAL EMERGENCIES OF PREGNANCY

The following is an outline of some of the problems occasionally encountered in pregnancy.

Vaginal Bleeding

An undiagnosed pregnancy may present with vaginal bleeding.

Bleeding from the vagina during pregnancy may be caused by a variety of disorders, including:

- miscarriage — spontaneous or induced;
- the fetus grows outside the uterus in either the fallopian tube, the ovary, or the abdomen (ectopic pregnancy);
- abnormally located placenta encroaching on the birth canal (placenta previa);
- placenta separates prematurely from the wall of the uterus (abruptio placenta).

Vaginal bleeding in non-pregnant women is usually caused by menstruation or a gynecological problem.

The amount of bleeding may vary. Abdominal pain or cramping, fever or shock may accompany vaginal bleeding.

Management of Vaginal Bleeding

Regardless of the cause, the patient must be transported to a physician. The severity of the patient's condition will dictate the urgency. During transport, the patient should be kept warm and comfortable and oxygen administered if necessary. Reassurance will also be helpful. The Attendant should not attempt to pack the vagina. It will not control the bleeding and it may be harmful.

Toxemia

The early stage of toxemia in pregnancy is called pre-eclampsia. It may include high blood pressure, headache, agitation or swelling. The advanced stages of eclampsia may include seizures and coma.

Management of Toxemia

If toxemia is suspected, refer the patient for medical attention urgently. Any stimulus may cause a seizure. Therefore, handle the patient gently and avoid excessive noise and bright lights.

If seizures occur, the patient must be protected from injury to herself or the fetus, and the airway must be kept open. Ideally, position on her left side. Alternatively, elevate the patient's right hip with a pillow and move the uterus to the left. Provide high-flow oxygen at 10 Lpm. TOXEMIA IS A LIFE-THREATENING EMERGENCY FOR MOTHER AND FETUS; THEREFORE, ALL THESE PATIENTS FALL INTO THE RAPID TRANSPORT CATEGORY.

Part IX, Section A

Skin and Soft Tissues Anatomy and Function

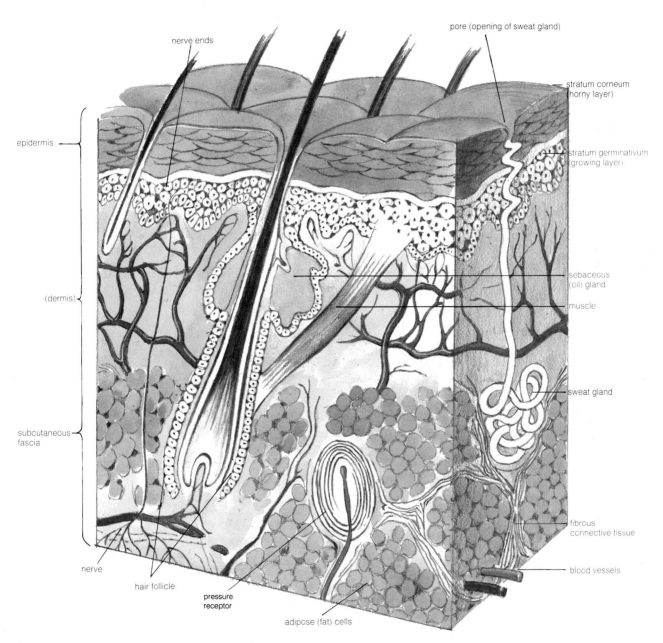

For purposes of this section, the skin and soft tissues include:
1. skin
2. subcutaneous tissue
3. muscle
4. tendon
5. ligament

SKIN

Skin is an extensive and complex organ, consisting of tough, elastic tissue which protects and covers the entire body.

The skin serves two main functions:
1. To protect the body from:
   - loss of body fluids;
   - bacterial invasion;
   - alterations in temperature.

2. To contain sensory receptors, which convey information about the environment to the brain.

LAYERS OF THE SKIN

There are two main skin layers: the epidermis and the dermis. Each layer differs in structure and function.

The epidermis is the outermost covering. It is made up of dead hardened cells which are constantly being rubbed off and replaced. Deeper in the epidermis are cells that constantly reproduce to replace the outer cells.

Some of the cells in the deeper layer also contain pigment granules. These cells, together with the blood in the small vessels of the skin, give the skin its colour.

The dermis has a framework of elastic connective tissue and is well supplied with blood vessels and nerves. Many special structures are found in the dermis, including sweat glands and ducts, oil (sebaceous) glands and ducts, hair follicles, blood vessels and specialized nerve endings.

Sweat glands discharge through sweat ducts onto the surface of the skin. Sebaceous glands produce an oily substance called sebum. Sebum is important in maintaining the water-proofing of the skin and in keeping it supple.

Hair follicles are the small organs from which hair grows.

Blood vessels and a complex array of nerves are also contained in the dermis.

THE SKIN AS AN AID TO ASSESSMENT

Part of every assessment should include an evaluation of the skin. The skin, like any other organ, reacts to injury or illness. Because it is on the surface, it is easily accessible and, obviously, very visible. It provides much information, which is easily obtained. Assessment of the skin should include the following:

* temperature
* colour
* moisture

1. Temperature

Skin temperature increases directly with increasing cutaneous blood flow. Conversely, skin temperature falls with vasoconstriction. This is part of normal temperature regulation. For example, in a hot environment, more warm blood is diverted to the skin, to allow it to lose some body heat to the surrounding air. Conversely, in shock, for instance, blood is diverted to the body core to minimize blood loss and to provide the vital organs with the available blood. Sweating also helps to regulate temperature.

2. Colour

Skin, to a greater or lesser degree, is transparent. How transparent it is depends upon the number of pigment (melanin)- containing cells. This varies considerably among different races. In fair-skinned people, the colour of the skin is an excellent indicator of the underlying circulation. In dark-skinned individuals, the mucous membranes are a more accurate guide (e.g. inside of mouth and eyelids).

If for any reason blood flow to the skin should be reduced, the skin will become pale or mottled. This might occur with loss of blood volume or with constriction (narrowing) of cutaneous blood vessels (e.g. shock, heart failure, cold). Pale skin may also occur in non-life-threatening situations as a normal reflex response (e.g. severe pain or vomiting).

FOR FIRST AID PURPOSES, PALE SKIN SHOULD BE CONSIDERED AS A SIGN OF SERIOUS ILLNESS OR INJURY.

If the cutaneous blood vessels should dilate (expand), resulting in increased blood flow to the skin, the skin will become pink (e.g. fever or blushing).

3. Moisture

Stimulation of the sympathetic nervous system (adrenalin and noradrenalin) also results in sweating (e.g. as in shock).

SUMMARY OF SKIN FINDINGS

COLOUR	POSSIBLE CAUSES
Increased redness	• Fever • Exercise • Allergic reaction • Warm environment
Pallor	• Significant blood loss (hypovolemic shock) • Severe pain • Fainting (syncope) • Fear

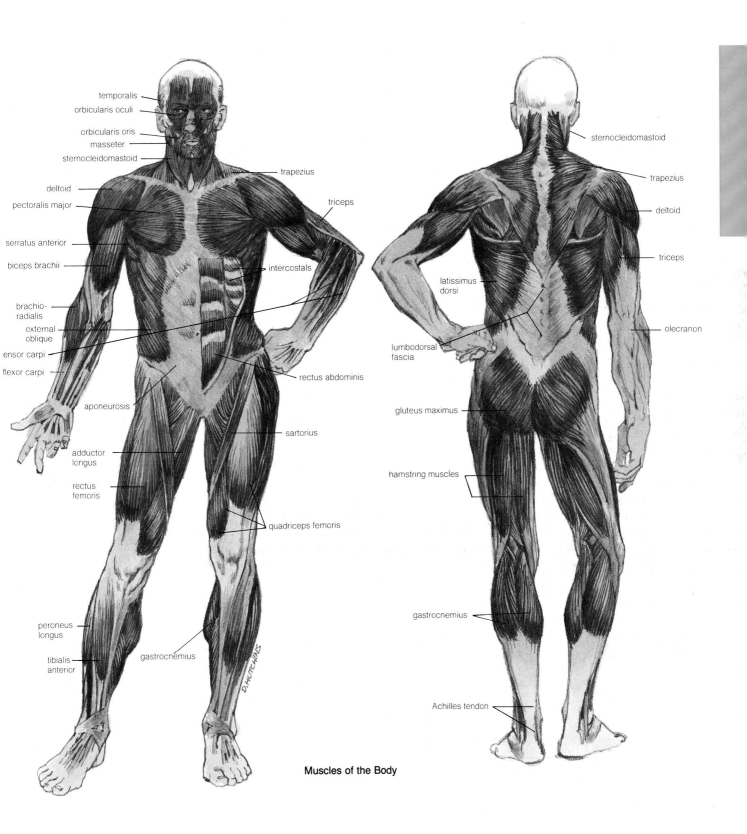

temporalis
orbicularis oculi
orbicularis oris
masseter
sternocleidomastoid
trapezius
deltoid
pectoralis major
triceps
serratus anterior
biceps brachii
intercostals
brachio-
radialis
external
oblique
ensor carpi
flexor carpi
rectus abdominis
aponeurosis
sartorius
adductor
longus
rectus
femoris
quadriceps femoris
peroneus
longus
tibialis
anterior
gastrocnemius

D. HUTCHINS

sternocleidomastoid
trapezius
deltoid
triceps
latissimus
dorsi
olecranon
lumbodorsal
fascia
gluteus maximus
hamstring muscles
gastrocnemius
Achilles tendon

Muscles of the Body

Bluish (cyanosis)	• Cold
	• Low oxygen in blood (hypoxia)
	• Shock
Mottled	• Cold
	• Shock

TEMPERATURE AND MOISTURE	**POSSIBLE CAUSES**
Hot and dry	Heat stroke
Hot and moist	Hot environment, fever
Cold and dry	Cold environment
Cold and clammy	Blood loss, heart failure, shock

SUBCUTANEOUS TISSUE

The subcutaneous layer is a combination of connective tissue and fat. This layer connects the skin to the surface muscles. The fat in this layer of tissue serves as the body's main insulation. Fat also functions as a reserve store of energy.

MUSCLE

Muscle is a special kind of tissue, capable of forceful contraction. There are different kinds of muscle tissue, each uniquely designed to carry out specialized functions. Types of muscle:

1. skeletal muscle — responsible for body movement;
2. smooth muscle — responsible for constriction of the blood vessels and peristaltic activity in the gastrointestinal and genitourinary systems;
3. cardiac muscle — responsible for the automatic pumping of the heart.

All muscles have arteries, veins and nerves. They cannot function without a continuous supply of nutrients, oxygen and the removal of waste products. Muscles are under the direct control of the nervous system.

1. SKELETAL MUSCLE

   Skeletal muscles are attached to the skeleton and are also known as voluntary muscles because they can contract on demand.

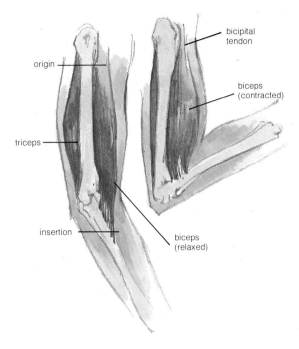

Muscle Movement

Muscle Movement

All types of muscle attachments are designed to harness the power of muscle contraction. Both ends of a muscle are usually attached to bone, either over a wide area but more often by a fibrous tendon.

A muscle acts on an appropriate impulse from its nerve supply. These nerves are called motor nerves.

In muscular contraction, the muscle is shortened. This pulls on the attachments at each end and brings them nearer to each other, causing movement.

Skeletal muscles pass over or across joints, permitting body movement. Most skeletal muscles exist in groups or pairs, which have equal but opposite functions. Voluntary contraction of one group of muscles is accompanied by automatic relaxation of the opposing group. This relaxation retains just enough tension to make the movement smooth and keep it under control. Muscles can only contract and relax, they cannot push.

Muscle Tone

Muscle tone is controlled by the nervous system and keeps the muscles in a constant state of readiness.

2. SMOOTH MUSCLE

Smooth muscles are involuntary and under the control of the autonomic nervous system. These muscles contract without conscious thought. This is where smooth muscles are found:

- digestive tract, where they move nutrients and waste materials along (peristaltic activity);
- blood vessel walls, where they regulate blood flow;
- tubes (ureters) that carry urine from the kidneys;
- walls of the bronchial tree, which regulates air flow.

3. CARDIAC MUSCLE

This muscle is highly specialized, possessing an intrinsic rhythm that allows it to contract and relax automatically. The rate and strength of contractions are controlled by the autonomic nervous system.

TENDON

A tendon is a band of strong, white fibrous tissue that connects a muscle to a bone. When the muscle contracts or shortens, it pulls on the tendon, which moves the bone. Tendons are so tough they are seldom torn.

LIGAMENT

Ligaments are fibrous tissue bands that connect one bone to another at a joint. They are found in all free-moving joints (e.g. knee) and also the less mobile joints (e.g. sacroiliac joint).

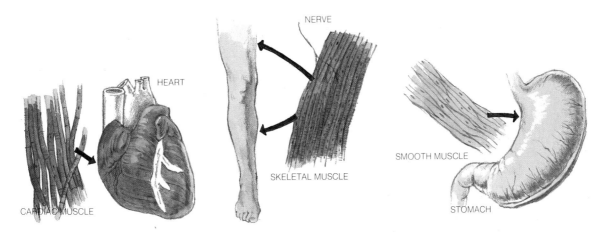

NERVE

HEART

SKELETAL MUSCLE

SMOOTH MUSCLE

STOMACH

CARDIAC MUSCLE

TYPES OF MUSCLE

Part IX, Section B
Inflammation, Repair and Healing

DEFINITION

Inflammation is a localized protective response of living tissue to an injury, or exposure to an irritant or infectious agent. In an attempt to isolate the offending agent, local blood vessels dilate, bringing in special cells to initiate healing and prevent further injury. The agents that may cause inflammation include:

1. infection (e.g. bacteria)
2. physical injury (e.g. contusion, crush, abrasion, foreign body, strain or overuse)
3. chemical injury (e.g. acid or alkali burn)

The stages of the inflammatory process are the same, regardless of cause, and can be summarized in the following steps:

1. The injured tissue cells release certain substances into the blood, which "trigger" the response.
2. The local capillaries dilate, greatly increasing the blood supply to the part. This can be easily observed as a reddening of the skin overlying the injury.
3. The local capillaries become relatively porous, allowing plasma to leak into the region of the injured tissue. This results in swelling and usually pain. The pain arises from both direct damage to the local nerves and stretching of the nerves due to swelling. That is why, in tissues where there is little room for swelling (e.g. fingertip, nose, ear canal), the pain can be so acute.
4. Cellular elements also accumulate (e.g. white blood cells). Some of the cells attack and kill infectious organisms; others carry away dead cellular debris and still others attempt to neutralize toxins.

The excess plasma, together with some of the cellular elements, make up "inflammatory exudate". It can often be seen to ooze from raw or open tissue (e.g. after a burn or abrasion) as a clear, straw-coloured fluid, called serum.

The local signs of inflammation are:

- heat
- swelling
- redness
- pain

Some infectious agents produce enough toxin to make the patient feel generally ill and may also result in fever.

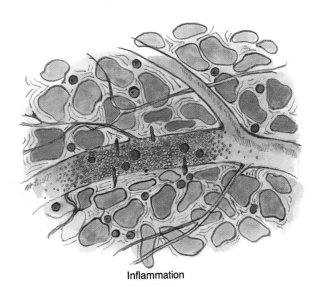
Inflammation

CLINICAL VARIETIES OF INFLAMMATION

Inflammation may run its course without destroying any tissue or there may be local tissue death.

Some bacteria produce tissue toxins powerful enough to actually kill the tissue in which they are concentrated (e.g. gangrene). This is especially true in tissues where there is no room for swelling, and the resulting collapse of the local capillaries hastens tissue death due to lack of oxygen.

Pus

Pus is an inflammatory exudate containing white blood cells, often dead, as well as cellular debris from dead tissue. Pus also contains germs, some of which are still alive, and therefore infectious.

Abscess (Boil)

An abscess (boil) is a localized collection of pus within the tissues, usually found in hair-bearing areas of the skin (e.g. back of neck, axilla).

For treatment, see Section E, First Aid Room Techniques, page 220.

Cellulitis

Cellulitis is an inflammation of a diffuse, spreading nature, lying between the skin and underlying tissues. It is caused by an infectious organism. It may spread from an abscess, but more often arises locally, following a penetrating skin wound — even a minor one.

The surrounding area is hot, red and swollen, and fades gradually at the edges. Mild local infections may be treated with hot compresses. More serious degrees of infection, as with abscesses, should be referred to a physician.

THE LYMPHATIC SYSTEM

We all know about the body's circulatory system, which is made up of the arterial system and the venous system, but there is a third network of vessels which make up the lymphatic system. They are less visible than the arteries and veins, but are present throughout the body and serve a very necessary function.

The body fluid that accumulates in the tissue spaces between cells at the site of an infection is collected by the lymph vessels and carried away to the local lymph nodes (glands). Here it is "processed" before eventually returning to the general circulation. The nodes effectively remove any infectious organisms before allowing the lymphatic fluid to return to the bloodstream.

In the days before antibiotics, if bacteria escaped into the general circulation, a condition known as "septicemia" could develop and was usually fatal. The lymphatic system helps protect the body from septicemia.

Lymphadenitis

In the lymph nodes, the bacteria are engulfed by white blood cells and other specialized cells. This process often results in the regional lymph nodes becoming swollen and tender (swollen glands). This condition is called "lymphadenitis". Occasionally, the lymph node itself may become abscessed by a particularly severe infection, but following most infections the lymph nodes usually return to normal.

Lymphangitis

"Lymphangitis" is an inflammation of the lymphatic channel leading to the lymph nodes from the original site of infection. It may be seen as a red streak overlying the path of the underlying lymphatic channel, which may also be tender and swollen.

Treatment

Both these conditions should be referred for medical follow-up by the family physician. In isolated areas, the treatment of a localized infection would be intermittent application of hot compresses to the affected area (see First Aid Room Techniques, page 220), until medical attention is available.

SPLEEN

In addition to the lymphatic channels and the lymph nodes, the spleen also makes up part of the lymphatic system.

The spleen is a solid organ, about the size of a small fist, located in the left upper quadrant of the abdominal cavity. It contains soft pulp called lymphoid tissue which filters out old red blood cells, as well as manufacturing certain types of blood cells.

The spleen has an unusually large blood supply and may bleed profusely if injured. It is particularly vulnerable to rupture with blunt trauma to the abdomen or left lower chest.

RUPTURE OF THE SPLEEN IS ALWAYS A LIFE-THREATENING EMERGENCY, AND FALLS INTO THE RAPID TRANSPORT CATEGORY.

Any patient who has suffered a blunt trauma to the abdomen or lower chest, and who shows signs of developing shock, should be suspected of having a ruptured spleen, until proven otherwise. They require immediate transport to the nearest hospital on an emergency basis. Minutes count! Follow the Priority Action Approach for abdominal injuries.

HEALING

Healing is the restoration of integrity to injured tissue, and follows any condition that can result in tissue injury or death.

Basically, healing occurs by formation of scar tissue. The process can be explained best by giving an example — the repair of a simple laceration:

1. The edges of the wound are loosely brought into contact with one another.
2. A thin layer of blood or plasma forms between the edges and produces a clot. This is essential.

3. New fibrous tissue cells begin to grow through the clot to "bridge the gap", forming a loose network of new tissue.
4. Blood vessels then grow across the wound in a similar manner.
5. The cells of the deep layer of skin (dermis) are now able to grow across the top and be nourished from below. Healing is then complete. The process usually takes 5-6 days but may not be structurally sound for another week, depending upon location.

   Fast healing occurs in areas of relatively good blood supply (e.g. face) and slow healing tends to occur over bony prominences (e.g. knee, elbow, knuckle).

If the wound edges are not brought together, a larger amount of blood clot is required to "fill the gap" and healing takes longer. It also results in a bigger scar.

Where the gap in the skin is large, and cannot be closed initially, a process called "granulation" occurs. Here, meaty-looking, rough-textured tissue grows up from the bottom of the wound to the level of the surface. Then the skin grows slowly in from the sides at a rate of approximately 1mm per day. Obviously, healing takes considerably longer this way.

Finally, because of the loss of integrity of the body's normal barrier to infection, any skin wound is more easily subject to infection until healing is complete. Infection is a common complication of skin wounds.

Part IX, Section C
Wound Infection

INTRODUCTION

The subject of "inflammation" has already been discussed in Section B, page 199. The term "infection" applies to an inflammatory reaction resulting from the presence of harmful microorganisms. Infections may be caused by several different types of microorganisms, including bacteria, viruses, fungi and parasites. Not all organisms are harmful. Many are present normally in different parts of the body, where they perform useful and necessary functions (e.g. in the bowel to aid digestion). However, if these organisms enter another part of the body, they may cause infection (e.g. fecal contamination of a skin wound). Most wound infections are caused by bacteria. Infections can develop in any tissue of the body, from a variety of mechanisms and from many different organisms.

In the course of their work, First Aid Attendants will most likely encounter wound infections which are frequently caused by bacteria.

Though infections can occur anywhere in the body, this section will discuss "wound infections" and their complications.

BACTERIA

Bacteria are living organisms and need the following conditions to help them survive and grow:

1. moisture;
2. nutrients;
3. oxygen — although some bacteria, such as tetanus (lockjaw) and gas-gangrene bacteria, live without oxygen;
4. temperature — normal body temperature, 37°C (98.6°F), is the best temperature for most bacteria to grow and multiply. Heat kills bacteria and can be used to disinfect objects.

Bacteria can enter the body in several ways: through a wound, through the nose and mouth, or through the genitourinary system.

Bacteria are found everywhere. Many are capable of producing infection if they are allowed to enter the body. The intact skin normally serves as an effective barrier to infection but, should the skin become broken (e.g. a laceration or abrasion), bacteria can then enter the body.

Bacteria can spread in many ways — especially by fingers and hands. From here, they can be carried to the eyes, nose, mouth and to other people, and especially to open wounds.

Bacteria may enter a wound:
- at the time of injury;
- after the injury.

At the Time of Injury

Bacteria are introduced into the wound both by the object which caused the injury and from the patient's own skin. In open wounds, dirt in clothing may be carried into the deeper tissues of the wound, carrying bacteria that are difficult to remove. Materials vary greatly in their capacity to carry bacteria. Metal fragments are often fairly free of bacteria. Soil and vegetable matter are usually heavily contaminated.

After the Injury

As soon as a wound is inflicted, it can become contaminated from bacteria on the patient's skin. Bacteria can also be introduced by someone who breathes or coughs into a wound or touches it. Unsanitary first aid techniques will contaminate the wound. Poor hygiene and improper handling of the wound dressings can also introduce bacteria.

WOUND INFECTION

Recognition

Signs of infection do not appear immediately after the injury because bacteria need time to grow and multiply. Signs may appear as early as one day after injury, or may be delayed for several days. Wound infections may be recognized by:
- redness around the area; red streaks extending from the area;
- swelling of the infected part and/or the lymph nodes that drain the part;
- heat around the affected area and, sometimes, fever;

- aching and local tenderness around the wound;
- pus beneath the skin or draining from the wound.

Signs of fever, swollen and sore lymph nodes, and red streaks extending from the area usually indicate lymphangitis (see Section B, page 200). A patient with suspected lymphangitis should be examined and treated by a physician as soon as possible.

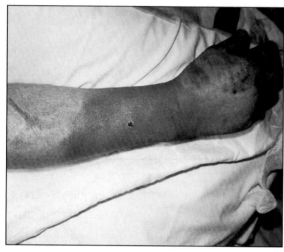

Wound infection with gangrene

Prevention

The aim of first aid treatment of open wounds is, first: to control hemorrhage and, next: to prevent or minimize the chance of a wound infection.

For instruction on proper handling, cleansing and dressing techniques, see Section E, page 216.

Treatment

Once a wound infection is suspected, the patient should be referred to a physician for follow-up care and appropriate treatment.

FROM THE MOMENT OF INJURY, THERE IS RISK OF INFECTION AND THIS CONTINUES UNTIL THE WOUND IS HEALED.

TETANUS

Tetanus (lockjaw) is a serious infectious complication of a wound. It is caused by infection from bacteria that inhabit the intestine of domestic animals. It is found in soil and dust, deposited there in animal feces. It is also found in human feces. It grows best in the absence of oxygen, so is most likely to complicate deep wounds that have not been adequately cleaned and have poor drainage. However, tetanus may occur as a complication in any size or type of wound, all the way from seemingly trivial puncture wounds and abrasions, through lacerations, burns and up to compound fractures. Approximately one-third of tetanus patients have an unrecognized wound or one considered insignificant by the patient.

The tetanus bacteria produces a powerful toxin, which greatly increases the irritability of the nervous system. It starts with local spasms in muscles around the wound site and these may become widespread generalized spasms. The spasms are usually triggered by external stimuli, such as noise, light, touch or changes in temperature. The stimulus may be minimal, such as a draft or cool air from an open door. Early in the course of tetanus, patients may complain of irritability, headache, low-grade fever or abdominal-wall muscle cramps. There may be tightness of the muscles of the jaw, which make it difficult to open the mouth (hence the term "lockjaw"). Spasms of the face muscles may cause a fixed half-smile and spasms of the throat muscles may make swallowing impossible.

The painful and fatiguing contractions may involve other muscles of the body and are usually separated by periods of relaxation. This leads to progressive exhaustion and death due to mechanical failure of the breathing mechanism, or from cardiac failure.

Signs of tetanus may develop from three days to three weeks following injury. The average time is seven days.

Specific treatment is not within the scope of first aid, but the Attendant should be able to recognize early signs of the condition. ANY PATIENT SUSPECTED OF HAVING TETANUS MUST BE CONSIDERED A MEDICAL EMERGENCY AND BE RUSHED TO HOSPITAL WITHOUT DELAY. That is very important because, once established, the mortality rate for tetanus is still about 40%, even with appropriate therapy.

TETANUS CAN BE PREVENTED IF ALL WOUNDS RECEIVE PROPER TREATMENT AND ALL PATIENTS WITH WOUNDS HAVE UP-TO-DATE TETANUS IMMUNIZATION. (See below.)

Wound Care and Tetanus Prevention

All wounds should be thoroughly cleaned as described in Section E, page 216. Dilute hydrogen peroxide (3%) is particularly useful in the first aid treatment of wounds where soil has been carried deep into the tissues.

Each patient with a wound should receive a tetanus toxoid injection as soon as possible after an injury, preferably within 24 hours. This applies to any individual, whether or not there has been a prior immunization, unless a "booster" was administered within the past five years.

Immunization must be given within 36 hours. If medical attention will be delayed, it is even more essential that the wound be properly cleaned and dressed.

The patient who is developing early signs of tetanus must be transported rapidly to hospital and be given supportive care with minimal external stimulus. Cotton-batting plugs may be placed in the patient's ears; adequate blankets should be used to keep the patient warm and the transport vehicle may be darkened. Oxygen may be administered if the patient has respiratory muscle spasms.

GAS GANGRENE

Gas gangrene, like tetanus, is caused by bacteria that thrive in the absence of oxygen. Wounds involving muscle, especially deep wounds with considerable muscle destruction, poor drainage and soil contamination, are the most dangerous. The earliest signs are usually sudden onset of pain and swelling in an area of wound contamination, with local tissue discolouration, and a brownish foul-smelling watery discharge. There may also be a low-grade fever and, sometimes, a generalized shock-like state. The most definitive characteristic is the presence of a crackling (crepitus) beneath the skin when the swollen tissue is pressed, due to tiny gas bubbles in the tissues. **The discharge is highly infectious.**

The first aid management includes local wound care as outlined in the wound section (see Section E, page 216). IF GAS GANGRENE IS SUSPECTED, THE PATIENT MUST BE TRANSPORTED TO A MEDICAL FACILITY AS RAPIDLY AS POSSIBLE. General supportive care for shock should be provided and oxygen administered. The wound may be lightly packed with gauze saturated with 3% hydrogen peroxide.

Part IX, Section D
Soft Tissue Injuries

Soft tissues include all body structures except organs and bones.

Most injuries involve soft tissue such as skin and muscle. Any break in the continuity of tissue is classified as a wound. Breaks in bones are also classified as wounds but are referred to as fractures and are dealt with in a separate section. (See Part X, Section B, page 245.)

In general, these injuries may be categorized as follows:
- wounds — open and closed
- muscle or tendon strains
- ligament sprain
- any combination of the above

This section will deal only with wounds and their management. The treatment of strains and sprains is discussed in Part X, Section B, page 245.

Wounds are of two types:

1. Closed wounds — Injury occurs to underlying structures with no break in the skin.
2. Open wounds — There is a break in the skin surface and underlying tissue may be exposed.

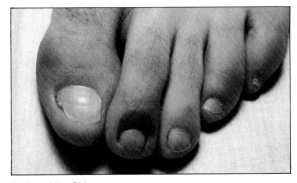

Bruise of the Skin

CLOSED WOUNDS

Closed wounds may result from the impact of blunt objects or from excessive pressure or force. There may be considerable crushing of tissues beneath the skin, accompanied by hemorrhage.

Closed wounds range from a small bruise (contusion) to ruptured internal structures. By their very nature, the extent of injury may be difficult to assess.

The force of the injury often ruptures small blood vessels. If the injury is close to the surface, the immediate leakage of blood and plasma causes swelling and pain. A bruise or discolouration of the skin (ecchymosis) may occur within hours or days. A bruise looks like a black and blue mark. As the wound heals, the bruised area becomes paler, greenish-brown and finally yellowish.

When large amounts of tissue are injured or when larger blood vessels are ruptured at the injury site, a rapidly forming hematoma will develop. A hematoma is a collection of blood and plasma in the damaged area (swelling).

A hematoma may give rise to complications that usually occur as a consequence of compression of blood vessels or nerves. This may cause circulation deficiencies, loss of use or feeling, or increasing pain of the affected extremity.

Closed Wound Management

Small contusions (bruises) usually require no emergency treatment. During the first 48 hours, the application of cold and modest pressure will limit localized swelling, thereby decreasing pain and disability.

Larger contusions and/or hematomas will require elevation of the injured part, and appropriate immobilization, as well as the application of cold.

Application of Cold

Cold will help to reduce pain and limit swelling. Initially, cold should be applied to the entire injured area for 10 minutes at a time. If applied for longer, it may have a reverse effect and the vessels may dilate instead of remaining constricted.

Cold should be applied for approximately 10 minutes, removed for 5 minutes, then reapplied. This procedure gives the best results in limiting swelling in the soft tissue area and can be initiated and continued for up to 48 hours after an injury.

Neither ice in plastic bags nor chemical cold packs should be applied directly to the skin. They should be wrapped in some form of material (one layer of moistened toweling or a drainage dressing) before being placed on the injury.

OPEN WOUNDS

By the very nature of open wounds, the continuity of the skin's surface is broken, and bleeding is present. Open wounds are susceptible to infection. There are several types of open wounds:

- abrasion
- laceration
- puncture
- avulsion
- amputation

Because of their importance and complexity, crush injuries (see page 211), burns (see page 287) and electrical injuries (see page 293) will be discussed individually.

Abrasion

This is the most superficial type of open wound, merely roughening the skin's surface. It may be a single, fine line (scratch) or a wide grazed area. Bleeding is usually very slight, but as dirt or other foreign material may be ground into the abraded area, they may become infected.

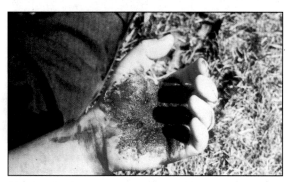

Abrasion

Laceration

A laceration is a cut that may have sharp or jagged edges. The subcutaneous tissue, the underlying muscles and associated nerves and blood vessels may be involved. The appearance and significance of the wound relate directly to the cause — utility knife, chain saw, etc. The extent of damage to underlying tissues may be difficult to assess. Blood loss and infection are the primary complications of lacerations.

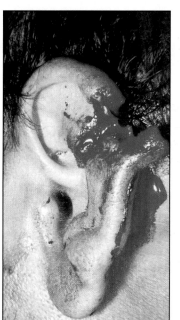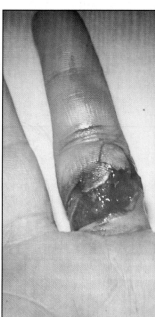

Laceration

Puncture

A puncture may vary in size and depth, depending on the cause.

Depending on their location, puncture wounds may pierce major blood vessels and organs, causing rapidly fatal internal bleeding. The Attendant should be especially wary of puncture wounds to the neck, chest, abdomen or groin.

External bleeding is usually not severe if the wound is small. Small puncture wounds may become infected quite readily, as they are difficult to clean.

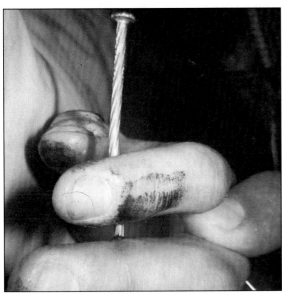

Puncture

Avulsion

An avulsed wound occurs when there is full thickness of skin loss, exposing deeper tissues. Complications of an avulsion injury may include loss of blood, infection and delayed healing.

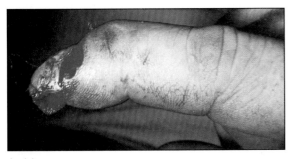

Avulsion

Amputation

An amputation occurs when there is a complete loss of a body part. Bone and other tissues are often exposed. Complications may include bleeding, shock, infection and disability.

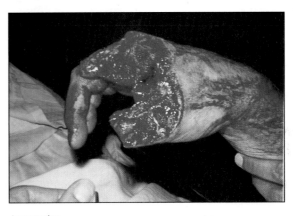

Amputation

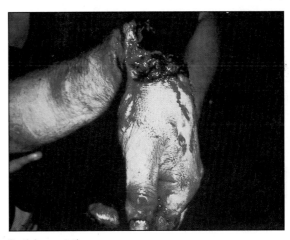

Partial amputation

TREATMENT OF MAJOR WOUNDS

The treatment of major open, soft tissue injuries is governed by the Priority Action Approach. The general principles outlined below must be followed:

- Control bleeding.
- Prevent infection.
- Immobilize the affected part and keep the patient at rest.

Controlling hemorrhage is the first priority. Once hemorrhage has been controlled, there may be justification for some wound cleansing. This particularly applies where a wound is grossly contaminated by animal or vegetable matter, such as with wounds sustained in meat and fish packing plants or those contaminated by soil. The risk of infection increases in proportion to the time it takes to obtain medical attention and close the wound.

Cleansing of major wounds must be limited to irrigating with sterile saline or tap water. The Attendant should not use chemical antiseptics or solvents, which damage or destroy healthy body cells. Further cleansing of major wounds is beyond the scope of the Attendant and must be left to the attending physician.

Priority Action Approach for the Treatment of Major Wounds

1. Check the scene for hazards.
2. Begin the primary survey. Assess the airway with careful C-spine control and, if necessary, assist ventilation.
3. Provide supplemental high-flow oxygen.
4. Assess circulation. Control all major external bleeding with direct pressure. Indirect pressure or esmarch bandages may be required.
5. Irrigate the wound with sterile saline or tap water, if available. **Do not delay the rapid transport of patients in shock to irrigate the wound.**
6. Cover the wound with sterile gauze and/or ABD pads.
7. Apply an appropriate bandage to cover the dressings and maintain adequate pressure.
8. Any objects protruding from the wound should be left in place. The objects may require support with additional dressings. If the patient falls into the Rapid Transport Category, the dressings should be done en route. For these patients, treatment at the scene should be limited to major external bleeding only. DO NOT LET THE APPLICATION OF COMPLICATED DRESSINGS DELAY RAPID TRANSPORT OF PATIENTS WITH SHOCK OR THOSE WITH PENETRATING INJURIES TO THE HEAD, NECK OR TORSO.

9. Immobilize all limbs with major wounds to minimize further bleeding or injury. These patients should be transported by stretcher. (See Part XVI, Section A, page 357.)
10. Notify the physician, nurse or ambulance attendant of any suspected foreign bodies in the wound.

Management of Severed Parts

When treating a patient with an amputation, the Attendant must be primarily concerned with the ABCs of patient care. However, the Attendant must take steps to keep the severed part viable, in case it can be reimplanted. A well-preserved part may be reimplanted up to 24 hours after injury. However, if the following procedures are not instituted, the amputated part may only be viable for a few hours.

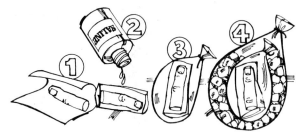

Management of a severed part

The following procedure applies to amputations, avulsed flaps of skin and tissue.
1. Find the severed part.
2. As carefully as possible, clean off any gross foreign matter. Pick off any large pieces of dirt but do not scrub the part.
3. Dress the part in sterile gauze, clean sheets or towels.
4. Moisten but do not soak the dressing with sterile saline. It is important that the amputated part not get water-logged. Do not place the part in soapy water, formalin or antiseptic solution.
5. Place the dressed part in a waterproof bag or container and seal it.
6. Place the bag or container inside another container that is filled with ice, preferably; if ice is not available, cold water. Do not freeze the part.

7. Transport the part with the patient.

DO NOT COMPROMISE PATIENT CARE. LIFE-SAVING PROCEDURES ALWAYS TAKE PRIORITY OVER MANAGEMENT OF THE SEVERED PART.

CRUSH SYNDROME

Most industrial injuries are caused by forces acting over a short period of time, i.e. a fall, heavy equipment accident, or an injury caused by a falling object. However, some crushing injuries cause damage to the body as a consequence of force being applied over a relatively long period. In addition to direct soft tissue damage, continued compression of the muscles and skin will cut off circulation leading to further tissue destruction. This type of injury is seen most often when the victim is trapped with the limbs compressed for several hours (e.g. in mine cave-ins, rock slides, collapsed buildings). Individuals whose legs are caught under heavy weight will continue to suffer tissue damage until the limbs are freed.

In tissues that are compressed this way, the cells become impaired and begin to leak watery fluid into the surrounding tissue. If the swelling is excessive, the resulting tissue pressure may compress already compromised blood vessels, leading to hypoxia and acidosis in the tissue with local cell death.

A syndrome is a set of symptoms or signs that occur together. The classic crush syndrome is an initial shock state caused by the prolonged compression injury and resultant generalized swelling, which may lead to kidney failure and death if not treated urgently and appropriately in a hospital.

The crush patient may seem to be uninjured when extricated. If possible, a history should be obtained as to the duration of compression. If the victim has been trapped for two hours or longer he/she most likely will complain of initial pain in the affected part, followed by numbness. Some patients are unable to give an adequate history due to the severity of associated injuries. A thorough examination is imperative, especially if there may be delays in transportation to hospital. As soon as the grime has been cleared away, look for patches of reddish skin, which indicates the area of compression. The victim's whole body must be examined for swelling, loss of sensation, pain on passive movement of muscle groups and loss of

power. In most cases the limbs are involved, but areas of pressure can also occur on the buttocks, trunk or neck. The reddish areas may progress to blister formation, which can be mistaken for a burn. Lacerations, dislocations and fractures may also be present.

Soon after it is released from compression, the affected limb becomes swollen and tense. The muscle is insensitive and paralyzed and superficial skin sensation is lost, usually in a patchy distribution. Later, the limb may go cold and blue and become pulseless. Such patients are often in shock. Severe thirst, generalized swelling and an elevated temperature may also be present.

Upon completion of the Priority Action Approach, and after attending to any life-threatening conditions, the victim should be treated as outlined for shock in Part V, Section B, page 102. These patients fall into the Rapid Transport Category.

The injured limb should be moved as little as possible. It should be kept cool with waterproof ice bags to decrease the rate of tissue and cell breakdown. Cold should be on for 10 minutes and off for 5 minutes, then reapplied. Cold may also help living tissue to survive despite a low blood supply. Immobilization may be useful to help delay absorption of the harmful muscle breakdown products.

LARGE EMBEDDED FOREIGN BODIES

Large embedded foreign bodies should be removed only by a physician.

When confronted with a patient with a large embedded foreign body, the Attendant must follow three general principles of management:

1. Do not move or alter the position of the foreign body. Attempt to control bleeding with direct pressure around the wound. If bleeding is arterial, a pressure point should be used. (See Part V, Section C, page 108 on Bleeding Management.)

2. A quick attempt should be made to stabilize the foreign body. Remember that penetrating injuries of the head, neck, chest, abdomen and groin fall into the Rapid Transport Category.

3. Patients with *LARGE* embedded foreign bodies who fall into the Rapid Transport Category should be comfortably immobilized on a long spine board, with the appropriate stabilization of the protruding foreign

body. The Attendant may have to shorten a very long object to facilitate transport. In these cases, the foreign body must be stabilized first.

PRESSURE INJECTION INJURIES

Pressure injections of any foreign material, such as paint, solvents, oil, grease, air or water into the body may produce devastating, disabling injuries. THEY MUST BE RECOGNIZED AND THE PATIENT REFERRED PROMPTLY TO A HOSPITAL. Delays in access to medical care may result in loss of an affected limb. An innocent-looking puncture wound to a finger or thumb may be the only evidence of a substance injected under pressure of 3,000 to 7,000 pounds per square inch (psi). The high pressure of industrial compressors can force the material along tendon sheaths, nerves and blood vessels. Damage is caused not only by the mechanical force but also by chemical irritation.

Important signs and symptoms:

- As with any other assessment, the Attendant must determine the mechanism of injury.
- A small puncture wound which may ooze grease, paint or other matter.
- Pain in the affected area, especially on movement; however, the onset of pain may be delayed for a few hours.
- Swelling and/or subcutaneous emphysema.

Part IX, Section E
First Aid Room Techniques and Procedures

Prevention of infection is an integral part of wound care. In the first aid room, handwashing is the most effective method for preventing transfer of infection to the patient, from one patient to another and from one part of the patient's body to another.

Clean equipment, a clean first aid room and good work habits are also important for infection control.

First aid procedures must be carried out with minimum risk to the First Aid Attendant. In some instances, the use of gloves is necessary to protect the First Aid Attendant from infection:

1. when touching secretions and excretions
2. when touching broken skin
3. when touching mucous membrane

HANDWASHING

Handwashing is essential to prevent infection and it must be practised by all Attendants. It is a procedure for cleansing the hands and wrists in order to remove foreign matter, including bacteria.

Handwashing Policies

1. Attendants should not wear jewellery on their fingers, with the exception of a simple wedding band.
2. Fingernails must be clean and trimmed.
3. Soap loosens dirt and grease, making it easy to remove them from the skin.
4. Running water carries dirt and debris away.
5. Use disposable paper towels.
6. A waste container for used paper towels should be near the washbasin.
7. The use of liquid soap is preferred (bar soap can contribute to transfer of infection).
8. Attendants must wash their hands:
   - when coming on duty
   - when the hands are visibly dirty
   - before and after contact with patients
   - before eating or going for break periods
   - after using the toilet
   - after blowing or wiping the nose
   - after handling soiled articles, instruments, dressings
   - before and after wound dressing procedures
   - before going home

Procedure

1. Wet hands thoroughly in warm, running water.
2. Add soap and make a lather, using a brisk scrubbing motion. Do not use a brush. Wash the fingers, palms, back of hands, wrists and under the nails. WASH SHOULD BE DONE FOR NO LESS THAN 10 SECONDS.
   Unlike an antiseptic, which inactivates bacteria, soap cleans by removing them and allowing them to be rinsed off. This is why it is necessary to wash vigorously when ordinary soap is used.
3. Rinse the hands thoroughly. The water should flow from the fingers back towards the wrists and arms.
4. Gently dry hands with a paper towel and USE THE TOWEL TO TURN OFF THE FAUCET. DISCARD THE USED TOWEL IN THE WASTE BASKET.
5. Frequent handwashing may lead to minor skin irritations. The Attendant is encouraged to use a protective lotion when off duty.

GLOVES

Whenever direct contact with any patient's blood or other body fluids is possible (e.g. care of open wounds), the use of gloves is MANDATORY! This serves to protect the First Aid Attendant from diseases carried by blood/body fluid. It does NOT take the place of infection control (i.e. handwashing).

Procedure

1. Wash hands.
2. Use disposable medical gloves.
3. Wear gloves while treating the patient and while cleaning up.
4. Discard gloves following each patient or procedure.
5. Wash hands.

CLEANING EQUIPMENT AND FURNITURE

The Attendant is responsible for clean equipment and a clean environment. This will require two steps: cleaning and disinfecting. Equipment and work surfaces must be cleaned and rinsed with a mild detergent and water to remove all organic material before they are disinfected. Sterilization, which kills all microorganisms, is rarely required in a first aid setting. If sterilization is required for some items, a small autoclave should be used, because chemical sterilization takes at least seven hours with the appropriate agent.

The Attendant will probably require two disinfectants, a non-rusting germicidal for soaking instruments and a chlorine-based solution for equipment and surfaces contaminated by blood or other body fluids.

Non-rusting Germicidals

Examples of these solutions are Sporicidin® and Cidex®. They should be mixed in a covered container because they can be reused for up to 28 days. The cover minimizes odour and evaporation. Specific directions will be found with each product. For example, instruments immersed in Cidex® (a glutaraldehyde) for 20 minutes will be thoroughly disinfected. They should then be rinsed with tap water and dried ready for reuse.

It is possible for an electrolytic type of corrosion to occur if two dissimilar metals are present in the same solution for 24 hours or longer. For this reason, it is recommended that the containers be plastic. Furthermore, instruments of different metals should each be soaked in their own separate plastic containers.

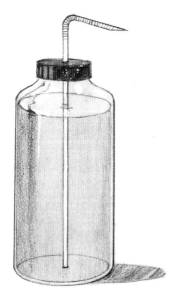

Sample cleaning bottle

Figure IX-2

Chlorine-Based Solutions

While chlorine bleach mixed in a 1:10 solution is an effective and inexpensive agent, it causes rust and damages plastic and aluminum. Sodium dichloroisocyanurate (NaDCC) is a buffered chlorine solution that is less corrosive. One example is Presept tablets, which dissolve in water. The solution remains stable for one week and can be effectively and safely used to wipe hard surfaces when mixed in a squirt bottle (see Figure IX-2). These bottles allow the solution to flow downward while the bottle itself is being held upright.

NOTE: Germicides may be considered a hazardous material under the Workplace Hazardous Materials Information System (WHMIS). It's important to cover container, consider ventilation and have an MSDS available.

PROCEDURES

Metal Instruments

1. Wear gloves.
2. Thoroughly clean the instruments with the mild detergent to remove debris. Rinse well with tap water. Shake off excess water.
3. Place equipment in the container of non-rusting germicide for the appropriate time (e.g. for Cidex®, a minimum of 20 minutes).
4. Rinse thoroughly with tap water, air dry and store in clean container.

Airway Equipment and Thermometers

1. Wear gloves.
2. Clean and rinse the airway equipment with the mild detergent to remove debris. Rinse well with tap water. Shake off excess water.
3. Immerse equipment in the buffered chlorine solution (e.g. Presept prepared in a 500 ppm solution) for 10 minutes.
4. Rinse thoroughly with tap water, air dry and store in clean plastic bag or container.

Large Equipment

A routine cleaning program (maintenance) must be in place. In addition, stretchers, treatment chairs, tables and counter tops, as well as the ambulance interior must be cleaned by the Attendant following any contamination.

1. Wear gloves.
2. Clean the surfaces with the mild detergent solution.
3. Spray and wipe the surfaces, using the buffered chlorine solution in the squirt bottle.
4. Use the squirt bottle on all hard-to-reach areas (e.g. stretcher frame).

First Aid Room and Ambulance

1. Keep the first aid room and the ambulance clean on an ongoing basis.
2. At least weekly, ensure that they receive a thorough cleaning.

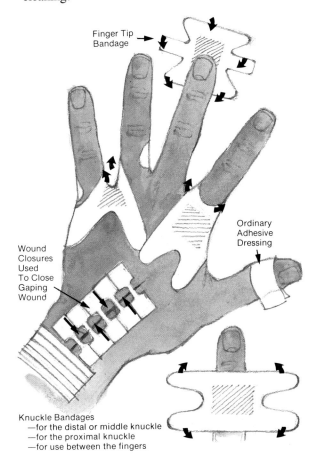

Finger Tip Bandage

Ordinary Adhesive Dressing

Wound Closures Used To Close Gaping Wound

Knuckle Bandages
—for the distal or middle knuckle
—for the proximal knuckle
—for use between the fingers

Typical hand and finger bandages

OPEN WOUND MANAGEMENT

Many minor injuries treated by the Attendant may not require medical attention. When treating minor injuries, the Attendant is accepting a serious responsibility. An Attendant must know one's own skills and limitations, and when to call for assistance.

Minor Wound Management

The following minor wounds are slow to heal and prone to infection. The Attendant should refer these patients to a physician.

1. Superficial wounds longer than 2 cm and wounds under 2 cm that gape when cleaned and are difficult to close.
2. Wounds that are jagged, irregular or where the flesh is destroyed or macerated.
3. Wounds that are deep or may have embedded foreign materials, such as glass, metal or wood.
4. Wounds that are cut so that there is a flap of full-thickness skin.
5. Wounds to the fingers, hands, toes or feet, even though small, may need suturing. Skin closures usually do not stay secure when the skin is mobile or under pressure. This applies particularly to the palms of the hands and soles of the feet.
6. Wounds over joints, such as knees or elbows, which cannot be easily immobilized for seven days.
7. Human bites and animal bites.
8. Wounds that are bleeding vigorously, such as scalp injuries, and that do not stop with pressure usually require sutures to arrest hemorrhage.
9. Facial wounds, unless the wound is very superficial and is not under tension when closed, may leave visible scars.
10. Wounds that are very dirty with ground-in dirt, asphalt, etc., or that are associated with large contaminated abrasions.

Once the Attendant decides to refer the patient to a physician, the worker should get to a medical facility as soon as possible, preferably within six hours.

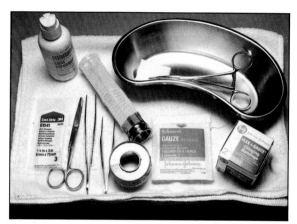

Equipment for minor wound management

Management of Minor Wounds and Lacerations

1. The Attendant must wash his or her hands and put on gloves.
2. The wound should be fully exposed. This may require removal of clothing.
3. The wound is assessed for type and mechanism of injury as well as the need for referral.
4. Wounds in hairy areas (scalp, limbs) that will be cared for by the Attendant should have the hair shaved approximately one centimetre back from the wound edges to facilitate treatment. EYEBROWS MUST NOT BE SHAVED AS THEY MAY NOT GROW BACK IN.
5. The cleansing solution is chosen. Recommended solutions to have available are:
   - Normal saline — non-irritating irrigating solution, can be used in any clean wound. THIS IS THE ONLY SOLUTION USED FOR A WOUND NEAR THE EYES.
   - Mild antibacterial, detergent solution (e.g. Savalon®, Hibidil) is used for most wound cleansing. It can be used full strength for wound cleansing but should be diluted in clean water, 10 ml of concentrated soap solution in 200 ml of water for soaking wounds.
   - Hydrogen peroxide (3%) — germicidal, useful for removing foreign material, dead or damaged tissues (e.g. for puncture wounds, animal bites or old infected wounds). Must not be used on wounds requiring sutures as the edges of the wound will be damaged, delaying healing.

   The following solutions are NOT recommended:
   - Alcohol — destroys healthy tissue.
   - Iodine — destroys healthy tissue.
   - Zephirin hydrochloride — loses potency in storage and becomes unsterile.
   - Mercurochrome or other coloured solutions — colours the wound, making identification of underlying structures and developing infection difficult.
   - Commercial first aid creams — of no value to the patient.
6. The area surrounding the wound is cleansed. The wound is covered with sterile gauze and held steady with one hand while the Attendant cleanses the surrounding skin with the other hand. Using sterile gauze dampened with the cleansing solution, the Attendant must work outward from the wound and discard the swabs often. An area of several centimetres around the wound is cleansed. ABSORBENT COTTON OR PAPER TISSUES MUST NOT BE USED; SHREDS OF THESE MATERIALS MAY REMAIN IN THE WOUND.
7. The wound is cleansed. The wound is gently spread apart and explored for blood clots and foreign material. Blood clots often contain specks of dirt. If dirt and grime are embedded in the wound, they may have to be gently removed using sterile gauze and a mild antibacterial, detergent solution. If the wound is especially dirty or contains blood clots that do not come out, the wound should be irrigated with one part three percent hydrogen peroxide to three parts sterile saline. This will help dissolve blood clots and clean the wound. Diluted hydrogen peroxide is especially helpful in removing blood clots from the hair. A three percent concentration of hydrogen peroxide will burn the wound and should not be left on the area for long.
8. THE NEED FOR REFERRAL SHOULD BE REASSESSED AFTER EXAMINATION OF THE WOUND. When the wound is clean, it should be irrigated with copious amounts of saline.
9. The wound area is prepared for the application of skin closures.

- To ensure adhesion of the closure, wound edges should be dried and hair removed.
- Tincture of benzoin (Friar's Balsam) may be applied sparingly around the wound to increase the stickiness of the surface. Cotton-tipped applicators are used to ensure that the compound does not get into the wound where it will irritate and burn.

  Tincture of benzoin takes about a minute to dry.

10. Lacerations and minor avulsions are taped.

  Butterfly bandages or other skin-closure tapes may be used to bridge the wound. They are available commercially in a variety of sizes.

- Apply one skin closure at a time. Apply half of the skin closure up to the wound margin and press it firmly into place.
- Close up the skin edges with clean fingers and press the free half of the closure firmly into place. A large skin closure may be applied temporarily to the centre of the wound as a holding device.
- Apply additional strips of butterflies to complete the closure.
- If any of the initial closures are incorrectly applied, they can easily be removed and repositioned.
- If a "holding" skin closure is used, it may be removed when the rest of the closures are in place. Lift the edges on the same side of each flap and gently pull them off along the long axis of the wound to avoid straining the other skin closures. Finally, a strip of adhesive may be laid over all the flaps on each side of the wound. This will lend strength to the closures and increase the surface area being used for adhesion.
- A large bandage may be applied to cover the entire wound dressing. The adhesive of the outer dressing should not touch the adhesive of any of the skin closures. The outer dressing should not touch the adhesive of any of the skin closures. The outer dressing may have to be changed, but the skin closures should stay in place for at least 10 days.
- Skin closures are not recommended in these situations. Medical referral is required:

  - wounds with irregular edges or lacerations with poor proximation of the skin edges;
  - areas affected by musculoskeletal movement, such as joints;
  - wounds with high skin tension or where there is marked retraction of the skin;
  - moist or hairy regions such as the axilla, groin, genitalia or perineum.

11. The Attendant must advise the patient to keep the dressings clean and dry in order to prevent infection. The patient is instructed to watch for signs of infection (see below).

  The Attendant advises the patient to make sure his or her tetanus immunization is up to date (for clean minor wounds, tetanus immunization within the past five years is considered adequate). This immunization should be obtained within 24 hours.

12. The Attendant should have the patient return in 24 to 48 hours for follow-up.

- The wound is checked for infection.

  The outer dressing should be removed after 24 to 48 hours to check for infection. A small amount of redness and swelling beside the wound is part of the normal healing process. Redness, heat, swelling and tenderness are signs of infection. Pus may be present. If there is infection, all the closures should be removed and the wound allowed to drain. It should be irrigated and the patient referred to a physician.

- Treatment continues until the wound heals.

  If no infection is found after the first dressing change, the wound should heal well. The skin closures should be left on for 10 days. Closures on the patient's face may be removed after five days.

A healing wound does not achieve its greatest strength for about two or three weeks. Even after the skin closures have been taken off, a dressing should be used until the wound is two weeks old. The outer dressing may be changed as often as necessary if it becomes soiled or wet. The dressing should be changed to check on progress of healing every two or three days.

The patient should be instructed to keep the dressings clean and dry in order to prevent infection.

SPECIFIC PROCEDURES

The following chart describes the specific procedures for managing minor wounds.

TYPE OF WOUND	DESCRIPTION/CAUSES	ASSESSMENT	MANAGEMENT/SPECIAL NOTES
ABRASIONS	• Loss of the outer protective layer of skin so blood vessels are exposed. • Usually due to rubbing on a hard surface, e.g. "rug burns" or "road rash". • Common in children, cyclists and motorcycle riders	• Major consideration is the amount of contamination, because small dirt and/or rock particles easily become embedded in these wounds.	• Cleanse the wound by scrubbing and irrigating the area. Referral may be required if abrased areas are extensive or if scrubbing is too painful for the patient. • Sometimes the cleansing process can cause small arterial bleeds. Apply pressure to the area to control bleeding. • Minor abrasions may be left undressed; large abrasions in areas where clothes will irritate them (e.g. knees, elbows) should be covered with a non-adherent dressing (e.g. Telfa® or Jellnet®). • Will require tetanus toxoid if indicated.
LACERATIONS AND AVULSIONS	• Open wound or tear in the skin. • May be deep or superficial. • Edges of lacerations may be jagged or neat. • Variety of causes.	NOTE: • Location of wound(s). • Mechanism of injury. • Apparent depth of wound. • Is bleeding controlled? • Are edges neat or jagged? • Possible contamination.	• *Lacerations that will require suturing should not be cleansed with peroxide.* • Use the anti-bacterial detergent to cleanse wounds except those around the eye, which should be cleansed with saline.
PUNCTURE WOUNDS	• A penetration of the tissues with a blunt or pointed object, which may result in underlying tissue damage. • Common causes are stab wounds, stepping on a nail, etc.	• These wounds may appear small on the outside but may have caused severe damage inside. • Note mechanism of injury, location and superficial appearance of wound. • May be minimal external bleeding.	• These wounds are not sutured due to the likelihood of contamination below the surface. • Clean the wound with soap and warm water. • Soak the wound in a diluted hydrogen peroxide solution or the detergent antibacterial solution (15-20 minutes). • Instruct patient to continue the soaks at home 3 or 4 times a day for 48 hours. Have patient return for reassessment after 2 days.

SMALL FOREIGN OBJECTS IN WOUNDS

Foreign bodies are very common and can be any material. They can vary in size from small slivers and pieces of glass to large impaled objects as in Part IX, Section D, page 211.

SLIVERS

Wooden Slivers

Locating a small wooden sliver is often difficult for two reasons:

1. The sliver may be flesh-coloured and completely embedded.
2. The patient may report for treatment after attempting to remove it.

Locating small wooden slivers

1. Cleanse the area thoroughly but gently with the detergent solution and dry it with gauze.
2. Paint the area with a coloured solution (e.g. Povidone-Iodine). Allow the area to remain wet for 15 to 30 seconds, then wipe the colour away with gauze.
   If the end of the sliver is close to the surface, it will soak up some of the coloured antiseptic and show up as a dark spot.

Removing the sliver

1. Determine the angle of the sliver.
2. Grasp the end of the sliver with a pair of sliver forceps. Withdraw the sliver in the same direction as it entered.
3. After removal, treat the wound as for a puncture or laceration (see page 216).

Metal Slivers

This type of sliver enters the flesh either:

1. while the worker is handling metal materials; or
2. from flying metal, such as a chip that breaks off the head of a chisel when it is struck by a hammer.

If metal slivers can be seen and easily removed, they are managed as wooden slivers. Staining is not helpful.

If the mechanism of injury suggests that the sliver was travelling with sufficient force to penetrate and damage deeper structures (e.g. joint), do not probe the wound.

Dress the wound, immobilize the area and refer the patient to medical attention.

Any sliver, whether wood or metal, which may have penetrated a joint or gone deep enough into the flesh to damage deeper structures, must be immobilized and referred to medical attention.

Glass Slivers

Glass slivers are commonly found in fingers or soles of feet. They are usually invisible to the naked eye and therefore difficult to remove with sliver forceps. After soaking the affected area with detergent solution in hot water for 20 minutes, the sliver may be removed with gentle scrubbing. A large piece of glass may be removed by the Attendant only if it comes out easily and does not involve a vital structure (e.g. neck). Bleeding, which may occur after removal, can be controlled by direct pressure. If the wound is large enough, it may require referral to a physician for suturing. Small wounds may be treated and closed as previously described.

FISH HOOKS

If a fish hook is caught in the soft fleshy part of the skin and the point is almost or actually poking through the skin, the hook can be pushed further through the skin and the barb cut off. The remaining portion can then be backed out.

If the fish hook is pointing towards deeper structures, the patient should be referred.

Patients with fish hook injuries must be observed carefully for signs of inflammation or infection for several days. They should soak the affected part in warm, salty (one level teaspoon per two litres) water four times a day for five to ten minutes. The patient should be questioned to make sure he has had a tetanus immunization or should be given immunization if his shots are more than five years old.

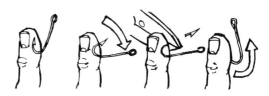

Fish hook removal

SUBUNGUAL HEMATOMA

A blow or crush injury to a finger or toe frequently causes a collection of blood to form under the nail bed. This condition, which is called a subungual hematoma, may cause throbbing and be very painful. If the blood is released, the patient feels some relief. The blood may be evacuated through a small hole in the nail at the centre of the collection of blood. If a nail drill is unavailable, the hole can be made with the red-hot end of an opened paper clip. The nail has no nerve endings so this procedure is painless. A pair of pliers or locking forceps should be used to hold the paper clip steady. The Attendant should ensure that the patient's hand or foot is on a firm surface. If releasing the blood does not stop the pain, a fracture of the distal phalanx should be suspected and the patient referred for medical attention. If there is initial relief, but the blood returns, instruct the patient to use a sterilized needle to reopen the hole.

PATIENTS WITH BADLY CRUSHED DISTAL PHALANGES OR DISTAL FINGER-JOINT INJURIES SHOULD NOT BE GIVEN THIS TREATMENT. THEY SHOULD BE REFERRED FOR MEDICAL ATTENTION.

RING REMOVAL

Injured fingers frequently swell. If the patient is wearing a ring proximal or near the injury, the swelling may impair blood circulation in the finger. Rings on fingers near an injury should be removed.

Most patients who have a swollen finger from a contusion, sprain, burn, insect bite or edema can have their rings removed by simple lubrication of the finger with soap or petroleum jelly. If this does not work, the string method can be used. Wrap the finger with string from the tip to the ring, then insert the string under the ring. The ring is pulled distally as the string is unwound. (See Fig-

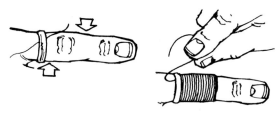

Ring removal
Figure IX-3

ure IX-3.) This method cannot be used where there are major lacerations or the finger is crushed. In these cases, the ring must be removed with diagonal cutters or a special ring cutter.

ABSCESS (BOIL)

An abscess (boil) is a localized collection of pus within the tissues.

They are usually found in hair-bearing areas.

Treatment usually involves draining the abscess. This will occur naturally if the abscess is left alone for a few days. The process can be hastened by local application of hot or warm compresses until, after a day or two, the skin bursts, allowing the pus to escape. Once the core is discharged, dry dressings should be applied. Clean the area intermittently with an alcohol swab as necessary. NOTE: Neither the patient or the Attendant should squeeze the abscess. This action is likely to cause the infection to spread to deeper structures.

If an abscess is large or very painful, or involves the face, neck, groin or buttocks, referral to a physician for surgical drainage is indicated. This should also apply if the patient is generally feeling sick, has a fever, or if local measures don't seem to be effective within 12 hours.

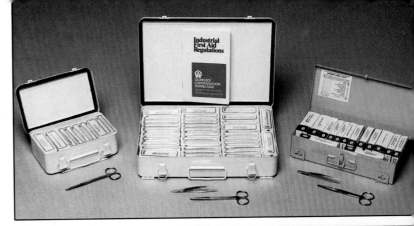

BANDAGES AND SLINGS

The Industrial First Aid Regulations list the various equipment and supplies for use in industrial first aid kits. This section describes those basic items the Attendant will be working with most of the time.

Dressings

Dressings and bandages differ in appearance and function.

Dressings are for use in the initial covering of open wounds to prevent further contamination.

First aid kits and rooms are usually equipped with a wide variety of dressings.

Dressings range from the common adhesive strips to very large bulky items, commonly known as abdominal dressings, ABD pads or drainage dressings.

Most commercially obtained dressings are individually wrapped for sterility.

Very large dressings, including abdominal or multi-trauma types, may be wrapped in plastic but not be sterile. Usually these types of dressings are used as soakers. A soaker is a pad that covers the sterile gauze dressing on a wound and soaks up excess blood.

A wound dressing must have these characteristics:

1. It must be larger than the wound.
2. It must be sterile, if possible.
3. It must be thick, soft and compressible to permit evenly distributed pressure over the entire area of the wound.
4. It should have a lint-free surface.

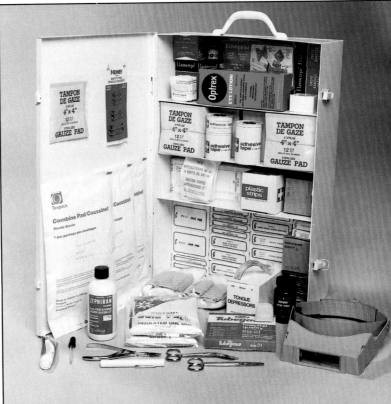

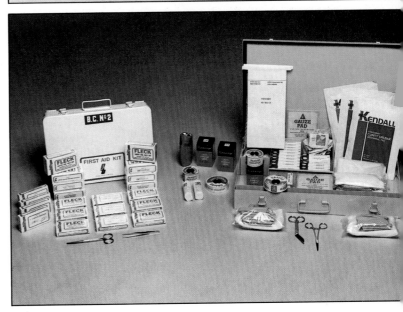

Industrial First Aid kits

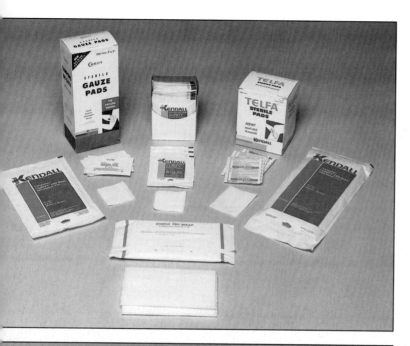

Bandages

A bandage is used to secure any dressing covering a wound. The most common types of bandages are:

1. crepe or tension elastic roller type, usually 5 cm to 15 cm wide and 4.5 metres long when stretched;
2. self-adhering, form-fitting roller;
3. elastic adhesive-backed roller;
4. gauze roller;
5. tubular gauze;
6. triangular.

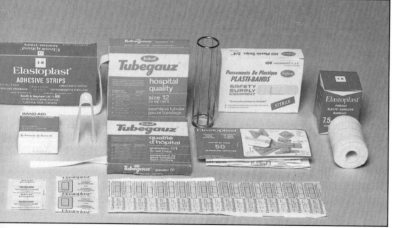

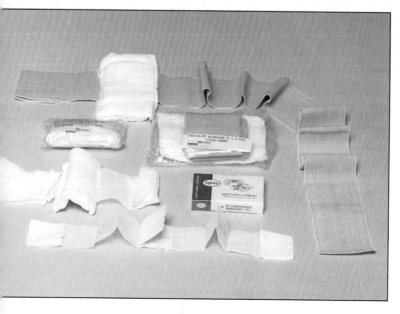

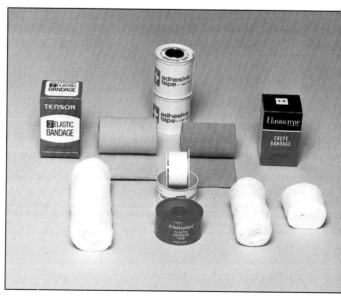

Typical bandages and dressings

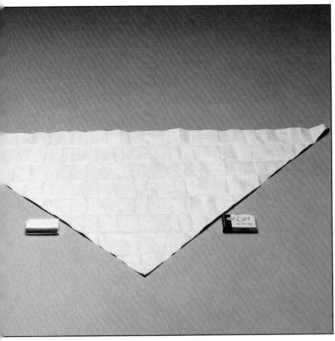

Open triangular bandage

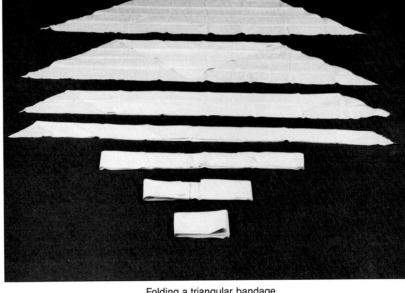

Folding a triangular bandage

The triangular bandage is the oldest type of bandage and one of the most versatile. It can be used:

- to secure dressings in place;
- to apply and maintain pressure to bleeding wounds, as with the loop tie;
- for slings to support upper limbs;
- to secure splints to the body or limb;
- as extra padding to fill body curves;
- to pad splints;
- to be folded or unfolded, making a narrow, broad or roller bandage;
- to be applied quickly and efficiently to any part of the body without moving the patient.

The triangular bandage is a piece of material 150 cm to 160 cm in length at the base and consists of the following parts:

- a base
- a point
- two sides
- two ends

A broad bandage is made by bringing the point down to the base and then folding it once. A narrow band-age is made by folding the broad bandage a second time. When not in use the bandage should be folded as follows:

- Make the unfolded bandage into a narrow band-age.
- Bring each end to meet in the centre.
- Double the bandage upon itself. When stored like this the triangular bandage can be unfolded to make a narrow bandage for immediate use.

Several methods can be used to secure the ends of a triangular bandage. The most common method is the square or reef knot. Square knots are recommended because they do not slip once tightened and they can be easily untied.

A surgeon's knot is sometimes used since it will not slip while being tied.

Bulky supports for large embedded foreign bodies can be made from triangular bandages. If there is hemorrhage and a protruding foreign body or bone fragment, a ring pad is recommended to provide pressure and prevent further tissue injury.

Slings

Slings may be used to support an injured upper limb. Four types of slings can be used. The large arm sling is used when full arm support is required. The small arm sling is used to support the wrist and hand, leaving the elbow free. The triangular arm sling holds the forearm with the elbow in acute flexion. The collar and cuff sling is used for the same purpose as a small arm sling. It will not slip off the patient's arm and is useful when the arm is flexed or extended more than 90 degrees.

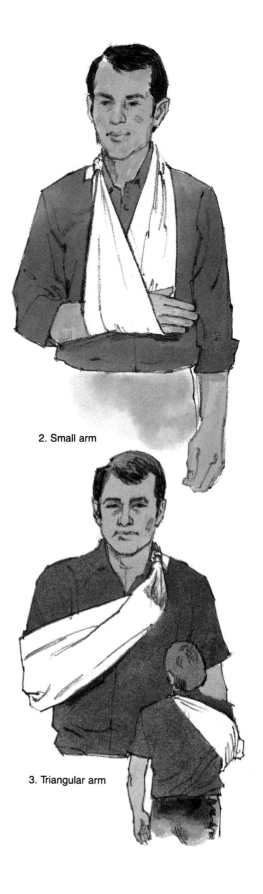

2. Small arm

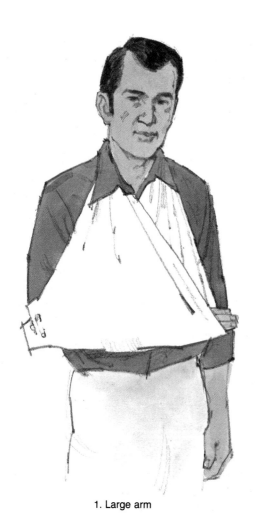

1. Large arm

3. Triangular arm

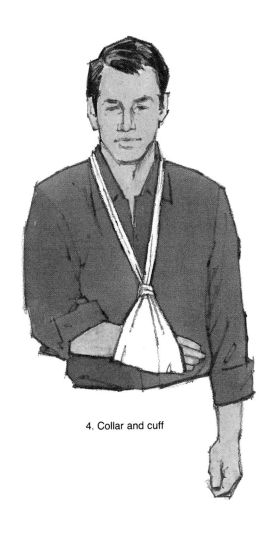

4. Collar and cuff

Principles of Bandaging

1. The bandage must be tight enough to control hemorrhage and immobilize the wound but not tight enough to constrict circulation to any parts distal to the injury.
2. The bandage must be applied so that pressure to the wound is evenly distributed over the entire area.
3. The bandage must cover the entire dressing.
4. Where possible, fingers and toes should be accessible for checking circulation and distal pulses.
5. Bandage knots must be accessible.
6. Bandage knots must not put pressure on the body, which may cause sores.
7. Roller bandages must not encircle a limb underneath splints; they may impair circulation.

NON-PRESCRIPTION DRUGS IN FIRST AID ROOMS

Periodically, an Attendant may have occasion to dispense a non-prescription drug (i.e. aspirin, antihistamine). The onus is on the Attendant to ensure that he or she is familiar with the common side effects of these medications, as well as the indications and contraindications for their use.

Aside from the issue of allergic reactions and other reactions of an adverse type, other issues should be taken into consideration. Specifically, there are some medications which may cause drowsiness, or interfere with the alertness and manual dexterity normally required by a worker in the performance of their duties.

RECORDS AND REPORTS

The Attendant's duties include keeping records of all first aid treatments given. It is very important that these records and reports are clear, concise and correct. Although prompt and effective first aid treatment is always the first priority, an accurate and factual account of the patient's condition, from the time of the accident until arrival at a medical facility, is also of great importance. Records and reports ensure the continuity of treatment to the patient and provide information vital to the worker's and employer's interest. All the necessary information may not be available to the Attendant at the time of the accident. It must be gathered and recorded as soon as possible afterward. With experience, the Attendant will learn to obtain most of the information required while giving care to the patient at the same time.

The first essential in any record is an adequate identification of the patient. If the person is conscious, ask for full name and be sure the spelling is correct. The person may be well known to you, but the name may be duplicated many times among the million claims on file with the Workers' Compensation Board. The inclusion of the patient's birth date or Social Insurance Number will ensure positive identification.

The Attendant in British Columbia must be familiar with the following forms and records:
• Treatment Record Book
• Form 7A — First Aid Report
• Form 7 — Employer's Report of Injury or Industrial Disease

- Form 6 — Application for Compensation and Report of Injury or Industrial Disease
- Form 8 — Physician's Report
- Form 9 — Employer's Subsequent Statement

Treatment Record Book

Any first aid report could provide information later on a worker's compensation claim, so it is critically important that the record is full and accurate.

THE DETAILS OF ALL INJURIES ARE TO BE ENTERED IN THE RECORD BOOK, USUALLY BY THE ATTENDANT. RECORDS MUST BE MADE OF ALL REPORTED INJURIES, COMPLAINTS OF ILLNESS, ALL TREATMENT AND FOLLOW-UP CARE GIVEN TO EACH PATIENT. Information given by the patient and signs and symptoms obtained by the Attendant upon examination must be recorded. The names and addresses of witnesses, if any, should also be noted.

The record should show the time and nature of the accident and the exact time that the patient was first seen by the Attendant. The actual injuries should be described precisely. Accepted medical terms should be used wherever possible, to avoid misinterpretation. Do not confuse symptoms with physical signs. Describe fully and accurately signs that are seen, felt or heard during examination of the patient. There must be an entry in the Treatment Record Book for every treatment rendered, every minor injury, each re-dressing and the application of every bandaid. The injury may not be disabling or need medical aid, but at a future point, this record may be the only material evidence that an accident had occurred.

Describe accurately the patient's complaints and any physical findings. If there is no visible mark, report that.

The time of the accident and of the examination should be reported as accurately as possible. An Attendant who goes to the scene of the accident should record the condition in which the patient is found. If the patient was treated at the first aid room, a description of the arrival should be recorded.

Treatment Record Books are provided by the employer and should be kept in the first aid room. When they are full, they should be kept for at least five years after the date of the last entry. WCB officers will want to see the record books when inspecting the work site.

First Aid Report — Form 7A

When first aid is given to an injured worker or the worker reports any injury or industrial disease and is sent to or advised to see a physician or qualified practitioner, the Attendant completes a Form 7A and gives it to the employer for submission to the Workers' Compensation Board.

All information recorded should be checked against the Treatment Record Book for errors or omissions.

Employer's Report of Injury or Industrial Disease — Form 7

The employer of a worker who has been, or claims to have been, injured or who has sustained an occupational disease that requires medical attention must file a Form 7 within three days, whether or not there was any time loss.

The Form 7 should be signed by a company official who is authorized to make expenditures on behalf of the employer. Where there are circumstances that require additional explanation, the explanation should be given in a letter, attached to the Form 7. All information on the Form 7 should be checked against the Treatment Record Book for any errors or omissions.

Application for Compensation and Report of Injury or Industrial Disease — Form 6

A Form 6 is sent directly to the worker by the Workers' Compensation Board. It is used by the injured worker to make a claim to the Workers' Compensation Board if the disability is likely to result in time loss of one or more working days. If the worker asks for help in completing the form, the Attendant may assist.

Employer's Subsequent Statement — Form 9

A Form 9 is completed by the employer when the injured worker returns to work or is able to return to work. Ordinarily the Attendant will not be involved in the completion of a Form 9.

Physician's Report — Form 8

A Form 8, Physician's Report, is the responsibility of the physician or qualified practitioner who attends the injured worker.

Ordinarily, neither the Attendant, the employer nor the worker will be involved in completion of the Form 8.

Patient Evaluation Chart

Copies of a patient evaluation chart should be kept handy in the first aid kit, the emergency transportation vehicle or the ambulance. It should be completed accurately and accompany the patient to medical aid whenever possible. It indicates the patient's condition when first examined by the Attendant and any changes in the condition over a period of time. An evaluation chart is especially necessary when there is a head injury, and it should always accompany the patient.

The Attendant's Responsibility

- Provide first aid care and treatment in the best interest of the injured worker to the best of the Attendant's ability.
- Keep accurate records.
- Complete and forward reports promptly.

When forms are not correctly filled in or are sent to the WCB late, there can be long and unnecessary delays in the processing of claims.

NOTE: COMPENSATION PAYMENT

The Attendant should never give an opinion on whether or not compensation will be paid. That is the decision of the Workers' Compensation Board.

Part IX, Section F
Occupational Dermatitis

Many people who have never before experienced "skin trouble" may occasionally develop some form of "dermatitis" relating to their work environment.

Taken as a group, the most commonly encountered type of occupational disease is that of dermatitis. Most occupational skin disease results from contact with a chemical substance, of which there are hundreds of thousands in common use today.

Chemicals can affect the skin in two ways:

- as a direct irritant
- by causing an allergy

"Primary irritant contact dermatitis" is by far the most common, making up about 75% of all occupational skin disease.

SIGNS AND SYMPTOMS

The first symptoms are usually redness, irritation and occasionally swelling. The patient may complain of itchiness and sometimes pain. Blistering may sometimes occur, to the point of weeping. Thickening and fissuring (cracking) may develop later. Superimposed bacterial or fungal infection can be a complication of the underlying condition. With long-term exposure, some substances are known to be carcinogenic (cancer-causing).

Any part of the body that comes into contact with one of those agents can be affected. Usually, it's the hands and forearms, but a dust, mist or fume can cause inflammation of the face, neck, ankles or other exposed areas. The belt area and anterior thighs adjacent to the pockets may also be affected.

Dermatitis is not contagious, unless secondarily infected, but can spread to other parts of the body if left untreated.

THE CORRECT TREATMENT — STARTED EARLY — IS ESSENTIAL TO THE CONTROL OF DERMATITIS.

PRIMARY IRRITANTS

A skin irritant is any substance that damages the skin by direct contact rather than by allergy.

Virtually any substance can be an irritant under certain circumstances, depending on a variety of factors that include the susceptibility of the individual and the circumstances of contact — such as concentration of the substance and length of time of exposure.

Acids and alkalis are examples of primary irritants.

SENSITIZERS

Sensitizers do not affect everyone, only those individuals who have a particular susceptibility to them. The symptoms may not arise until some time after the initial exposure, even developing on parts of the body that were not exposed to the sensitizing agent. Once an individual has become sensitized to a substance, he or she probably will remain so. Also, it is not unusual for the reaction to occur with progressively smaller amounts of the sensitizer with each subsequent exposure. The sensitivity may also develop with exposure to other chemicals of a similar nature. Other individuals may exhibit a sensitivity initially, only to develop a tolerance over time, and eventually not react to the sensitizing agent at all.

Some substances can be both an irritant and a sensitizer.

CHEMICAL CAUSES OF DERMATITIS

The following groups of compounds are recognized as the main causes of industrial dermatitis:

1. Mineral oils
2. Solvents
3. Other chemical groups
   - Acids and alkalis
   - Oxidizing/reducing agents (e.g. hydrogen peroxide)
   - Protein precipitants (e.g. formalin)
   - Allergens (e.g. cedar dust)

1. Mineral Oils

Mineral oils often cause "oil acne", due mainly to the blocking of the hair follicle by dirt. Symptoms: blackheads and pimples wherever there is frequent contact with oil and oily clothing. Normal skin function is prevented and inflammation follows. The next stage is likely to be infection.

The condition can become worse through prolonged contact with mineral oils. The presence of wart-like or other swellings, ulcers and sore patches that do not heal can be early warning signs of cancer and should be checked by a doctor.

Covered parts of the body may be affected, as well as exposed areas such as the hands and face. Workers should understand the importance of protecting the skin in their genital areas.

In the early stages, such conditions respond well to treatment with little personal inconvenience or time lost from work. However, treatment must not be delayed.

The same dangers and precautions as for mineral oils apply to workers who come in contact with pitch, tar and some of their derivatives. Furthermore, some of those substances are known to be carcinogenic.

2. Solvents

Solvents like kerosene, turpentine, acetone and trichloroethylene remove the natural oils from the skin, leaving it vulnerable to damage by other substances.

It may take several hours or longer to replace the natural surface coating removed by solvents. Long periods of immersion in water-based fluids can also weaken the protective action of the skin.

HOW TO PREVENT OCCUPATIONAL DERMATITIS

It is far easier to prevent occupational dermatitis than to cure it, but effective prevention requires full cooperation between management and employees.

The following guidelines are designed to eliminate contact between irritant and skin where possible and to care for skin that has been exposed.

A Safer Workplace

Wherever a material in use is known to be harmful, every effort should be made to eliminate it or to switch to a safer substance.

A Safer Worker

Despite all the precautions taken to provide a safer working environment, contact with dermatitis-causing substances will still be necessary in certain industries. The worker must be protected with suitable apparel. THE IMPORTANCE OF PERSONAL CLEANLINESS CANNOT BE OVEREMPHASIZED.

A GUIDE TO PERSONAL PROTECTION

Personal Cleanliness

Personal cleanliness is vital in the prevention of occupational dermatitis. It is extremely important to remove all dirt and contaminants from the skin at the end of the work day, as well as before breaks (e.g. eating or smoking).

Effective cleansing facilities must be provided by the employer wherever irritating substances are a hazard, and the employees should use those facilities.

For maximum protection against dermatitis after exposure to irritants:
- Use the cleanser or soap provided.
- Rinse thoroughly with running water.
- Dry completely on clean towels or with hot air dryers.
- Use baths or showers when provided.
- Where possible, change clothing (including socks and underwear) at the end of the day, preferably at the work site.
- Ideally, all contaminated work clothing should be washed professionally. If washed at home, work clothing must be laundered separately from the family clothing.
- Always wash hands before and after using toilet facilities.
- Do not smoke a cigarette when there is a contaminant on the hands.

Selecting Cleansing Agents

Washing with soap and water is simple and usually sufficient. The quality of the soap is important.

A good quality super-fatted soap (liquid, gel or tablet) that lathers well is safe and adequate, but some soaps and domestic detergents can be harsh on sensitive skin. Some of the popular face and bath soaps are not pure soap at all but non-fatted chemical detergent. Dermatologists have found this soap particularly damaging to irritated skin and sometimes even to normal skin. In some cases, soap may not be enough to cope with deeply ingrained dirt and water-repellent substances like paint and tar.

Special skin cleansers, usually in gel form, have been developed to control dermatitis by keeping the skin healthy. The gel is rubbed in well to loosen all dirt and then washed away in running water. Waterless skin cleansers are available for use where there is no water supply. Liquid and gel skin cleansers and creams should be in specially designed dispensers, to reduce the risk of cross-infection.

Conditioning cream should be applied at the end of the work day, especially when the activity or frequent washing tend to remove the skin's natural secretions.

Avoid the use of solvents such as methyl hydrate, kerosene, paint thinners and acetone. They remove too much of the skin's natural oils and they, too, can cause dermatitis. Repeated use of coarse abrasives (pumice stone or dry powders) can also be harmful to the skin.

Protective Clothing

Depending on the nature of the job, protective clothing can include overalls, aprons, gloves, footwear, leggings and face shields. They should protect exposed skin and the worker's own clothing, which may absorb an irritant and prolong the skin's exposure to it.

The following advice can be given to workers who are exposed to dermatitis-causing substances:

Wash all clothing frequently. There is no point in washing the skin thoroughly, then covering it with a contaminated coverall.

NOTE: THIS IS ESPECIALLY IMPORTANT FOR THOSE WHO WORK WITH MINERAL OILS. PROLONGED CONTACT WITH OILY MATERIALS MAY RESULT IN CANCER OF THE SKIN.

- Wash protective clothing frequently.
- Regularly inspect all protective apparel for excessive contamination, holes or worn areas. This especially applies to gloves, which wear out quickly.
- Non-fabric gloves such as rubber, PVC and neoprene should be used only when necessary, or as recommended for specific chemicals. They provide no ventilation and can themselves cause irritation.
- Never change into oil-stained coveralls.
- Do not put an oily rag into pants pockets; it may affect the skin underneath.

Barrier Creams

Where protective clothing cannot be used and exposure to an irritant is unavoidable, protect the skin with barrier cream. The cream will shield the skin from contact with the hazardous substance and make cleansing easier. However, other preventive measures should still be followed, even though a barrier cream is used.

It is important to choose the correct cream for a particular situation, because some promote absorption of certain substances rather than hinder it. A safety equipment supplier or industrial supply house should be able to advise on the proper cream.

When using barrier creams:

- Be sure the skin is clean and dry before application.
- Remove the cream by washing after each work session, and before meal time and coffee breaks.
- Apply fresh cream to clean skin to provide continuous protection.
- Read and follow the manufacturer's directions.

Treatment

For serious skin injury resulting from highly caustic or irritant chemicals, see the section on Poisons, Part XII, Section A, page 316, and also the section on Management of Chemical Burns, Part XI, Section C, page 290.

Injuries or dermatitis, however minor, should be protected with a suitable dressing. Signs of skin irritation of any kind should be reported to a physician. Early advice and treatment can prevent a minor case from becoming serious, and will reduce the chance of long-term disability. It may also minimize the chance of a recurrence for those who cannot completely avoid exposure to an offending agent.

HIVES (URTICARIA)

Hives is a common skin reaction, affecting as much as 20% of the population at some time during their lives. It can be considered as a skin response that follows exposure of the affected person to a substance to which they are allergic. Though not invariably due to allergy, that is by far the most common cause likely to be encountered by the IFA Attendant.

The exposure may occur by several routes:

- Direct contact
- Inhalation
- Ingestion

The response may be:

- Localized (e.g. mosquito bite)
- Generalized (e.g. drug reaction)

Other, rarely encountered causes for urticaria might include certain types of infection, cancer, sunshine, scratching and even emotion.

Signs and Symptoms

1. Raised, reddened, swollen wheals with sharply defined map-like borders. Diameter can range from less than one centimetre to several centimetres in size.
2. Intense itching or prickly sensation.
3. May be associated with chest tightness, wheezing and cardiovascular collapse (anaphylaxis). See Part V, Section C, page 101.

Treatment

Local

- Cool compresses
- Antipruritic (anti-itch) lotions (calamine, oatmeal)

Orally

- Antihistamines (chlorpheniramine, astemizole, terfenedine)

Injection

- Adrenaline — to be used only in case of anaphylaxis (see Part V, Section C, page 101).

Part IX, Section G
Cumulative Trauma Disorders

TENDONITIS AND TENOSYNOVITIS

Definition

A tendon is a band of strong white fibrous tissue that connects a muscle to a bone. A tendon is often surrounded by a sheath of specialized tissue called the synovial sheath, which lubricates the tendon and allows it to glide smoothly through the surrounding tissues.

Inflammation of the tendon (tendonitis) and of its synovial sheath (tenosynovitis) often occur simultaneously. For the purposes of the IFA Attendant, the two conditions can be considered the same. They may also be confused with bursitis (see below) because they are often situated close to one another anatomically, and the symptoms and signs may be identical.

The cause of these inflammatory conditions is often obscure. A number of factors have been identified:

- Age — the conditions are more common in middle or older age groups, perhaps because of changes of blood supply and aging of the tissues.
- Direct trauma — may occur following blunt trauma or with sudden stretching of the tendon.
- Excessive use — RSI (repetitive strain injury), also known as CTD (cumulative trauma disorder) tend to occur where there is frequent repetitive use of a limb. The activity is usually forceful and often unaccustomed (see risk factors below).
- Associated with systemic disease — (e.g. arthritis) the tendonitis develops as a primary feature of the underlying disease and is not just an increased susceptibility to injury in the diseased tissue.
- Infective — bacterial invasion may follow a penetrating injury.

Specific Types of Tendonitis

- Hand/Wrist:
  a) extensor tendonitis — pain with extension of fingers or wrist;
  b) flexor tendonitis — pain with flexion of fingers or wrist;
  c) de Quervain's disease — pain with use of wrist or thumb at base of first metacarpal, radially;
  d) trigger finger — a snapping movement of a finger due to swelling and restricted gliding of the flexor tendon.

- Elbow:
  epicondylitis — tennis elbow (laterally) or golfer's elbow (medially) — this is a localized inflammation of the muscle and tendon where they attach to the bone at either side of the elbow (the epicondyles).
- Shoulder:
  a) rotator cuff tendonitis — painful rotation of the shoulder;
  b) supraspinatus tendonitis — painful abduction of the shoulder;
  c) bicipital tendonitis — pain in the anterior shoulder with flexion of the shoulder or elbow.
- Hip:
  a variety of tendons can become symptomatic in the hip region. They are difficult to distinguish from one another. They are characterized by pain in the hip region with specific movements.
- Knee:
  patellar tendonitis — tender just distal to the patella anteriorly and pain with kneeling or knee extension.
- Achilles tendonitis — tender heel cord posteriorly with pain on walking.

Risk Factors in Overuse Injuries

The most common type of tendonitis to be encountered by the IFA Attendant will be the "excessive use" type. Areas frequently affected will be wrist tendonitis, elbow epicondylitis and shoulder rotator cuff tendonitis. Several important risk factors have been identified:

- Repetition — where the physical activity is not only repetitive in nature but also the cycle is repeated frequently.
- Excessive force — the more forceful the activity, the more likely an injury may occur. The use of excessive force or an unnecessarily tight grip on hand tools or the need for "jerky" work movements may contribute to the development of tendonitis. A relaxed, smooth working rhythm does much to protect against tendonitis. Power tools should be available when excessive force is needed.
- Unaccustomed — where the worker is new to the job, the job function has recently changed or the worker has recently returned to work after an absence (vacation, other injury). Injury results when there has been

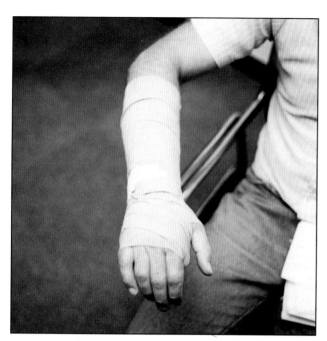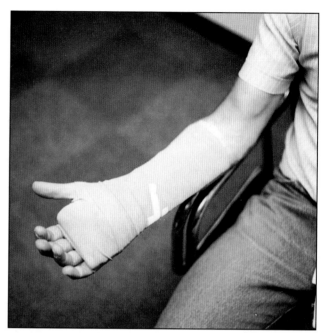

Immobilization for tenosynovitis of the wrist

insufficient time for the body tissues to become acclimatized to the activity.
- Posture — where the job requires sustained or awkward limb postures.
- Vibration — the presence of vibration, especially low frequency, may contribute to injury (e.g. pneumatic tools, chainsaws).
- Temperature — cold tissues may be more subject to injury.
- Mechanical factors — inadequate ergonomic design of tools and/or work stations can contribute to injury.

Signs and Symptoms

- Pain — with motion of affected tendons
- Tenderness — along the course of the tendon
- Swelling
- Redness
- Crepitus (a "leathery" creaking sensation palpable over the involved tissues, with minimal movement)

Management

- Rest — mild cases will often recover spontaneously with a few days of rest or with a temporary change in work activities.
- Splinting — immobilization of the affected part by splinting the part in the position of function will eliminate movement of the tendons and allow them to heal. Hot soaks for 10 to 15 minutes, four times a day, may also be helpful. If, after three days of immobilization there is no improvement, the patient should be referred for medical attention. For a significant tendonitis, the patient must be advised NOT to try to exercise the tendons or "work out" the inflammation.
- Physiotherapy — many methods are available on the advice of a physician.
- Medication — ASA or prescription anti-inflammatories.
- Injection of steroids — should be reserved for resistant cases.

Principles of Prevention

- Hand tools, machines and work stations should be designed to employ sound ergonomic principles — the worker should use tools that allow the job to be done without excessive muscle activity. Heavier work needs bigger and heavier tools with comfortable hand grips. The workplace should be designed so that the person can perform work activities without excessive stretching. Movement that carries the hands away from the body should be avoided. A good posture allows the worker's elbows to be by the side and the forearms to be horizontal or inclining slightly downward. The wrists should not be flexed and the fingers not too widely spread or tightly clenched. Tasks should be performed at a correct height in relation to the worker. If the worker is seated, there should be a stable seat with adequate back support. Seating should be adjustable to suit the individual. The worker's feet should be firmly supported on the ground or on an adequate foot rest.
- Rotate tasks — repetitive use of the same group of muscles over long periods of time (e.g. several hours) should be avoided. It may be helpful to rotate workers through a variety of jobs in the course of their regular shift, so that they will use a variety of movements as the day progresses. Occasional rest periods are also helpful.
- Pre-employment screening — when possible, it is preferable to try to suit the physical characteristics of the worker to the job requirements.
- Automation — this has the effect of reducing the need for manual tasks of a repetitive nature.
- Proper work techniques — beginners should be shown clearly how to do the work without physical stress. They should be counselled on the general rules of reducing body strain. A worker's body build should be considered in relation to the demands of the job. It is unlikely, for example, that the seat used by the previous worker will be at the right height for a new worker. It is also likely that the various tools will need to be adjusted for the new worker's comfort. Supervisors should be able to identify when an employee is performing in an awkward or uncomfortable way, so that they can counsel the worker accordingly.
- Allow for conditioning of the new worker or for the established employee assigned to a new job. This is also important for the worker returning from vacation or from an absence due to illness. Workers should be given a chance to acclimatize to the task by having a varied work schedule for the first few days.
- Workers often continue working until their injuries become so severe that further work is impossible. They should be encouraged to report tendonitis pain at an early stage, so that they may be temporarily moved to a different activity.

BURSITIS

A bursa is a sac-like cavity lined with a slippery synovial tissue. Bursae are found at sites of potential friction between tendons and muscles and bony prominences lying beneath them. Their purpose is to reduce friction between the tissues. "Wear and tear" on the tendons and muscles are reduced in this way.

In bursitis, the bursae have become inflamed. The causes of bursitis are varied:

- acute trauma;
- chronic overuse;
- infection;
- in association with systemic disease (e.g. arthritis, gout).

Sites of involvement of bursitis include:

- shoulder — most common site — known as subacromial or subdeltoid bursitis;
- elbow — olecranon bursitis;
- knee — prepatellar or suprapatellar bursitis — house maid's/carpet layer's/tile setter's knee;
- hip — trochanteric and others.

Signs and Symptoms

The clinical presentation of bursitis is so similar to that of tendonitis that it is often difficult to differentiate between them. The Attendant may note:

- pain — especially with movement;
- swelling;
- redness;
- warmth.

Note that the signs are also similar to infection (cellulitis), especially in the knee area. Because it is extremely important not to delay treatment of an acute infection near a joint, early referral to a physician is indicated. Fever, if present, is an indication of infection.

Treatment

- Uncomplicated acute bursitis — treat as for tendonitis with rest and immobilization. If there is no response within two or three days, refer to a physician.
- Suspected infected bursitis — refer urgently to medical aid.

NERVE ENTRAPMENT SYNDROMES

There is a group of syndromes characterized by compression/entrapment of peripheral nerves at a variety of typical sites. They include:
- carpal tunnel syndrome — median nerve compression at the wrist;
- cubital tunnel syndrome — ulnar nerve compression at the elbow;
- radial tunnel syndrome — radial nerve compression at the mid-arm level laterally.

Typically, the patient will complain of:
- numbness and tingling;
- pain;
- muscle weakness;

in the pattern of the affected peripheral nerve.

The most commonly encountered condition is that of carpal tunnel syndrome.

CARPAL TUNNEL SYNDROME (CTS)

This condition is caused by compression of the median nerve at the flexor side of the wrist as it passes into the hand. Typical symptoms include numbness, tingling or burning of parts of the thumb, index, long and ring fingers, with pain and occasional muscle weakness of the thumb. The condition often arises spontaneously but certain work activities may precipitate symptoms. It is more likely to occur when the work involves frequently repetitive, forceful movements of the affected wrist and hand. The worker may also be unaccustomed to the activity. When work is a factor, patients are usually young and the onset is usually rapid. Vibrating equipment may also be involved.

Treatment includes rest, splints and medication. Surgery is sometimes necessary.

In milder cases, the symptoms can come and go over a period of many months. They can safely be observed initially but, for severe or persistent symptoms, refer to medical aid.

HAND-ARM VIBRATION SYNDROME
(Vibration White Finger Syndrome)

In industries where vibrating tools are used regularly over a period of years (e.g. forestry, hard-rock mining), a condition known as VWF syndrome can arise.

The worker will experience sudden, repeated, painful blanching of the finger tips, usually of both hands and precipitated by cold weather. This is due to interference with the blood supply of the fingers as a result of arteriolar spasm of the digital arteries. The condition tends to progress gradually over several years, where there is continued exposure to vibration.

There is really no effective treatment available, other than to minimize exposure to cold and to vibrating tools.

Part X, Section A
Skeletal System Anatomy and Function

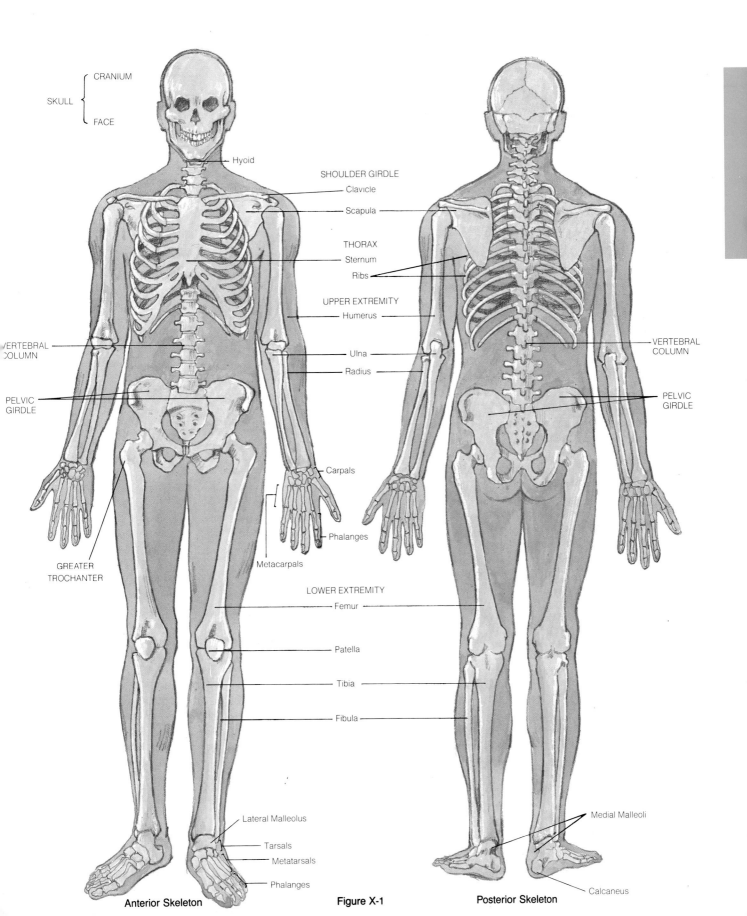

SKULL
CRANIUM
FACE

Hyoid

SHOULDER GIRDLE
Clavicle
Scapula

THORAX
Sternum
Ribs

UPPER EXTREMITY
Humerus

VERTEBRAL COLUMN

Ulna
Radius

PELVIC GIRDLE

Carpals

Phalanges

Metacarpals

GREATER TROCHANTER

LOWER EXTREMITY
Femur

Patella

Tibia

Fibula

Lateral Malleolus

Tarsals

Metatarsals

Phalanges

VERTEBRAL COLUMN

PELVIC GIRDLE

Medial Malleoli

Calcaneus

Anterior Skeleton   Figure X-1   **Posterior Skeleton**

THE SKELETON

The skeleton is the bony framework of the body. The skeleton's function is to give shape, strength and rigidity. It protects organs and acts as a movable framework so that muscular contraction may move the body. The framework of the skeleton allows an erect posture against the pull of gravity and gives form to the body. Bones are living tissue, like muscle and skin. Most bones have a central hollow space called the medullary cavity. It contains a fatty substance called bone marrow, which is involved in the formation of blood cells. The outer hard shell of the bone is the cortex. The external surface of all bones is covered by a connective tissue layer, the periosteum. It is very rich in nerve endings and very sensitive to trauma. Blows to the bone are usually very painful.

JOINTS

To permit movement of the body as a whole or in part, many of the bones are connected by joints.

A joint consists of the ends of two or more bones and the surrounding connecting and supporting tissues. Joints may be slightly movable or freely movable.

Slightly Movable Joints

These are joints that have a pad of fibrocartilage between two bones. The intervertebral discs function as pads between adjacent vertebral bodies that allow some flexibility in the vertebral column. The symphysis between the pubic bones is also of this type, although there is practically no movement.

Freely Movable Joints

Articulations of the ball-and-socket type are the most mobile. Hinge joints permit free movement in a single plane. Pivot joints permit rotary movements, such as the proximal end of the radius pivoting around the ulna.

Joints are held together by a capsule and supporting ligaments, which are bands of tough fibrous tissue. Muscles and their tendons pass around and across joints. The bone ends are covered with very smooth tough connective tissue, the articular cartilage. The joint is enclosed in a fibrous articular ligament. The capsule is lined by a synovial membrane, which secretes synovial fluid, lubricating the joint.

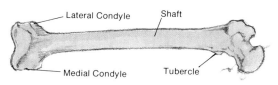

Anatomy of bone

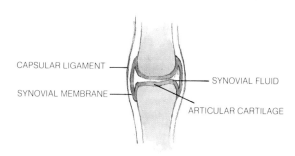

Joint structure

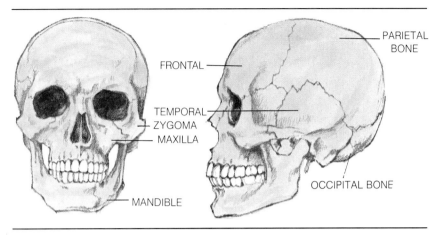

Bones of the face and skull

THE HEAD

The bones of the head are:
- the skull, which forms the cavity containing the brain;
- the facial bones.

Skull

The bones of the skull consist of two firm layers and a sponge-like, bony core. This gives the skull great strength in proportion to its weight. The dome-like shape of the skull also contributes to its strength. An infant's skull is made up of separate bones, which eventually fuse.

The large bone forming the forehead is the frontal bone and the large bone forming the back and base of the skull is called the occipital bone. The occipital bone contains the foramen magnum, a large opening through which the spinal cord passes. The vault and sides of the skull are made up of the parietal and temporal bones. The floor and anterior portions of the skull contain a number of small openings for vessels and nerves.

The Face

The face is made up of multiple bones, most of which are fused together. Some of these facial bones are the zygoma (cheek bone), the maxilla (upper jaw), the mandible (lower jaw) and the nasal bones. The mandible is the only movable facial bone.

SPINAL COLUMN

The vertebral spinal column serves two purposes:
- supports the head and upper part of the body;
- provides rigid protection for the spinal cord.

The spinal column has 33 individual bones, the vertebrae. These are separated from each other by pads of cartilage, the intervertebral discs. These discs not only serve as cushions between each vertebra but also allow for movement in the spinal column.

Individual vertebrae consist of a body which supports weight and an arch through which the spinal cord passes. Each vertebra has a spinous process projecting posteriorly. Each vertebra also has two transverse processes projecting laterally. Ligaments and muscles are attached to these projections.

At the upper end of the spinal column are seven slender cervical vertebrae. Below these are 12 more heavily constructed thoracic vertebrae, the upper part of the back. Below the thoracic vertebrae are five more massive lumbar vertebrae, which form the lower part of the back and carry the weight of the upper body. Below is the sacrum, which is part of the pelvis and consists of five fused vertebrae. Just below the sacrum are four vertebrae called the coccyx, or tail bone.

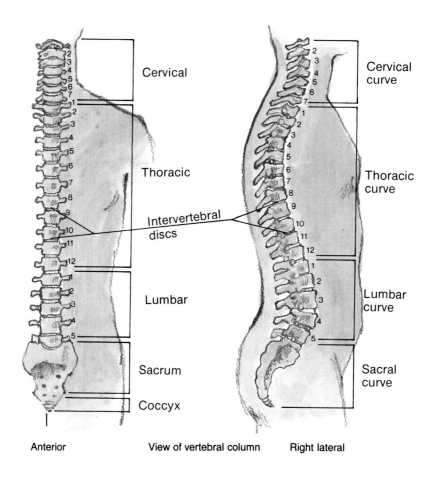

Cervical

Thoracic

Intervertebral discs

Lumbar

Sacrum

Coccyx

Cervical curve

Thoracic curve

Lumbar curve

Sacral curve

Anterior   View of vertebral column   Right lateral

THORAX

The thorax is formed by the thoracic vertebrae, the ribs, the costal cartilages and the sternum. The thorax protects the heart, thoracic blood vessels and lungs. The diaphragm forms the floor of the thoracic cavity and the roof of the abdominal cavity.

Ribs

There are 12 pairs of ribs, which are long, slender, curved bones. The ribs articulate with the thoracic vertebrae posteriorly and curve around to form the rib cage. The first seven ribs are attached to the sternum by the costal cartilages. The eighth, ninth and tenth pairs of ribs are each attached to the cartilage of the rib above. The 11th and 12th pairs of ribs do not attach to any bones at all in the front. They are called floating ribs.

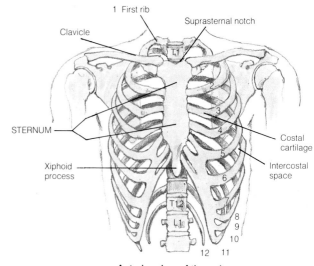

1 First rib

Clavicle

Suprasternal notch

STERNUM

Xiphoid process

Costal cartilage

Intercostal space

Anterior view of thoracic cage

PART X, SKELETAL SYSTEM 241

Sternum

The sternum, or breast bone, is a thin, flat bone located in the anterior part of the thorax, along the midline of the body. The sternum is approximately seven inches long and two inches wide. The xiphoid process is the small protrusion at the inferior part of the sternum.

UPPER EXTREMITY

The shoulder is formed mainly by the scapula (shoulder blade), the clavicle (collar bone) and the upper end of the humerus. These bones and their muscular attachments are called the shoulder girdle.

The clavicles can be felt anteriorly just above the thorax on either side. They are slender, curved bones forming the anterior part of the shoulder. They join with the sternum medially and with the scapula laterally.

Scapula (Shoulder Blade)

The scapula is a flat, triangular bone which is supported against the rib cage posteriorly by large muscles. The upper and outer part of the scapula forms the socket of the shoulder joint. This joint is a ball-and-socket joint. Muscles pass from the scapula across the shoulder joint to the arm.

Upper Arm

The upper arm has only one bone, the humerus. The proximal end of the humerus is ball shaped and fits into the socket of the scapula at the shoulder joint. The distal end of the humerus forms the upper half on the hinged elbow joint.

Elbow

The elbow is a hinge joint. It is formed by the distal end of the humerus articulating with the proximal ends of the ulna and radius.

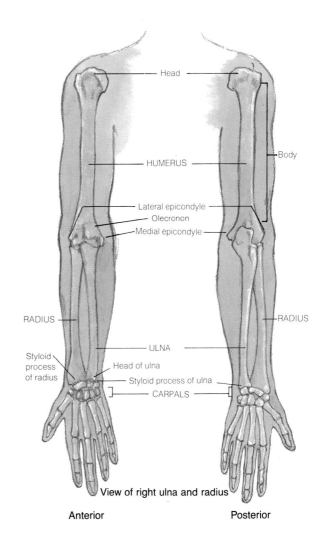

View of right ulna and radius

Anterior   Posterior

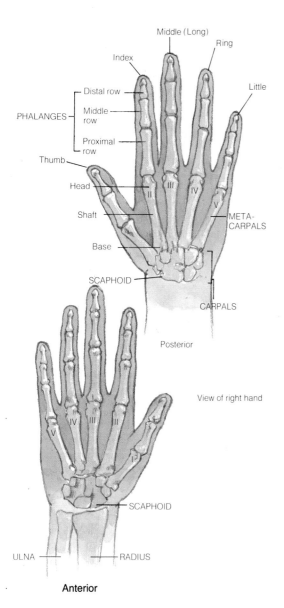

Forearm

The forearm consists of two bones, the radius and the ulna. The proximal end of the ulna forms one half of the elbow joint, while the distal end acts as a pivot around which the radius moves when the forearm is rotated. The upper part of the radius is joined to the ulna below the elbow joint. The larger, distal end of the radius forms part of the wrist joint. The ulna is on the little finger side of the forearm or medial side of the forearm when the forearm is in the anatomical position. Conversely, the radius is on the thumb side of the forearm or on the lateral side of the forearm in the anatomical position.

Wrist

The wrist is composed of eight small bones, the carpal bones, arranged in two rows of four. The carpal bones join with the distal ends of the radius and ulna to form the wrist joint. The wrist joint is capable of motion in four directions — extension, flexion and side to side. Distally, the distal row of carpal bones articulate with the five metacarpal bones of the hand.

Hand

The five metacarpal bones and 14 phalanges (three for each finger and two for the thumb) make up the skeletal framework of the hand. The metacarpal bone of the thumb has a special joint for flexion, extension and rotation. The distal ends of the metacarpal bones articulate with the proximal row of finger bones, the phalanges.

PELVIS AND LOWER EXTREMITY

The lower extremity includes the pelvis, hip joint, thigh, knee joint, leg, ankle and foot.

Pelvis

The pelvis forms the floor of the abdominal cavity. The pelvis or pelvic girdle is a bony ring formed by the sacrum and the two large, wing-like pelvic bones (innominate bones). Each of these two bones has three separate components, the ilium, ischium and pubis. The pelvic bones join in front to form the pubic symphysis. Posteriorly, each pelvic bone articulates with the sacrum (sacroiliac joint) and is connected to it by broad, very strong ligaments.

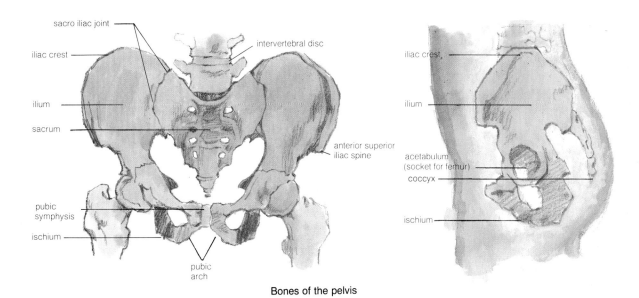

Bones of the pelvis

The pelvic bones contain the sockets (acetabula) for both hip joints. The entire weight of the upper body is transmitted through this bony ring through the hip joint and into the legs.

The pelvis surrounds and provides protection for the pelvic cavity. In this cavity lie the bladder, the rectum and, in the female, the reproductive organs.

Thigh

The femur is the long bone of the thigh and extends from the hip to the knee. It is a strong, heavy bone, the longest in the body. At the proximal end of the femur, there is a rounded head which forms the ball of the ball-and-socket joint of the hip. Between the head and the shaft of the bone is a stout neck. At the base of the neck on the lateral side, where it joins the shaft, there is a heavy mass of bone called the greater trochanter (see Figure X-1).

The distal end of the femur widens into two bony prominences, the lateral and medial condyles. The smooth articular surfaces form a hinge joint with the tibia.

Knee Joint

The knee joint is the largest joint in the body. It is formed by the distal, medial and lateral condyles of the femur that articulate with the proximal end of the tibia, which has corresponding medial and lateral plateaus. Its ligaments are very complex and quite susceptible to injury.

The patella, or knee cap, is a flat bone embedded in the tendon of the quadriceps muscle. It is about 5 cm long and 5 cm wide and has three bursae (pad-like sacs), one above, one in front and one below. When the knee is bent, the patella becomes fixed against a notch in the condyles of the femur. The patellar ligament is a strong ligament that attaches the quadricep muscle and patella to the anterior tibia.

Lower Leg

The lower leg extends from the knee to the ankle and contains two bones: the tibia and fibula. The tibia, or shin bone, is the larger bone of the lower leg and is responsible for weight bearing. The upper (proximal) end of the tibia widens and flattens to form the lateral and medial plateaus. The condyles of the distal femur roll on the tibial plateaus when the knee is flexed or extended. The distal tibia is narrower and articulates with the talus.

The fibula is a long, slender bone lateral to the tibia. Proximally, it articulates with the tibia below the knee joint. Distally, it articulates with the talus and is joined to the tibia by a tough fibrous membrane.

Ankle and Foot

The ankle joint is made up of the distal ends of the tibia and fibula articulating with the talus. At the ankle joint, the distal end of the medial tibia forms the medial malleolus. The distal end of the fibula forms the lateral malleolus.

The two malleoli strengthen the ankle joint, by completing the bony mortice and by giving attachment to the strong collateral ligaments. The foot has seven tarsal bones. The talus fits into the mortice formed by the tibia and fibula to complete the ankle joint. The heel bone is called the calcaneus. The five metatarsals correspond to the metacarpals of the hand and are numbered from the medial side. There are two phalanges for the big toe and three for each of the other toes.

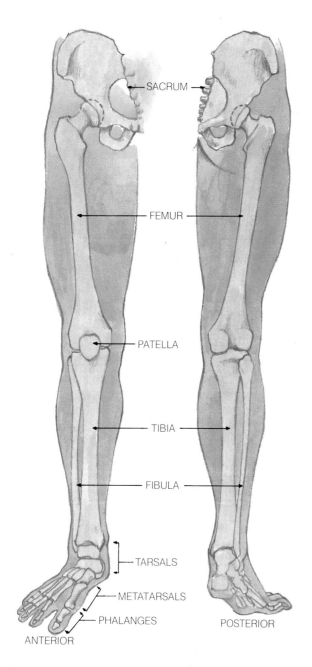

Bones of lower limb

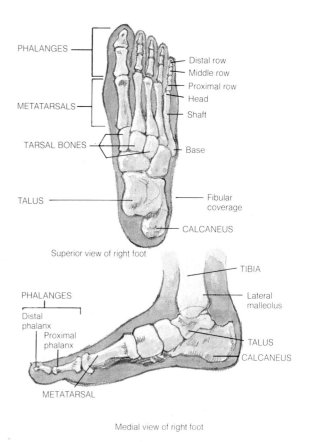

Bones of the foot

Part X, Section B
Sprains, Dislocations, Fractures

Proper management of a patient with a sprain, dislocation or fracture will not only minimize pain but will also promote the patient's recovery.

MECHANISM OF INJURY

- Angular force (e.g. fall on outstretched hand)
- Direct blow (e.g. skull fracture)
- Compression force (e.g. fall from ladder, landing on feet)
- Crush (e.g. log on pelvis)

SPRAINS

A sprain is stretching, partial or complete tear of a ligament at a joint.

Sprains may vary in severity from partial tearing of a single ligament to a complete disruption of multiple ligaments of one joint. If in doubt as to whether the injury is a sprain or fracture, always treat it as a fracture.

The signs and symptoms of sprains are similar at all movable joints:

- History is usually one of twisting or stretching of a joint beyond its normal range of motion.
- Swelling from hemorrhage commences immediately after injury and is always accompanied by pain.
- Point tenderness at ligament attachments or along the length of the ligament.

DISLOCATIONS

A dislocation is a displacement of one or more bones so that the joint surfaces are no longer in contact. When force is applied near a joint, one bone may become displaced from the other, instead of the bone giving way, as with fractures.

A compound dislocation is where air and bacteria have access to the injury site, just as with a compound or open fracture.

The signs and symptoms of a dislocation are essentially the same as for a fracture. Dislocations usually demonstrate:

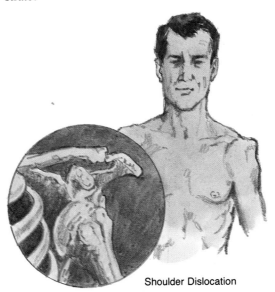

Shoulder Dislocation

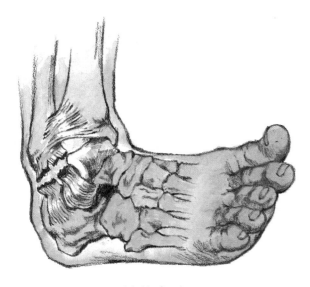

Lateral Ankle Sprain

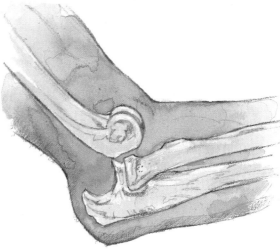

Elbow Dislocation

- severe pain, especially about the ligaments;
- obvious gross deformity and irregularity;
- a complete or near-complete inability to move the affected joint;
- the joint is often locked in a deformed position.

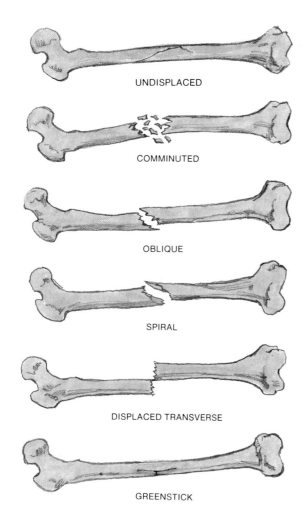

Types of Fractures

FRACTURE-DISLOCATION

A fracture dislocation is a dislocation associated with a fracture.

FRACTURES

A fracture is a break in the continuity of a bone. Fractures are classified as:

- Closed (simple) Fractures — The surface of the skin is intact.
- Open (compound) Fractures — The surface of the skin is broken, usually by the bone. Contaminants have access to the fracture site. Therefore, foreign material and bacteria may enter and infect the bone and soft tissue.

Signs and Symptoms of Fractures

It is important to be able to recognize fractures for proper management.

The signs and symptoms of fractures are:

1. History — Mechanism of injury will tell the Attendant what forces have been applied to the patient.
2. Pain — Pain is generally sudden, may be extreme, and is usually localized to the site of the fracture.
3. Deformity — The limb may be angulated or appear shorter than the other one.
4. Tenderness — Point tenderness at the fracture site is the most reliable indicator of a fracture.
5. Swelling — An increase in the size of the part. Swelling may occur with soft tissue injuries, fractures or dislocations.
6. Loss of Stability — The inability to use the extremity. The injured limb may not be able to support any weight.
7. Discolouration (ecchymosis) — Unless blood vessels close to the surface are ruptured, black and blue marks may not be evident until some hours or days after the injury.
8. Crepitus or a Grating Sound — The sound or feeling when the ends of bones rub on each other. This sign should not be purposely brought about but may have occurred at the time of injury.

PRIORITY ACTION APPROACH TO LIMB INJURIES

The evaluation and management of the injured worker with limb injuries follows the Priority Action Approach outlined in Part III, page 20.

1. Assess the scene.
2. Perform a primary survey.
3. Ensure an open airway with C-spine control.
4. Assess for adequate breathing and, if necessary, assist ventilation.

---

5. Administer high-flow oxygen by mask if necessary.
6. Assess circulation and control life-threatening external bleeding.
7. Perform a secondary survey.
8. ALWAYS MANAGE LIFE-THREATENING CONDITIONS BEFORE ATTEMPTING TO MANAGE ANY FRACTURES OR DISLOCATIONS.

PRINCIPLES OF EXAMINATION OF LIMB INJURIES

Listen to the patient's story and to any bystanders who may have witnessed the accident. Knowing the mechanism of the injury can be of great value in making an accurate diagnosis. Ascertain whether the patient can move the injured limb. *If time permits* AFTER all injuries have been attended to, the main features of the history should be recorded.

Look — Compare the injured limb with the normal limb. The patient usually can help locate the area injured.

Feel — If necessary, remove clothing by cutting it away from the injury. Feel (palpate) gently for deformity, swelling and point tenderness. Check for nerve damage by inquiring if feeling is present distal to the injury site. Compare with the other limb. Numbness, tingling and loss of movement may indicate nerve damage. Check circulation by pressing on the nail beds or tips of the fingers or toes, then watch for the colour to return. Check the distal pulses and compare them with those of the other limb.

The finding of a weak or absent pulse distal to the injury site indicates either of the following conditions:
- shock;
- vascular injury at the injury site.

To differentiate the two conditions, the Attendant must assess the pulses in the opposite limb. The finding of decreased or absent pulses in all limbs indicates shock. If the pulses are normal in the opposite limb then a vascular injury must be suspected. The finding of a cold, white, pulseless limb from a vascular injury is a *limb*-threatening emergency. The finding of shock is a *life*-threatening emergency; therefore, both conditions fall into the Rapid Transport Category.

A PATIENT WITH A LIMB-THREATENING INJURY SHOULD HAVE THE SECONDARY SURVEY CONDUCTED, QUICK IMMOBILIZATION OF THE LIMB AND BE UPGRADED INTO THE RAPID TRANSPORT CATEGORY.

Support the limb as much as possible during examination and treatment to reduce pain and avoid further injury. Look for any hidden injuries, such as a fractured pelvis. Extreme pain from an injury may override or mask other injuries.

All the findings of the examination should be noted and, if time permits, recorded. This is valuable information.

Part X, Section C
Principles of Immobilization

When there is a break in the continuity of tissue, the tissue loses its ability to support itself. The basic problem is the same whether the break is in the continuity of soft tissue or bone.

Soft tissue damage is damage to muscles, ligaments, tendons, blood vessels and nerves. It may be more serious than damage to the bone because healing may be prolonged or incomplete.

Immobilization means any method that holds a body part still and prevents movement. For example, a pressure bandage applied to a break in soft tissue tends to immobilize the injured tissue and aids in the arrest of bleeding by squeezing the injured blood vessels and keeping the tissue still. Joint movement near a soft tissue injury will tend to move the tissue and encourage further bleeding, so it may be necessary to immobilize nearby joints as well as the break in the soft tissue. Therefore, some soft tissue wounds will require splinting as well as dressing.

REASONS FOR SPLINTING

All fractures are complicated to some degree by damage to the soft tissue and structures surrounding the bone. The major cause of tissue damage at a fracture site is movement of the broken bone ends. Normal elasticity of the muscles, as well as spasms of the muscles and their response to trauma, tends to pull the jagged bone ends into the surrounding tissue. The broken end of bone may be comparable to the broken end of a bottle. It is important therefore to prevent a fractured bone from rotating or further penetrating the soft tissues. Overriding bone ends will allow shortening of the limb.

TYPES OF SPLINTS

The most common and suitable splints are:

Prepared Wooden Splints

Wooden splints must be well padded, preferably with foam.

Wooden splints are primarily used to immobilize lower limb injuries. There are two common sizes:

- Long splints are 1 cm x 10 cm plywood notched at one end, 158 cm long, covered with 2.5 cm thick foam.
- Short splints are 1 cm x 10 cm plywood notched at one end, 104 cm long, covered with 2.5 cm foam.

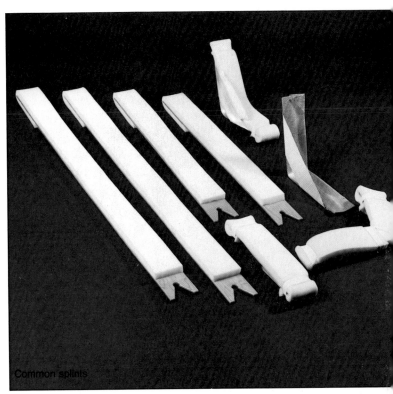

Common splints

Expanded Metal Splints

Metal splints are usually used for upper limb injuries or for extra support at the ankle. This type of splint is lightweight and can easily be formed or folded to match the contour of the injured limb. One layer is usually not sufficient to provide adequate support and a minimum of four thicknesses must be used. If more support is required, use more layers. Expanded metal splints are approximately 10 cm x 60 cm.

Fracture Boards

Fracture boards are commonly called spinal boards and are used primarily when full body immobilization is required.

The long board is approximately 2 cm x 45 cm x 182 cm, with strap and hand holds along each side.

Air Splints

Air splints were introduced to emergency care work several years ago and have gained popularity where short-term minor immobilization is required, such as for a closed injury to the foot, hand or wrist. They have several disadvantages:

- If too much air pressure is applied, circulation may be impaired.
- They are unsuitable for use on an angulated limb.
- Air transportation may decrease the pressure within the splint when flying from the accident site to a lower altitude.
- They may develop air leaks, especially if stored in extremes of temperature over an extended period.
- They prevent application of cold to the injury site.

Traditional methods of splinting are preferred over air splints when time is not critical and there are no potentially life-threatening conditions.

Traction Splints

A traction splint is a device which has been designed to hold lower extremity fractures, particularly fractures of the femur and upper tibia (not involving the knee joint), in alignment through constant, steady traction on the lower extremity. THEY SHOULD NOT BE APPLIED FOR FRACTURES OF THE HIP, KNEE, ANKLE OR FOOT.

The traction splint acts as an effective splint by providing countertraction. The device is seated proximally against the ischial tuberosity of the pelvis and attached to the foot by way of an ankle hitch.

As traction is applied to the foot, a countertraction force is exerted by the proximal end of the splint, where it is seated against the ischial tuberosity.

This type of device is not suitable for upper extremity injuries because the application of countertraction in the axilla could damage the complex of nerves and blood vessels passing through the axilla.

There are several varieties of traction splints available but the basic principles of application are the same for all traction splints. PROPER APPLICATION OF A TRACTION SPLINT IS NOT EASILY ACCOMPLISHED AND REQUIRES FREQUENT PRACTISE.

Splints described in the Industrial First Aid Regulations are most effective. Only if the patient falls into the Rapid Transport Category or if those splints are unavailable should alternative methods of splinting (such as pillow splints or blanket immobilization) be substituted.

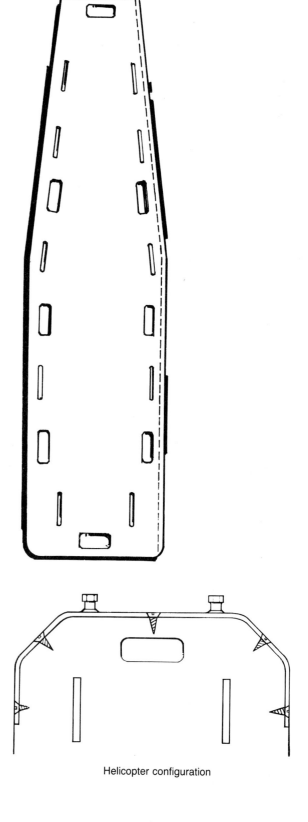

Helicopter configuration

PRINCIPLES OF SPLINTING

- The evaluation and management of the injured worker with limb fractures follows the Priority Action Approach outlined in Part III, page 20.
- If the patient falls into the Rapid Transport Category, modified immobilization techniques for limb fractures must be carried out prior to transport. If the Attendant is waiting for the transport vehicle and all life-threatening conditions have been managed and are being regularly reassessed, the following, more elaborate splinting techniques, may be used.
- *Cut away any clothing* from the injury site, if necessary.
- *Cover open wounds,* if any, with sterile dressings and bandage appropriately.
- *Check the circulation* and motor and sensory functions distal to the injury site before and after splinting.
- *Steady and support* the injured limb before and during the splinting.
- *Apply cold* if the part is swelling and circulation is not deficient. Control of swelling must be instituted as outlined in Management of Soft Tissue Injuries, Part IX, Section D, page 207.
- *Apply traction,* if required.
- *Straighten* severely angulated fractures of long bones. The patient may experience severe pain while the long-bone fractures are being aligned, but will usually be more comfortable after splinting is complete.

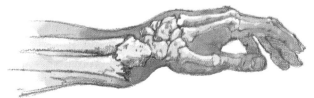
Skin under marked tension

- *Splint joint injuries as found* unless the following conditions are present:
    - Obvious dislocation or fracture dislocation where there is marked angulation and the distal limb is pale, cold and pulseless. The fracture may be opened or closed.
    - There will be more than a half hour between the time of injury and the patient's arrival at hospital.

Following the guidelines outlined in the Traction Section (page 253), grasp the distal portion of the injured limb firmly and, with increasing traction, put the distal portion in line with the proximal part of the limb. This may require a considerable amount of traction and will be facilitated if another Attendant gives countertraction to the limb proximal to the injury. The object is to align the distal and proximal parts of the limb — that is, to place the limb in a natural position. The patient may feel severe pain during this manoeuvre. When the limb has been placed in a normal position, it must be maintained in that position by appropriate immobilization.

When an injured limb fulfils the criteria outlined above, the patient should be transported to hospital with haste. Whether the Attendant elects to attempt a reduction or not, it is important that a physician be notified as soon as the patient reaches hospital. If manipulation is attempted, it is also important that the physician be notified, whether or not the circulation has been restored.

A more detailed description of these complications is discussed under the specific joint injuries.

- *Select the proper length of splint to effectively immobilize the joints above and below the fracture.* To determine the length of a splint, use the rule of thirds. Each long bone is divided into thirds. If the injury is located in the upper or lower third, assume the nearest joint to be unstable. Therefore, splints should extend

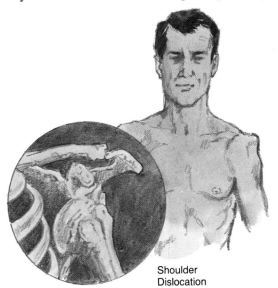
Shoulder
Dislocation

to immobilize the joint above and below this unstable joint (e.g. for fractures of the upper third of the tibia, the splint must extend to include the hip because the knee is unstable). Avoid splinting over open wounds or gross deformities, if possible.

- *Pad the entire splint,* paying particular attention to the natural body hollows and any deformities. It is often necessary to use extra padding to make the limb comfortable. The padding will shape the splint to the limb and prevent pressure sores from developing.

- Always anchor the splint to the stable part of the body first, then the part distal to the injury and, finally, the injured site. This avoids unnecessary movement of injured tissue or bones. Splint-securing material should be tight enough to support the limb and prevent movement but not so tight that it interferes with circulation.

- *If direct pressure is maintained over a wound* by loop tie bandages (see Figure X-2), do not release the pressure of the loop tie bandage when applying bandages over the splint. Do not trap a tied or wrapped bandage under splints. It may cause a dangerous constriction and interfere with access to wounds. The exceptions to this rule are:
  - a loop tie bandage with the knot exposed;
  - partial amputation necessitating the application of an Esmarch bandage.

- *Elevation of the injured limb* after immobilization will often provide comfort for the patient. The limb should be elevated approximately 12 inches and supported throughout its length with blankets and sandbags. If circulation is impaired, it is likely due to swelling, and elevation would be beneficial. However, if there is no detectable pulse distal to the injury in the affected limb, it should be managed in the horizontal position.

PROVIDING THERE ARE NO INDICATIONS FOR RAPID TRANSPORT, ALL FRACTURES AND DISLOCATIONS MUST BE IMMOBILIZED BEFORE THE PATIENT IS TRANSPORTED.

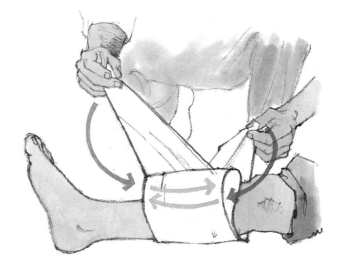

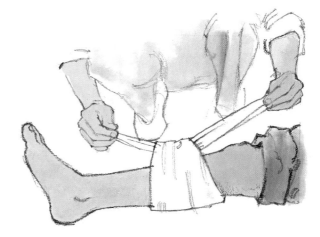

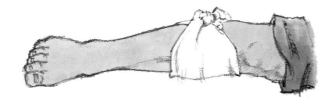

Figure X-2 Tying a loop tie bandage

TRACTION IN LIMB FRACTURES

Soft tissue injury during immobilization and transportation procedures can be eliminated by the application of moderate traction.

Traction is a firm and steady pull to improve the position of a badly deformed, shortened or angulated limb in order to achieve a more normal alignment. Identical traction techniques are used in open and closed fractures. Traction, for first aid purposes, should only be applied for mid-shaft long-bone fractures except as outlined in Joint Injuries, page 251.

Traction is also applied to help prevent further soft tissue injury. It may improve circulation and relieve pain.

NOTE: THE APPLICATION OF TRACTION WILL NOT BE FEASIBLE ON INJURED LIMBS OF PATIENTS IN THE RAPID TRANSPORT CATEGORY. IT WOULD BE UNSAFE TO APPLY THIS MANOEUVRE IN A MOVING VEHICLE.

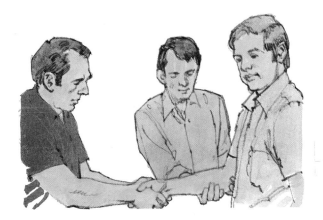

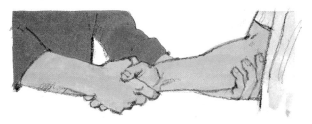

Traction for the upper extremity

The application of traction consists of the following steps, in the order listed:

1. Once the Priority Action Approach is completed, and providing there are no other serious injuries, traction should be applied as soon as possible.
2. Traction must be applied to that portion of the limb distal to the fracture site.
3. Firmly grasp the distal portion of the injured limb and, with increasing traction, place the distal portion in line with the proximal part.
4. Once it is applied, traction should be maintained by splinting techniques.
5. Traction straps must not interfere with circulation.

THE USE OF COLD IN DISTAL CIRCULATORY IMPAIRMENT

Cold packs or ice packs should *not* be applied, either locally or distally, to fractured limbs when distal pulses are absent or circulation is impaired.

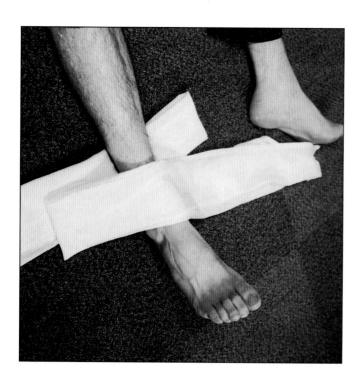
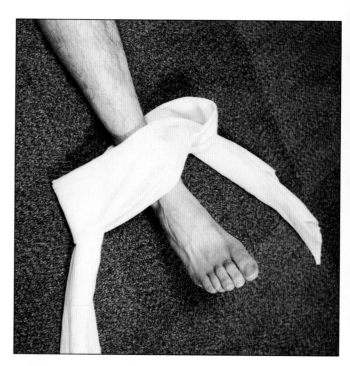
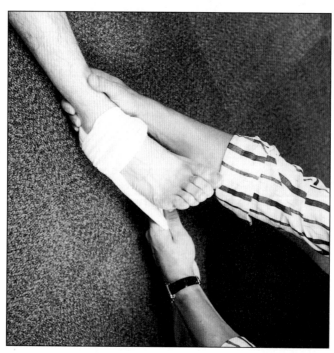

Traction applied to a lower limb using two narrow triangular bandages

Part X, Section D
Management of Upper Limb Injuries

PRINCIPLES OF IMMOBILIZATION

The general principles of immobilization should be followed when dealing with patients who have upper limb injuries (see Section C, page 251).

Additional Specific Upper Limb Management Principles:

1. Measure and mould metallic splints to the uninjured limb before putting them on the injured limb. If a longer splint is required, extend the splints as shown in Figure X-3.

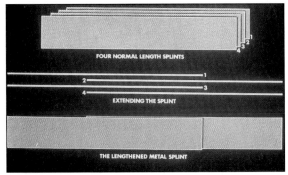

Figure X-3 Extending metallic splints

2. An injured hand must be placed and maintained in the POSITION OF FUNCTION — with some dorsiflexion of the wrist, the hand relaxed and fingers slightly flexed (see Figure X-4). Maintain this position with a pad in the palm of the hand or a suitably formed splint. If the fingers are markedly displaced, splint in position found.

3. Crepe bandages are recommended to secure metallic splints to the upper limb.
Immobilization with splints should begin from the sound part of the limb. Consequently, the crepe bandage should be applied from the proximal to the distal part of the limb.

4. Assess and reassess circulation.
For upper limb injuries, the radial pulse is the most reliable indicator of circulation. The injured limb must be compared with the uninjured limb. The ulnar artery also provides blood supply to the hand but it is usually not palpable. If the radial pulse cannot be palpated but the fingers are warm, or there is good capillary refill in the nail beds, adequate circulation is being provided by the ulnar artery.
Assess circulation before and after splinting and every 30 minutes thereafter. Any impairment should be brought to the attention of the attending physician.

5. Assess neurological function.
With upper limb injuries, the Attendant should assess the motor and sensory functions in the hand before and after splinting. If impairment is found, reassess every 30 minutes. Any impairment should be brought to the attention of the attending physician.

Slings

Slings are used quite extensively to immobilize upper limb injuries. They are normally used with rigid splints but sometimes slings and broad transverse bandages are used for complete immobilization.

Some injuries requiring sling-only treatment:
- scapular fractures
- clavicular fractures
- shoulder dislocations
- upper-third humerus fractures

TRACTION FOR UPPER LIMB INJURIES

If possible, all upper limb fractures should be immobilized in the thumb-up position (see Figure X-5). This allows the radius and ulna to remain in the anatomical position.

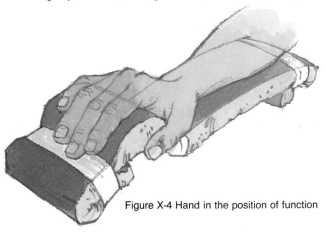

Figure X-4 Hand in the position of function

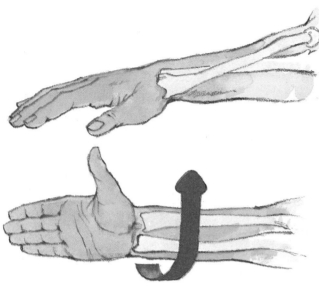

Figure X-5 Bottom diagram shows the upper limb
in the thumb-up position

FOREARM FRACTURES

- To apply traction, an Attendant and an assistant should grasp the arm above and below the fracture site. Traction should be a gentle extension to rotate and position the forearm.

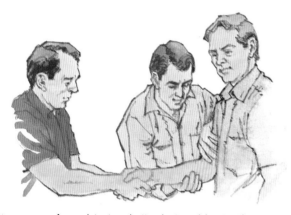

An assistant and attendant applying traction

- Another method is to grasp the patient's hand and with the Attendant's other hand grasp the arm above the fracture site. Apply gentle extension and rotation, positioning the arm in the thumb-up position. (See Figure X-6.)

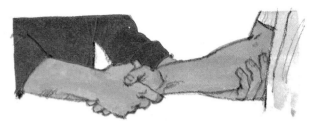

Figure X-6 Applying traction to a forearm

FRACTURES AT OR NEAR THE ELBOW

Upper-third fractures of the radius and ulna, elbow fractures or dislocations or lower-third humerus fractures are normally immobilized in the position found. Altering the position of these injuries may damage blood vessels or nerves. In the presence of a cold, pale, pulseless forearm and hand, a reduction should be attempted. To improve the position and circulation, follow the guidelines for forearm traction and gently increase the flexion of the elbow until the radial pulse is restored but do not exceed 90 degrees. However, if the joint is locked and cannot be flexed easily, discontinue reduction. If the radial pulse is present, even if weak, do not attempt any manipulation. Altering the position of the limb may increase the pain but, once traction has been completed, the patient should be more comfortable.

The Attendant must maintain the traction until the limb is fully secured to the splint.

If circulation does not return or it is deficient, keep the limb as close to horizontal as possible while keeping the patient comfortable.

SCAPULAR FRACTURE

Cause

- A substantial force applied directly over the scapula.

Signs and Symptoms

In addition to the general signs of a fracture, a scapular fracture may be indicated by:
- Tenderness over the immediate area of the scapula, which can be mistaken for a bruised muscle.
- Limited range of shoulder motion.
- Local swelling.

Possible Complications

• The scapula is embedded in muscle and is a substantial bony structure. An injury to the scapula that would cause a fracture may often also cause rib fractures and internal chest injuries.

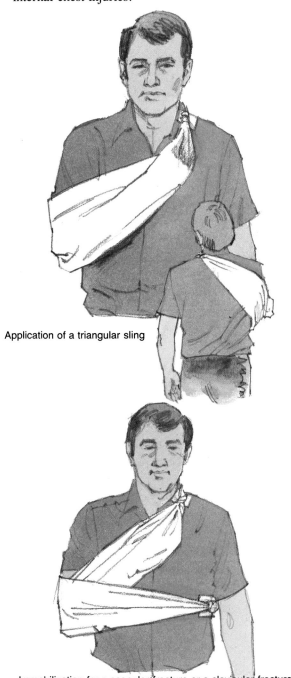

Application of a triangular sling

Immobilization for a scapular fracture or a clavicular fracture

Management

1. Ambulatory Patient
   • Place the affected arm in a triangular arm sling.
   • Apply a transverse broad bandage to limit the movement of the arm on the affected side.
   • Transport to medical attention.
2. If Patient Is Recumbent
   • If rib fractures or internal chest injuries are suspected, treat the patient as outlined for chest injuries, Part IV, Section C, page 57. Providing support to the affected arm may make the patient more comfortable.

CLAVICULAR FRACTURE

Cause

• Direct blow to the clavicle or shoulder.
• A fall on the outstretched arm.

Signs and Symptoms

In addition to the general signs of a fracture, a clavicle fracture may be indicated by:
• Irregularity of the clavicle.
• The patient may hold the arm against the chest with the other hand.
• The patient may be reluctant to move the arm on the affected side because of pain.

Possible Complications

• Complications are rare, although if the injury is severe enough, other chest wall structures (ribs), the lungs or the major vessels and nerves of the thoracic outlet may be damaged.

Management

• Apply a triangular arm sling.
• Place the centre of a broad bandage over the elbow on the injured side and tie off on the uninjured side.
• Transport to medical attention.
Apply a triangular arm sling to keep the weight off the injured clavicle. The sling should be tightened from the back to draw the shoulder slightly upward and backward.

BILATERAL CLAVICULAR FRACTURES

If both clavicles have been fractured, using slings could irritate the fractures and should be avoided.

In the absence of associated chest or other system injuries, the best treatment for bilateral fractured clavicles is to lay the patient on a stretcher with a firm pad between the shoulder blades.

SHOULDER DISLOCATION

Cause

• The patient may have fallen on the point of the shoulder.
• The arm may have been forcefully externally rotated or abducted.
• The patient may have a history of recurrent shoulder dislocations. They may reoccur with minimal trauma or abduction movements.

Signs and Symptoms

• The patient may hold the dislocated arm with the other hand to stabilize it.
• Pain, sometimes extreme.
• Possible deformity.
• The dislocation is most often anterior but it may be posterior. In an anterior dislocation, the humeral head comes out of the shoulder joint and lies anterior and below the shoulder joint. This means that the roundness of the shoulder is lost and there is usually a hollow below the point of the shoulder.
• The arm may be fixed in a position away from the trunk.

Possible Complications

• Circulation impairment and/or nerve injury.

Management

• Support the injured area with a blanket or pillow. The patient will often immobilize the dislocated arm by holding the wrist with the other hand.
• Pad between the arm and chest and secure the arm against the body without making it hard for the patient to breathe.
• If the patient is sitting or semi-sitting, a large arm sling can be used, secured with a broad transverse bandage.

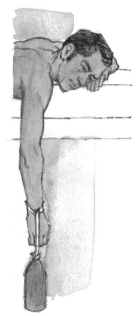

Reducing a dislocated shoulder

• Check the radial pulse before and after treatment. Check and record the movement or loss of sensation in the fingers before and after management. Compare the results to pulse and sensation in the uninjured limb.
• The Attendant should not attempt to relocate a dislocated shoulder if there is distal circulation because of the danger of causing a nerve or blood vessel injury. If transportation is delayed more than two hours and a fracture is unlikely (i.e. patient with a recurrent shoulder dislocation and minimal trauma), a relocation may be considered. A physician must be contacted to obtain specific instructions to attempt to reduce the dislocation. The simplest effective method is to place the patient face down on a high bed or bench with the affected arm dangling over the side and the bed supporting the upper lateral chest. Fix a weight of approximately 4 kg to the dangling wrist. Keep the patient in this position for up to ¾ of an hour or until the dislocation is reduced. The patient must still be assessed by a physician even after a successful reduction.

HUMERAL FRACTURES — UPPER THIRD

Fractures of the upper humerus may have similar signs, symptoms and complications to dislocations of the shoulder joint.

Because of the similarity between these two injuries, they are very difficult to differentiate without an x-ray. For details of management, follow "Shoulder Joint Dislocation Management".

HUMERAL FRACTURE (MIDDLE THIRD)

Cause

• A twist or fall on the outstretched arm.
• A direct blow.

Signs and Symptoms

In addition to the general signs of fracture, the patient may demonstrate:
• Possible inability to flex or extend the wrist and fingers.
• "Wrist drop" caused by damage of radial nerve, with inability to extend the wrist.
• Possible shortening of the arm.

Possible Complications

• Swelling may impede circulation.
• Radial nerve damage as demonstrated by inability to extend the wrist.
• Blood vessel damage.

Management

• Support the arm and assist the patient to a position of comfort.
• Check the distal circulation and motor and sensory function.
• Apply a full arm splint, extending from the armpit past the fingertip.
• Secure the arm to the splint with crepe bandage.
• Check circulation and motor and sensory function.
• Secure the arm to the body or apply the appropriate sling.
• Apply cold to the injury site.
• Transport to medical attention.

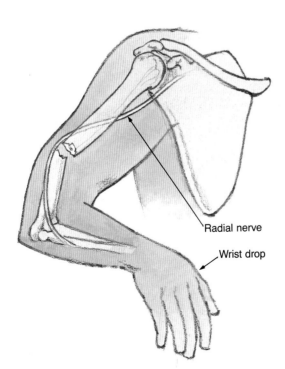

Radial nerve

Wrist drop

Wrist drop caused by radial nerve damage

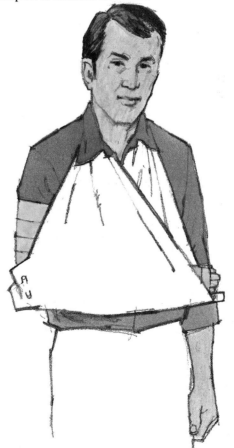

Full arm splint and large arm sling immobilization
for fractured humerus

HUMERAL FRACTURE NEAR THE ELBOW JOINT (LOWER THIRD)

Cause

- Fall on the extended arm.
- Fall on the flexed elbow.
- Force applied at the elbow.

Signs and Symptoms

In addition to the general signs of fracture, the patient may demonstrate:
- Possible instability of the elbow joint.
- Possible decreased circulation.
- Possible nerve involvement with weakness of muscles of the hand.

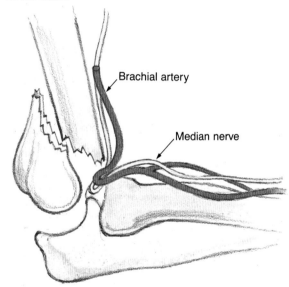

Brachial artery

Median nerve

Possible complication of lower third humeral fractures

Possible Complications

- This is often a very serious fracture due to the possibility of major blood vessel damage and nerve involvement.

Management

- Support the arm in the position found.
- Check the pulse of the limb distal to the injury. Check movement of fingers and wrist.
- Form a metallic splint to fit the contours of the arm from the axilla to past the fingertips.

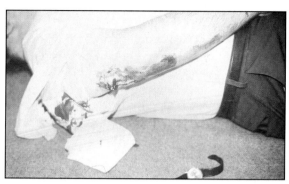

Open fracture

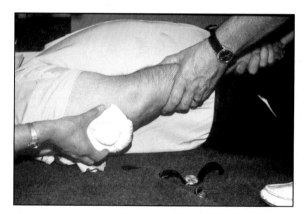

Dressings and ringpad

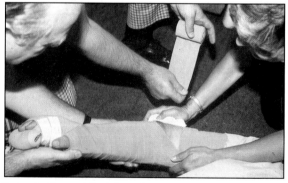

Separate Crepe at the injury site

- Remove any jewellery that may impede circulation. Pad the splint and secure to the limb with crepe bandage. If necessary, use extra padding to make the limb comfortable.
- Maintain the hand in the position of function, either with extra padding in the palm of the hand or by shaping the end of the splint.

- Tips of the fingers should be left exposed and the radial pulse should be accessible for continued circulation assessment.
- Support the immobilized limb, either in the appropriate sling if the patient can walk or fully supported at the side if the patient is lying down.
- Apply cold to the injured area.
- Transport to medical attention.

ELBOW DISLOCATION

Cause

- Fall on the outstretched hand.
- Direct blow.

Signs and Symptoms

- As for lower-third humeral fractures.

Management

- As for lower-third humeral fractures.

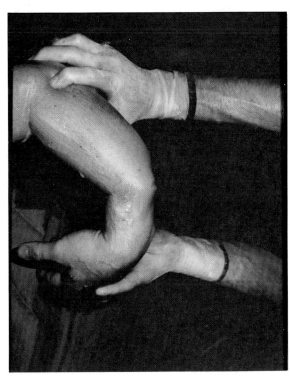

Fracture of Radius and Ulnar

RADIAL/ULNAR (MIDDLE THIRD) FOREARM FRACTURES

Cause

- A direct blow.
- Fall on the outstretched hand.

Signs and Symptoms

In addition to the general signs of fracture, the patient may demonstrate:
- Shortening.
- Limited range of wrist or finger movement.
- Limited range of forearm movement.

Possible Complications

- Circulation impairment.
- Possible nerve involvement.

Management

- Check circulation and movements of the fingers before and after traction.
- Apply gentle but supportive traction to the limb. If the forearm is angulated, apply manual traction and maintain traction until the limb is fully secured in a splint. In the absence of shortening or angulation, traction is usually not necessary.
- If possible, position the hand in the thumb-up position.
- Apply a formed and well-padded splint from the axilla to past the fingertips.
- Secure the splint to the whole arm with a crepe bandage snug enough to maintain support.
- Secure the arm at the patient's side or in a position of comfort.
- Apply cold to the fracture site.
- Transport to medical attention.

RADIAL/ULNAR (LOWER THIRD) WRIST FRACTURES AND DISLOCATIONS

Cause

- Fall on an extended arm and open hand.
- Direct blow.
- Twisting injury.

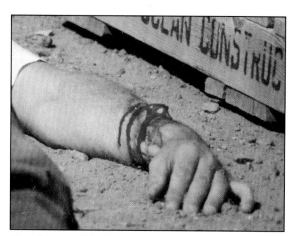

Open fracture of Radius/Ulnar lower third

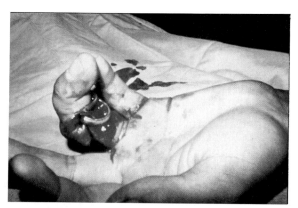

Fractured ring finger

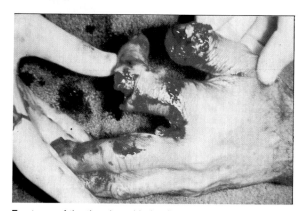

Fractures of the thumb and index finger

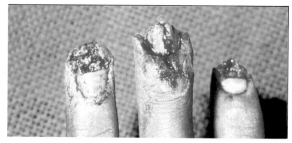

Fingertip fractures

Signs and Symptoms

In addition to the general signs of fracture, the patient may demonstrate:

- Inability to flex or extend the wrist.
- Inability to use the hand.
- The most common injury in this area is the Colles' fracture with a deformity which has the shape of a "dinner fork".

Possible Complications

- Blood vessel damage.
- Nerve involvement.
- Tendon damage.

Management

- Check circulation and motor and sensory function of fingers and support the injured area.
- Apply a formed, well-padded splint from the axilla to past the fingertips.
- Maintain the hand and wrist in the position of function, if possible, with extra padding in the palm.
- Secure the splint to the arm snugly enough to give support.
- If the patient is ambulatory, apply a large arm sling. If the patient is lying down, support and elevate the arm at his/her side.
- Apply cold to the injury site.
- Transport to medical attention.

HAND AND FINGER FRACTURES AND DISLOCATIONS

Cause

- Direct blow.
- Fall.
- Twisting injury.

Signs and Symptoms

- As for general signs of fracture.

Possible Complications

- Blood vessel damage.
- Nerve involvement.
- Tendon damage.

Management

- Check circulation and support the injured area.
- Do not apply traction to injuries at or near a joint.

- Apply a formed, well-padded splint from the elbow to past the fingertips.
- Maintain the hand and fingers in the position of function, if possible, with extra padding in the palm.
- Secure the splint to the arm snugly enough to give support.
- If the patient is ambulatory, apply an appropriate sling.
- If the patient is lying down, support and elevate the arm at the patient's side.
- Apply cold to injury site.
- Transport to medical attention.

Part X, Section E
Management of Lower Limb Injuries

PRIOR TO THE EVALUATION AND MANAGE-MENT OF LOWER LIMB INJURIES, THE ATTEND-ANT MUST FOLLOW THE PRIORITY ACTION APPROACH AS OUTLINED IN PART III, PAGE 20.

PRINCIPLES OF IMMOBILIZATION

The general principles of immobilization should be followed when dealing with lower limb injuries.

Additional Specific Lower Limb Management Principles

1. Always place splint-securing ties before placing the splints.
2. Use broad-fold bandages wherever possible. Place the chest tie high on the chest so it does not restrict breathing. The pelvic tie should be around the hips. The top of the tie should be just inferior to the iliac crest to avoid squeezing the abdomen.
3. Always attempt to use at least two wooden splints to immobilize the limb.
4. Splint-securing knots should always be against the splint or padded so they do not press on the patient's skin. Empty the patient's pockets of objects that may cause pressure sores.
5. Plantar splints for added ankle and foot support should conform to the natural shape of the foot and be well padded and braced.
6. The following tables list the order for tying splint-securing ties to ensure adequate support of the limb during splinting.

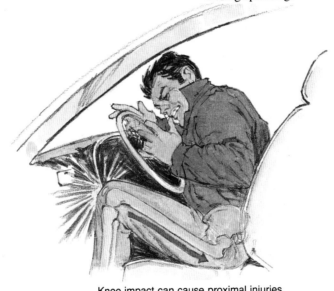

Knee impact can cause proximal injuries

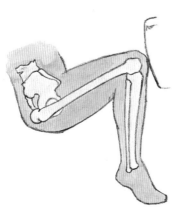

Dislocated hip

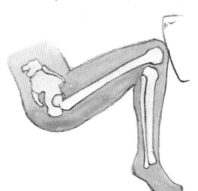

Dislocated knee joint

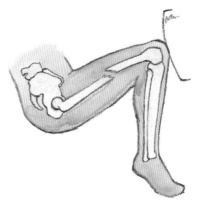

Femur fracture

TABLE X-a

Long Splinting Technique
1. Chest (trunk)
2. Hip (trunk)
3. Ankle (figure of eight)
4. Thigh
5. Just above knee
6. Knee
7. Lower leg
8. Traction (if necessary)

TABLE X-b

Short Splinting Technique
1. Thigh
2. Ankle (figure of eight)
3. Above the knee
4. Above the injury site
5. Below the injury site
6. Knee
7. Traction (if necessary)

PELVIC FRACTURE

Cause

- Fractures of the pelvis are most often caused by direct compression. Such injuries may occur in a fall from a height, crushing or violent impact to the pelvic area. Indirect force, such as the force transmitted along the femur when the knee strikes the dashboard in a head-on MVA, can also cause pelvic fractures. Suspect pelvic fractures in any high-velocity injury.

Signs and Symptoms

In addition to the general signs of a fracture, a patient with a pelvic fracture may demonstrate:
- Pain in the groin on the affected side.
- Increased pain in the pelvic region on compression of the iliac crest or pressure over the pubic symphysis (see Figure X-7).

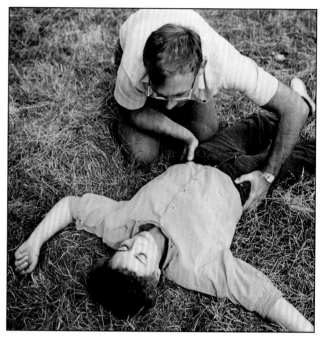

Figure X-7 Assessing for pelvic fracture

- Inability to move the lower limbs.
- Possible shock symptoms.

Possible Complications

- Internal hemorrhage may often cause hypovolemic shock as large blood vessels lie adjacent to the pelvis and may be easily lacerated. The extent of bleeding is often not obvious because bleeding occurs within the pelvic cavity.
- Tearing or rupture of the bladder or urethra (with possible blood at urethra opening).
- Fracture or dislocation of the femur.
- Open (compound) fractures of the pelvis are rare because of large adjacent muscles.

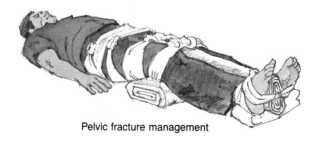

Pelvic fracture management

Management

- If the victim falls into the Rapid Transport Category, immobilize as outlined in Part XVI, Section A, page 356.
- Check circulation, sensation and motor nerve response of the lower limb.
- It is preferable that the patient not void (urinate). If there is a urethral tear, voiding may allow urine to leak into adjacent tissues.
- Place adequate padding between the legs and support them by tying the ankles (figure eight), knees and thighs together.
- Support the pelvic area by applying three overlapping broad triangular bandages around the pelvis. The top of the superior bandage should be just inferior to the iliac crest. Tie the bandages tightly enough to support the pelvis but not cause pain. Do not roll the patient when applying the bandages.
- Place the patient on a firm, well-padded stretcher or spine board.
- Support body curves with appropriate padding.
- A blanket or pillow may be placed under the patient's knees to maintain flexion. This will usually make the patient more comfortable although it should not be done if it causes pain or the patient has a suspected lower extremity fracture.
- Once the presence of a pelvic fracture is suspected, monitor the patient's general condition and vital signs closely and watch for hypovolemic shock.
- Transport the patient promptly to medical aid.

FRACTURES AND DISLOCATIONS OF THE HIP (UPPER-THIRD FEMUR)

A fracture of the upper third of the femur is called a hip fracture. The damage may occur in the head or neck of the femur.

Dislocations and fractures of the hip have similar consequences. The first aid treatment is the same for either injury and this section covers both types.

Cause of Dislocations of the Hip

- Any strong impact that forces the femur into the pelvis (e.g. when a flexed knee strikes a dashboard).
- Twisting force exerted on the femur which may occur in a fall.

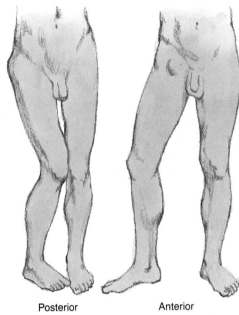

Posterior   Anterior
Dislocations of the hip

Possible Complications

- Nerve and vessel damage to the affected lower extremity.
- Fracture of the joint socket.
- Fracture of the pelvis.
- Injury to the knee.

Signs and Symptoms

- Usually severe pain at the site of injury.
- Deformity of the hip, anterior or posterior.
- Inability to move the affected leg.

1. Posterior Dislocations
   a) Leg turned inward with the knee slightly flexed and lying against the opposite knee.
   b) There may be a hard lump in the buttock of the affected side.
   c) The affected leg may be shortened.
   d) The patient may not be able to raise his toes or foot because of damage to the sciatic nerve. This is called "foot drop".
   e) There may be absent distal pulses in the affected limb.

2. Anterior Dislocations (occur very rarely)
   a) Limb rotated outward and abducted.
   b) The affected leg may be longer.

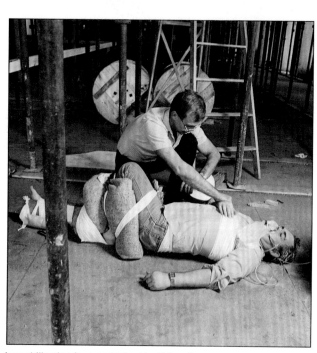

Management

- Check for circulation, sensory and motor functions distal to the injury.
- Immobilize the limb in the position of most comfort to the patient, as for femur fracture.
- If the limb is angulated and cannot be immobilized, support it with rolled blankets or pillows. Splint the uninjured limb and tie the injured leg to it with triangular bandages.
- Move the patient onto a firm, blanketed stretcher or spine board. Secure the patient to the stretcher or spine board to eliminate motion in the affected hip. Ensure prompt transport to a hospital. Early medical reduction of this dislocation is essential to avoid serious long-term complications. Once the dislocated hip has been *quickly* immobilized, the patient is placed in the Rapid Transport Category.
- Maintain a regular check of the vital signs, the patient's general condition and the state of distal pulses and neurological function in the affected limb.

If a dislocation is suspected and if the hip spontaneously reduces during treatment or transportation, notify the attending physician. Do not attempt manipulation if circulation is absent.

FEMORAL FRACTURES

Cause

- An accident involving stress or violent impact to the femur.

Signs and Symptoms

- Severe pain.
- Possible deformity.
- The foot of the injured limb may lie on its outer side (eversion) due to rotation of the entire limb distal to the fracture site.
- The injured limb may be shortened.
- The range of movement is limited by pain.
- Swelling at the injury site whether the fracture is closed or open.

Immobilization for a posterior hip dislocation

Possible Complications

- The blood vessels may be damaged and a patient may lose one or two litres of blood into the thigh. There may be external hemorrhage if the fracture is open. Consequently, patients with such fractures may often develop hypovolemic shock. Therefore, monitor for signs of shock (see Part V, Section B, page 100).
- There may be loss of blood supply or nerve damage to the distal limb, particularly with lower-third femoral fractures.
- Muscles in the thigh are powerful and, when stability of the femur is lost, these muscles contract, causing the bone ends to override.
- There may be foreign bodies (i.e. dirt or clothing) in the wound or bacterial contamination if the fracture is compound.

Management

- Support the injured limb.
- Check for circulation, sensory and motor function distal to the injury and repeat every 30 minutes.
- Apply firm traction before improving the position of the limb. Traction is applied in the long axis of the leg and the limb is gradually moved from the deformed position to a more normal alignment. Owing to severe muscle spasms, the Attendant may be unable to align the femur in a normal position and, consequently, the limb should be immobilized as close as possible to the normal position. A compound fracture should be covered with a dry sterile dressing and then traction should be applied as for a closed fracture (see Principles of Traction, Section C, page 253). Maintain the traction until the limb is completely immobilized.
- Apply two appropriate-length splints but, if possible, avoid placing them over wounds, swelling or obvious deformity. The joints above and below the site of the fracture must be immobilized.
- Secure the traction bandage to the splints, keeping the traction bandage ends in line with the leg and foot.

NOTE: A patient with lower limb fractures who falls into the Rapid Transport Category may have to be moved before the limb can be fully splinted. For appropriate immobilization in these circumstances, please see Part XVI, Section A, page 356.

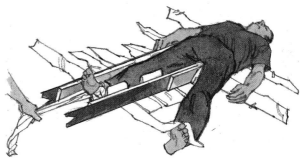

Applying traction and splints for a femur fracture

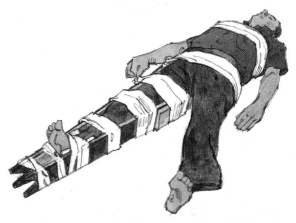

Completed immobilization for a femur fracture

When the patient is found prone with multiple injuries and cannot be fully assessed for vital system function (such as with a chest injury), with C-spine control log-roll the patient into a more suitable position (supine). The patient must be log-rolled to the supine position with C-spine control as the prime concern. The lower limb is of secondary concern in this situation. If help is immediately available, the injured limb should be supported during this move.

The patient who is found supine with an obviously fractured femur, but whose airway is compromised, will have to be moved into the lateral position for drainage. See Part IV, Section B, page 44.

INJURIES TO THE KNEE

Many types of injuries may occur at, or around, the knee, including sprains, dislocation of the joint, patellar dislocations, fractures to the distal femur, proximal (upper third) tibia and patellar fractures. All knee injuries are managed as for a femoral fracture, BUT WITHOUT TRACTION.

FRACTURE OF THE PATELLA

Cause

Fractures of the patella usually are the result of direct trauma and, therefore, separation of the fragments cannot be palpated.

Possible Complications

- Intra-articular fractures of the femur or tibia.
- Nerve and vessel injury if there is knee joint damage.

Signs and Symptoms

- Severe pain at the front of the knee.
- Inability or reluctance to flex the knee or move the limb.
- Broken fragments may be felt (they may be widely separated).
- Tenderness and marked swelling over the anterior knee.

Management

- Support the limb in the position of most comfort. Maintain the flexion of the knee with padding placed behind the knee.
- Apply cold. Cover the entire area of the knee joint (on for 10 minutes, off for five minutes).
- Check for circulation, sensory and motor function distal to the injury every 30 minutes.
- Splint the limb as for a femur fracture, with one of two splints positioned posteriorly (Figure X-8).
- Secure the limb to the splint.
- Move the patient onto a firm, padded lifting device.
- Transport to medical attention.

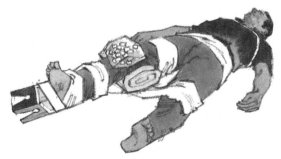

Figure X-8   Immobilization for a fracture of the patella

TRAUMATIC DISLOCATION OF THE PATELLA

Cause

- Dislocation of the patella may occur as a result of a direct force applied to the anterior medial aspect of the patella, driving it laterally. However, it most frequently occurs in the absence of trauma, in individuals with developmental weakness of the patellar mechanism. Incomplete dislocations usually reduce spontaneously when the knee is extended; this may also occur with complete dislocation. After spontaneous reduction, there is usually swelling of the anterior knee with marked tenderness along the medial border of the patella.

The typical deformity of acute traumatic dislocation of the patella:

- The knee is semi-flexed.
- The patella is displaced laterally.
- The quadriceps and patella tendons are taut.

Management

If it will take more than 20 minutes to get the patient to a physician, one or two attempts may be made to reduce the dislocation:

- Cool the knee with ice to reduce discomfort.
- Extend the knee gradually while applying pressure medially, pushing the patella over the lateral femoral condyle.
- Reapply cold and refer the patient to a medical facility, whether reduction has been achieved or not.

SPRAIN OF THE KNEE

The knee is very prone to injuries of the ligaments, which may range in severity from simple sprains to a complete tear of one or more of the major ligaments.

The four main ligaments of the knee in order of their vulnerability to injury are:

- Medial collateral
- Anterior cruciate
- Lateral collateral
- Posterior cruciate

Causes

- Fragment injuries occur when abnormal twisting or bending forces are applied to the knee. Thus, excessive rotation may tear any or all of the ligaments.

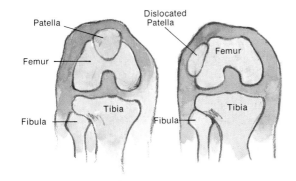

Front view of the knee, bent at a 45° angle.

Patella

Dislocated Patella

Femur

Femur

Tibia

Tibia

Fibula

Fibula

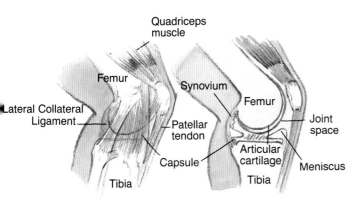

Quadriceps muscle

Femur

Synovium

Femur

Lateral Collateral Ligament

Joint space

Patellar tendon

Capsule

Articular cartilage

Meniscus

Tibia

Tibia

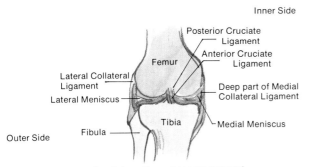

Inner Side

Posterior Cruciate Ligament

Anterior Cruciate Ligament

Femur

Lateral Collateral Ligament

Deep part of Medial Collateral Ligament

Lateral Meniscus

Tibia

Medial Meniscus

Fibula

Outer Side

Front view of knee, kneecap removed

- Knee forced inward may damage the medial collateral ligament.
- Knee jerked forward may damage the anterior cruciate ligament.
- Knee forced outward may damage the lateral collateral ligament.
- Knee forced backward may damage the posterior cruciate ligament.

It is not uncommon for injury of the medial collateral ligament, the anterior cruciate ligament and the cartilage to occur together, as excessive rotation can cause all of these structures to be injured.

Signs and Symptoms

Sprains to the knee range in severity from mild to severe.

- In a mildly sprained knee, the pain may be relatively insignificant. There will be little or no swelling. There are usually no complications and treatment consists of application of cold and tensor bandage.
- In a moderate knee sprain, where there is more pain and some swelling in the knee with possible hematoma formation, the patient may experience a brief loss of function at the time of the injury or within the next 24 hours as the swelling takes place. First aid treatment for a moderate knee sprain includes the application of cold and a tensor bandage. Have the patient use crutches; if possible, refer to medical attention.
- A severe knee sprain is one in which the pain, swelling and loss of function are immediate and any movement can increase the pain. Sometimes severe sprains are associated with dislocation of the knee or patella or tears of the ligaments of the knee. First aid treatment includes the application of cold, immobilization in the position of greatest comfort and transport to medical aid.

The most frequently injured ligaments of the knee are the medial collateral ligament and the anterior cruciate ligament. This injury can occur when the foot is planted firmly and the knee is struck from the lateral aspect. The condyle of the femur is driven into the semilunar cartilage, the cruciate ligament becomes overstretched and the medial collateral ligament is torn. Swelling is immediate. Damage to the surrounding bursae, blood vessels and nerves may occur.

CARTILAGE TEARS

The medial and lateral semilunar cartilages (menisci) lie on the superior surface of the tibia. In cartilage injuries, the point of tenderness is likely to be on the joint line. In ligamentous injuries around the knee, the point of the tenderness may be above or below the joint line.

Cause

- Semilunar cartilage injuries may be caused by a compression or grinding action of the femur on the tibia, with some cartilage interposed between. The injury that damaged the ligaments may also cause injuries to the cartilage. Once torn, the cartilage will not repair itself.

Signs and Symptoms

- Patient may have felt a clicking, snapping or tearing sensation in the knee.
- A torn cartilage usually has swelling, caused by increased synovial fluid or blood in the joint. The swelling may take a few hours to appear.
- The knee may be locked or may give way. Chips of cartilage may float loosely in the joint and form wedges which will lock the joint in a certain position.
- A patient who has had a knee cartilage injury that was not treated may find subsequently that the knee will lock spontaneously, usually in a flexed position. Sometimes patients can unlock it themselves. If the condition develops, such patients should be referred for medical attention.

Management of Suspected Knee Ligament and Cartilage Injuries

- Cool the knee with ice to reduce discomfort.
- Elevate in position of comfort (usually semi-flexed).
- Discourage weight bearing.
- Refer for medical attention.

BURSITIS OF THE KNEE

There are numerous bursae in and around the knee joint. They secrete fluid and lubricate the joint, absorb shock and prevent wear by friction. When irritated, the bursae may fill with a thin liquid called synovial fluid.

Irritation of the bursae of the knee is commonly referred to as housemaid's knee.

Cause

- A blow to the knee.
- Prolonged pressure on the bursae of the joint, such as from prolonged kneeling.

Signs and Symptoms

- Superficial synovial swelling on or just inferior to the patella.
- Local pain especially when kneeling.

Possible Complications

- Continued irritation and continued swelling may damage the bursae and joint structures.

Management

- Control swelling with elevation.
- Ensure minimal knee movement and do not allow the patient to continue to kneel.
- Apply crepe for support.
- Refer to medical attention, if required.

DISLOCATION OF THE KNEE

Knee dislocations are VERY SERIOUS INJURIES.

Cause

- A force strong enough to tear ligaments and displace bone ends.

Signs and Symptoms

- Pain, usually severe.
- Marked deformity and swelling. The proximal end of the tibia is completely displaced from its articulation with the femur.
- Loss of stability and often inability to move the joint.

Possible Complications

- The most serious complication of this injury is an injury to the popliteal artery, loss of distal circulation may occur due to blood vessel damage or compression.
- Nerve damage, as evidenced by paralysis and/or numbness of the foot.
- Ligament tears and joint capsule damage.

Management

- Management of a knee dislocation is essentially the

same as for any joint injury where the tissue cannot support itself.

- Dislocation may result in a number of different limb and joint positions. For this reason, there is no specific treatment for dislocations, apart from the general principles of management.
- No attempt should be made at reduction unless distal circulation is lost (see section on Dislocations). Because of the high incidence of blood vessel damage, which may ultimately result in the loss of the lower leg, patients with these injuries must be promptly transported to a hospital. Treatment before transportation should be confined to the Priority Action Approach and *quickly* immobilizing the limb.
- If a dislocation reduces spontaneously during treatment or transportation, the attending physician must be notified that a dislocation had occurred.

FRACTURES OF THE TIBIA AND FIBULA

Fractures of the lower leg may involve the tibia or the fibula or both. Because of the relatively large amount of soft tissue support surrounding the fibula, fractures of this bone are generally closed. The tibia lies immediately under the skin of the shin and, consequently, these fractures are more often compound.

Management

In the management of these fractures, the Attendant should immobilize the knee and the ankle. Two short

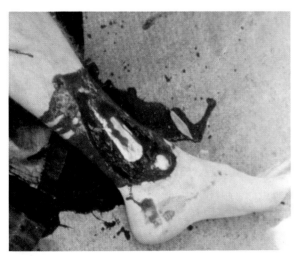

Fractured ankle and lower third tibia and fibula

splints, applied correctly, stabilize the lower leg, while allowing hip flexion and elevation of the injured part.

ANKLE FRACTURES/DISLOCATIONS

Ankle injuries (fractures or dislocations) are managed as for any other joint injuries. A plantar splint, braced as shown, is recommended for added support to the joint. Ankles that are badly deformed usually have a fracture dislocation of the joint. The distal circulation must be carefully monitored. If there is no circulation, manipulate as outlined in Section C, page 251. Fracture dislocations of the ankle are unstable. After manipulation, they must be maintained in the new position or they will redislocate. This reduced position must be splinted or they may be maintained manually by the Attendant. After immobilization, swelling can be minimized by elevating the ankle and applying cold.

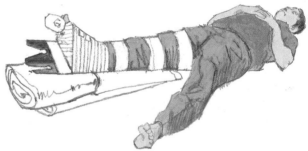

Ankle fracture management

ANKLE SPRAINS

The ankle joint is one of the most frequently injured joints. It may be difficult on initial examination to differentiate a simple sprain from an undisplaced ankle fracture.

Cause

- Ankle injuries are usually caused by inversion or eversion of the foot.

Signs and Symptoms

- Pain more acute on the injured side.
- The patient is reluctant to place weight on the injured ankle.
- Swelling usually appears shortly after the accident.
- If there is tearing of ligaments, discolouration will appear in one to two days.

Management (Severe Sprain)

- If x-ray facilities are reasonably close, the patient should keep off the injured ankle and go for x-ray diagnosis.
- In isolated or semi-isolated areas, the patient should keep weight off the injured ankle for 24 hours. The swelling should be controlled with elevation, cold and a tensor bandage, as required. If there is no improvement after 24 hours or if significant discolouration is present, the patient should be referred to a physician. If there is improvement and little or no discolouration, support the ankle with strapping and a tensor bandage.

Management (Simple Sprain)

- The swelling should be controlled with elevation, cold and a tensor bandage as required.
- Moderate activity should be encouraged if the patient can maintain weight on the injured ankle.
- Work activity may be altered if necessary (i.e. light duty).

INJURIES OF THE FOOT AND TOES

Injuries of the foot and toes are very common. The most frequent mechanism of injury includes a crushing force, direct trauma, inversion injury to the lateral foot and puncture wounds. Other less common injuries include a fall from height onto the heels and lacerations.

It may be difficult to distinguish between sprains and fractures of the foot. Regardless, injuries of the foot usually have significant swelling. Fortunately, vascular injuries are uncommon. As in the upper extremity, lacerations about the foot and ankle may have associated nerve and tendon damage. A simple puncture wound of the foot, especially if the puncturing object is contaminated (e.g. a pitchfork), may cause serious and rapidly progressive infections. All of these injuries should be assessed medically if the patient is at all incapacitated or their injury may have any complications (e.g. tetanus contamination).

Any fall from a height where the patient lands on the heels may result in a fracture of the calcaneus (heel bone). These injuries are very painful and associated with marked swelling. The skin about the fracture may blister in the first 24 hours. Immediate elevation and the intermittent application of cold is usually very helpful. In such falls, be sure to assess for an associated knee, pelvic or lumbar spine injury.

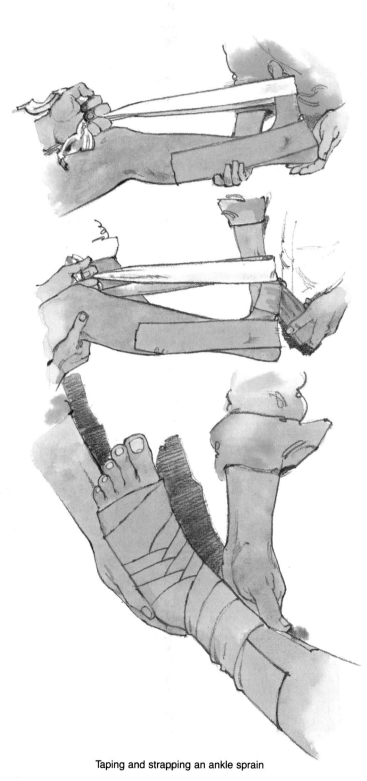

Taping and strapping an ankle sprain

Management of Foot Injuries

- Lay the patient in the supine position (if not contrain-dicated).
- Remove shoes and socks with care (they may have to be cut off).
- Check for deformity, sensation, motor function of the toes and circulation.
- Elevate the limb and apply appropriate dressings.
- The intermittent use of cold may be helpful.
- A pillow splint may provide excellent immobilization of the foot for isolated suspected foot fractures. Otherwise, use the splinting techniques as outlined in Ankle Fracture Section.

Generally, injuries of the foot will be disregarded when the patient falls into the Rapid Transport Category.

Part XI, Section A
Heat Exposure and Heat-related Emergencies

The human body is able to maintain a steady core temperature of 37°C (98.6°F) despite exposure to a wide range of environmental conditions. As discussed in the section on hypothermia, the human body has a number of mechanisms to stabilize internal body temperature. In this section, the disorders associated with heat exposure will be reviewed.

The body has to dissipate heat when working or exercising in a hot climate. Working muscle generates considerable amounts of heat. Heavy exertion on a very hot day could theoretically raise the body's core temperature to a fatal level were it not for the body's capability to dissipate heat.

Heat dissipation (loss) occurs through the following mechanisms:
- radiation;
- convection;
- evaporation.

Radiation is an effective means of heat loss provided that the surrounding temperature is less than the body's core temperature (37°C). When the outside temperature is close to the body's core temperature, heat loss through radiation is very minimal. When the outside temperature exceeds the core temperature, the body actually absorbs additional heat from the environment rather than losing heat.

Convection directly transfers heat only if cooler air passes over the warm body. On a windless day, or if the patient is well insulated with bulky windproof clothing, heat loss by convection is minimal or non-existent.

When the surrounding temperature is close to or higher than the normal body temperature, evaporation of sweat is the body's only effective mechanism for heat loss. However, if the humidity is very high, evaporation is reduced. Individuals who exercise or work hard on hot, humid, windless days are especially prone to those disorders associated with heat exposure.

If the body is unable to dissipate heat, core body temperature may rise to critical levels. Mild or moderate elevation of core temperature commonly occurs as fever, and is usually associated with infection and other illnesses. Heat stroke (hyperthermia) is a life-threatening elevation of the body's core temperature above 41°C (106°F), usually associated with a decreased level of consciousness and cardiovascular collapse.

Workers and athletes can produce as much as 2.5 to 3 litres of sweat per hour during periods of extreme exertion. Sweat is a solution of water and salt. As a result of profuse sweating, an individual may become dehydrated and salt-depleted. The problem is further complicated when the individual replaces the fluid loss with beer or salt-free fluids (e.g. plain water). The other major disorders associated with heat exposure are heat cramps and heat exhaustion. They are caused by salt depletion and fluid dehydration.

HEAT CRAMPS

Heat cramps result from salt imbalances in muscle. They occur when patients sweat profusely during a period of heavy exertion and replace their fluid losses but not their salt depletion.

Clinically, severe intense muscle cramps occur in those muscles that have performed the most work (usually the arms or legs). The onset is often delayed — cramping usually occurs during the resting period. There is no evidence that muscle injury occurs as a result of cramps. The core body temperature measured rectally is usually normal. The patient's vital signs are typically normal and there is no change in the level of consciousness.

Treatment focuses on fluid and salt replacement. Commercially available oral solutions or fruit juices are useful. A solution of one teaspoon of salt per half litre (500 cc's) or one pint of water is also recommended. Pure water or alcoholic beverages are contraindicated. Salt tablets alone are not recommended. They often pass through the bowel undigested and may induce vomiting.

If the patient has abnormal vital signs or a decreased level of consciousness, the Attendant must consider other heat-related disorders or other medical problems.

HEAT EXHAUSTION

Heat exhaustion is caused by both water and salt depletion associated with sweating during prolonged periods of exertion. Fluid replacement has not been sufficient to match the losses. The signs and symptoms may develop over a relatively short period of time (workers during extreme exertion who do not drink fluids) or take a few days to develop (for example, elderly patients in nursing homes may develop heat exhaustion during prolonged heat waves because of their inability to maintain adequate fluid replacement).

Signs and Symptoms of Heat Exhaustion

The patient may complain of weakness, fatigue or dizziness. Headache and nausea are also common features. The patient may faint. Muscle cramps also occur. Assessment of the vital signs may reveal a weak rapid pulse. Respirations may be shallow and the respiratory rate increased. The signs and symptoms of heat exhaustion are essentially those of mild hypovolemic shock. It occurs because salt and fluid losses have been excessive. Examination of the skin usually reveals it to be pale, cool and clammy. The process of sweating is preserved. This can be assessed by examining the skin of the forehead and the armpits. It is an important finding because the presence of sweating is often the only way to differentiate heat exhaustion from the life-threatening emergency of heat stroke. If untreated, heat exhaustion may progress to heat stroke.

Management of Heat Exhaustion

The essentials of treatment are to move the patient to a cooler environment and lay the person down. Excessive or tight-fitting clothing should be removed or loosened. The patient may be cooled by sponging with cool water and fanning. Care must be taken not to cool the patient too much. If the patient begins to shiver, the Attendant should stop sponging.

Only if the patient is fully alert and not nauseated should oral fluids be provided. Juice, soft drinks or a solution of salt water (1 teaspoon of salt in 1 pint or 500 cc's water) are best. Alcoholic beverages and coffee are not recommended.

In most cases, the patient's symptoms will improve dramatically within 30 minutes. However, it is best that these patients still be transferred to hospital for medical evaluation.

HEAT STROKE

Heat stroke (hyperthermia) occurs when the body's mechanisms for heat dissipation are overwhelmed and fail. Heat stroke must not be confused with thermal injury (i.e. burns). As a result of the heat exposure, core body temperature rises to critical levels approaching or exceeding 41°C (106°F). At these high temperatures, the cells of the brain, heart and kidneys are unable to survive and organ dysfunction develops. Heat stroke typically develops during periods of extreme exertion in a hot, humid environment. During long heat waves, elderly patients living in non-air-conditioned, poorly ventilated buildings are also at risk. The risk of heat stroke is also increased by inadequate fluid and salt intake. Certain medications may also increase the risk of heat stroke. Some drug overdoses or occupational exposures (e.g. pentachlorophenol) may cause heat stroke as a symptom of the poisoning.

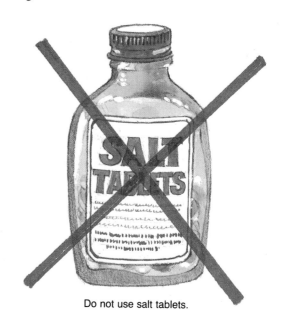

Do not use salt tablets.

Signs and Symptoms of Heat Stroke

As the body's core temperature rises to critical levels, organ dysfunction develops — especially in the heart and the brain. Therefore, most of the signs and symptoms of heat stroke relate to the cardiovascular and nervous systems. Patients may display some or all of the following signs and symptoms.

- hot, dry, flushed skin
- absence of sweating
- agitation, confusion
- decreased level of consciousness
- headache
- nausea and vomiting

- seizures
- increased respiratory rate
- irregular pulse
- shock
- cardiac arrest

The presence of hot, dry, flushed skin without any evidence of sweating is one of the important findings that differentiate heat stroke from the other heat-related illnesses. The lack of sweating attests to the body's inability to compensate for the heat stress because its compensatory mechanisms have been overwhelmed.

Recognition of severe heat stroke is not difficult when a patient exhibits the classical signs of elevated body temperature and altered level of consciousness in the midst of a heat wave or after heavy exertion on a very hot day. However, in our temperate climate, the signs and symptoms may not be typical and may not be recognized. Other medical illnesses may resemble heat stroke.

Priority Action Approach to the Patient with Suspected Heat Stroke

HEAT STROKE IS A LIFE-THREATENING MEDICAL EMERGENCY. Without prompt and aggressive treatment, the patient may die. Such patients are in the Rapid Transport Category but the Attendant must make every effort to lower the body's core temperature while awaiting transport and continuing en route.

1. The patient must be moved to the coolest spot available (e.g. placed in the shade).
2. All outer clothing should be removed.
3. The patient should be placed supine unless there is active vomiting or seizures. In this situation, the ¾ prone or lateral position is recommended.
4. Supplemental high-flow oxygen at 10 Lpm must be provided.
5. Cold water should be applied to the patient either by dousing (being careful not to drown the patient) or applying wet, cool sheets. Spraying or sponging the entire body with cold water is also effective. Fanning the patient promotes evaporation and increases the cooling rate.
6. If the patient is fully alert and not nauseated, give cold water or juice to drink. Alcoholic beverages are definitely not recommended.

7. If a core temperature can be measured without too much inconvenience or embarrassment, a rectal temperature should be recorded (a special rectal thermometer is required). Cooling measures should be stopped when the temperature falls to 38.5°C rectally.
8. Vital signs should be reassessed every 10 minutes during treatment and while en route to the hospital.
9. The seizing patient should be protected from further injury while cooling continues. An oral airway and assisted ventilation may be required, especially in the postictal period (see Part XIV, Section B, page 337 on seizure management).

SUMMARY

The most important aspect of heat stroke and other heat-related illnesses is prevention. The First Aid Attendant has an important role to play in preventing these medical problems. By teaching co-workers about the risk of heat-related illness and encouraging adequate salt and fluid replacement on hot summer days, the Attendant may prevent such emergencies from happening.

Part XI, Section B
Cold Injuries

COLD INJURY, FROSTBITE AND HYPOTHERMIA

Extreme cold, just like extreme heat, has the potential to cause injury and damage to tissue. Body cells can function only within a narrow temperature range. If the core temperature falls below a critical point, severe organ dysfunction begins.

Hypothermia is defined as a core body temperature of less than 35°C (95°F). Normal body temperature is 37°C (98.6°F). Frostnip is defined as a minor cold injury without soft tissue damage. Frostbite is defined as a cold injury with damage to the soft tissues, most commonly involving the lower extremities.

COLD INJURY AND TRENCH (IMMERSION) FOOT

These injuries are mild and no damage to the soft tissue occurs. Cold injury occurs as the result of prolonged exposure to cold (not necessarily freezing temperatures). Trench (immersion) foot occurs from prolonged exposure to cold water and is particularly common with hikers or hunters. The skin of the affected part is pale and cold to touch but does not feel frozen. Sensation is usually preserved to some extent. These signs and symptoms distinguish milder injuries from frostbite.

The emergency treatment of mild cold injuries focuses on removing the patient from the cold wet environment and rewarming the affected part. Wet and/or constrictive clothing must be removed. Contact with a warm object such as the Attendant's hands, or placing the affected hand in the patient's armpit, is all that is usually required. Tingling, mild pain and redness of the affected part usually occur during rewarming. The affected part usually heals completely on its own without further treatment. The patient should be referred for medical assessment if the symptoms persist.

FROSTBITE

Frostbite occurs when soft tissue is subjected to freezing temperatures. Tissue injury results when tissue temperature falls below a critical point. The tissue temperature is affected not only by the outside temperature and wind-chill factor but also by the blood flow to the tissue. Patients with pre-existing circulatory disorders are more susceptible to frostbite. Workers wearing constrictive clothing or who must work in cramped positions have reduced blood flow to the extremities and are also more susceptible to frostbite.

Frostbite occurs when ice crystals form within tissues. In addition, as the hands or feet (the most common sites) are cooled, the blood vessels of the skin constrict and blood flow is reduced significantly. Ultimately, the affected tissue, including its blood vessels and nerve fibres, is damaged.

Signs and Symptoms of Frostbite

The toes are the most commonly affected site. The symptoms will vary with the individual and the outside (ambient) temperature. Generally, symptoms begin with pain and redness. The redness represents the body's efforts to increase tissue temperature by increasing its blood flow. As the cold progresses, the affected part becomes pale and the pain is replaced by tingling and numbness. It is often described that the affected part feels like "a block of wood". The frozen extremity may appear completely white or be mottled with blue and white patches. The affected tissues feel frozen solid.

It is impossible to determine the full extent of injury at the initial assessment. A superficial mild injury may initially resemble severe frostbite, ultimately requiring amputation.

Treatment

The Attendant uses a Priority Action Approach to assess and prioritize the patient's injuries. The ABCs are obviously the Attendant's first priorities. Frostbite by itself does not cause alteration to the ABCs. Therefore, if the patient has abnormalities of the airway or breathing, signs of shock, or a decreased level of consciousness, the Attendant must diligently search for other injuries and also consider the possibility of severe hypothermia. The Attendant must not let a frostbite injury distract attention from other potentially life-threatening injuries.

The Attendant should remove any wet or constrictive clothing from the affected extremity. Care should be taken not to expose the extremity to further cold. Even if the patient cannot be moved indoors, the extremity should be wrapped in dry blankets after the appropriate dressing has been applied. The use of snow or ice packs is not appropriate as it increases the extent of the frostbite injury.

Management

The affected part should be covered lightly with a gauze dressing. Blisters should not be broken. The limb should be elevated (heart level) and immobilized with a well-padded, supportive dressing. The limb must be handled gently. The patient should not be allowed to walk or bear weight on the affected foot.

THE ATTENDANT MUST NEVER RUB FROST-BITTEN TISSUE. IT INCREASES THE EXTENT OF INJURY.

The mainstay of therapy is to rewarm the affected part. However, rewarming should be done once and only once, and as quickly as possible. Therefore, rewarming is usually best done in the hospital. Equipment limitations and time factors are the major problems with rewarming by IFA Attendants in the field.

ONLY IF TRANSPORTATION TO A HOSPITAL IS DELAYED FOR ONE TO TWO HOURS, AND ONLY IF ALL THE NECESSARY EQUIPMENT IS AVAILABLE, SHOULD THE ATTENDANT INITIATE REWARMING THERAPY.

Technique for Rewarming Frostbitten Tissue.

1. Immerse the part in a large basin or bath of warm water 38°C to 43°C (100.5°F to 110°F). The bath or basin has to be large enough so the affected part does not touch the sides and there is still sufficient room to stir the water.
2. The initial water temperature must be checked with a thermometer and monitored closely. The water will cool rapidly and additional hot water must be added to maintain the temperature within the desired range.
3. The thawing or rewarming process usually requires 30-40 minutes.
4. If the ears or nose are affected, the Attendant should apply hot-water-soaked dressings at the appropriate temperature for 30-40 minutes.
5. After rewarming, the affected part should be carefully dried and lightly dressed with dry sterile gauze and the affected limb kept elevated.
6. Frostbitten tissue must never be thawed by an open flame or radiating heat source (e.g. engine exhaust, radiator).

7. Rewarming must never be initiated if there is any chance that the affected part may freeze again before the patient reaches hospital.

As the part rewarms, the patient may experience considerable pain. THE AFFECTED PART MUST NOT BE RUBBED. The patient should be reassured that this is normal and a good sign that the affected part will recover. Swelling and blisters may also form within a few hours after rewarming. The Attendant should not be overly concerned about this.

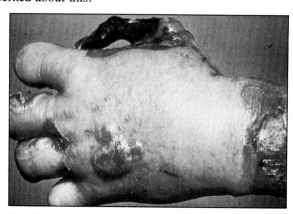

Frostbite approximately 10 days

HYPOTHERMIA

Hypothermia occurs when the body's core temperature falls below 35°C (95°F). Under normal circumstances, the body maintains a stable internal core temperature by balancing heat loss and production. The body loses heat by four mechanisms:

1. radiation;
2. conduction;
3. convection;
4. evaporation.

1. **Radiation:** All objects radiate heat. Radiation is the transfer of heat without direct contact. Radiation accounts for 50-65% of our heat loss.
2. **Conduction:** The transfer of heat by direct contact is called conduction. Air is a poor conductor of heat but water conducts heat very well. Heat loss by conduction increases 5 times in wet clothing and up to 25 times in cold water. This explains why falling into cold water rapidly cools the body. Anyone who has touched cold metal with bare skin on a cold day may

painfully remember this particular effect of conductive heat loss.

3. **Convection:** Heat loss by convection occurs whenever air or water contacts a warm surface and then moves away. A hot cup of coffee is cooled by convection when an individual blows on it. The wind-chill factor represents the additional heat loss by convection from the wind on a cold day.

4. **Evaporation:** Evaporation of sweat or water results in a net loss of heat from the body. This accounts for most of the remaining heat loss by the body in a normal environment. Evaporation is the major mechanism by which the body prevents excessive temperature rise (hyperthermia) when working in a hot environment (see Section A, page 277).

The body prevents heat loss by constricting the blood vessels to the skin and reducing the skin's blood flow. The body increases its internal heat production by shivering. The energy generated by shivering is used to maintain the body's core temperature. However, in moderate and severe hypothermia, with the onset of the changes in the level of consciousness, shivering is inhibited. Therefore, heat loss continues unabated.

There are many different causes of hypothermia. Outdoor workers are particularly at risk if they are not wearing adequate clothing or if the weather changes suddenly. Exhaustion from hard work and exercise in a cold, wet environment will also increase the risk. Immersion hypothermia may occur when an individual falls into cold water. Patients who are intoxicated with alcohol or drugs are also at risk of developing hypothermia if they lose consciousness in a cold environment. Alcohol and drugs also interfere with the body's shivering mechanism and induce vasodilation, thereby increasing blood flow to the skin. Trauma patients may also develop hypothermia as a complication of their injuries. Patients with shock or brain and spinal cord injuries are particularly at risk. Young children and babies are more susceptible to hypothermia because of their larger surface-area-to-weight ratio. Old people are prone to develop hypothermia because they are often chronically ill and their bodies cannot regulate temperature as well.

Stages of Hypothermia

As the body's core temperature falls, the patient will exhibit various changes. The brain and cardiovascular system are primarily affected in hypothermia.

Table XI-a illustrates the clinical stages of hypothermia as the core temperature drops. Note that mild hypothermia refers to a core temperature between 33°C and 35°C. Moderate hypothermia occurs at 32°C and severe hypothermia at 28°C. The Attendant should be able to use the patient's physical findings to classify the level of hypothermia. For example, the patient who is confused but still shivering has moderate hypothermia.

TABLE XI-a

Stage of Hypothermia	Temp	Physical Findings
	37°C	
	36°C	
MILD	35°C	Hypothermia occurs with a core temperature below this point.
	34°C	Shivering is present to maximize heat production.
	33°C	Vasoconstriction of the peripheral arteries (decreased pulse) in an attempt to minimize further heat loss and protect the core.
MODERATE	32°C	Confusion, decreased level of consciousness, inappropriate behaviour.
	31°C	Progressive decrease in the level of consciousness. Shivering is inhibited.
	30°C	Heart rate slows, irregularities of the heart beat may be detected. Respiratory rate falls.
	29°C	The pulse may become difficult to palpate. High risk of developing cardiac arrest, especially with rough handling. Pupils are dilated.

	28°C	Coma may develop, increased muscular rigidity. Slow heart rate. Pupils may be dilated and poorly reactive. Further decrease in respiratory rate.
	27°C	Patient may appear to be in cardiac arrest with absent pulses and no respirations. There may be no response to painful stimuli.
SEVERE	26°C	Victims are usually comatose, cardiac arrest may develop spontaneously.
	24°C	Frothy sputum may become apparent. This represents fluid congestion in the lungs.
	22°C	Maximum risk of cardiac arrest.
	20°C	Heart activity usually ceases.
	16°C	Lowest accidental hypothermia survivor.
	9°C	Lowest induced hypothermia survivor.

Diagnosing Hypothermia

Using Table XI-a, the Attendant should be able to estimate the degree of hypothermia. Patients who are cold but alert, fully oriented without any signs of confusion or inappropriate behaviour may be classified as mildly hypothermic. It is not usually necessary to record the patient's temperature. Oral temperatures are inaccurate and do not reflect core temperatures. The Attendant must never rely on an oral temperature to diagnose hypothermia. Rectal temperature is usually the only reliable method to measure core temperature. Taking a rectal temperature may be difficult, inconvenient or embarrassing to Attendant and patient. Nevertheless, documentation of a rectal temperature by the Attendant would be useful. Furthermore, ordinary thermometers only accurately record temperatures down to 35°C. Special low-reading thermometers are required. If there is a risk of hypothermia in your work environment, a low-reading thermom-

eter must be available. Recently, specially designed thermometers that fit into the ear canal have become available commercially. The temperature recorded from these devices accurately reflects the core temperature. They eliminate many of the problems associated with taking a rectal temperature. If one of these devices is available, the recording of core temperatures by the Attendant would be useful.

Priority Action Approach to the Patient with Hypothermia

The treatment of the patient with suspected hypothermia follows the Priority Action Approach beginning with the scene assessment and the primary survey.

Scene Assessment: Because of dangerous conditions (weather, avalanche, etc.) the victim may have to be rapidly extricated to a safe environment prior to the initiation of any assessment or treatment.

Primary Survey: The Attendant conducts a rapid primary survey focusing on the ABCs. The airway must be assessed and cleared if necessary. Patients not responding to verbal stimuli usually require the insertion of an oral airway to maintain patency of the airway. In moderate and severe hypothermia, there is a progressive decrease in the rate and depth of breathing. Assisted ventilation may have to be provided but the patient must *not* be hyperventilated. Assisted ventilations, if required, should be provided at a rate of 10-12 breaths per minute with supplemental oxygen. Supplemental oxygen must be provided to all victims with a decreased or altered level of consciousness. If available, heated, humidified air or oxygen should be provided. Heated, dry air or oxygen is of no benefit. Portable heating devices are now commercially available, which provide heated, humidified air/oxygen at 40°C to 45°C. This technique of airway rewarming has been shown to be very safe and effective with minimal risk of complications. Do not withhold oxygen from those patients who require it even if not heated.

Peripheral pulses become progressively difficult to palpate as the patient develops vasoconstriction and slowing of the heart rate. This occurs as the degree of hypothermia increases. Ultimately, these patients may appear to be in cardiac arrest with absent pulses and respirations. The Attendant must carefully feel for the carotid or femoral pulse. Because of the slowing of the heart rate and intense vasoconstriction, the Attendant should spend at least one minute feeling for a pulse over the carotid or femoral artery.

The patient with moderate or severe hypothermia is particularly at risk of developing cardiac arrest from rough handling. Unnecessary application of external chest compressions for suspected cardiac arrest in a patient with hypothermia may actually induce a cardiac arrest. Therefore, the Attendant must spend the extra time (up to one minute) looking for evidence of pulse or respirations. If no pulse and no respirations are detected then CPR must be initiated. Hypothermia also has a protective effect on the brain and heart, and these patients may survive long periods in cardiac arrest once they are rewarmed.

HYPOTHERMIC PATIENTS WITH CARDIAC ARREST ARE NEVER DEAD UNTIL THEY ARE WARM AND DEAD.

Obviously, any severe external bleeding must be controlled with direct pressure. Hypothermia victims often have associated injuries or other medical emergencies which must never be overlooked.

Management of Mild Hypothermia

The Attendant follows these general principles:

1. Assess and correct the ABCs.

   A — Maintain an adequate airway.

   B — Maintain adequate ventilation.

   C — Support the circulation as necessary.

   Patients with mild hypothermia alone should not have abnormalities of the ABCs. If any signs of deterioration develop in the patient's status, i.e. decreased level of consciousness, respiratory distress, decreased peripheral pulses, the Attendant must consider the presence of other injuries that may not have been initially apparent. The Attendant must frequently reassess these patients and upgrade them into the Rapid Transport Category if necessary.

2. Minimize further heat loss. The Attendant should remove all wet clothes and replace with dry clothing if available. Wrap the patient in warm blankets and/ or a sleeping bag. The patient should be moved to a warm environment as soon as possible. In the first aid room, turn up the heat as high as possible. In the ambulance or other vehicle, turn up the heater and warm the vehicle.

3. Handle the patient gently. Do not allow any exertion by the patient.

4. Do not suppress shivering even if it appears violent. This is the most effective way that the body has to generate heat. Calmly reassure the patient.

5. Do not give the patient any stimulants (coffee, tea) or any alcohol. Hot, non-alcoholic drinks containing sugar given by mouth are not useful in rewarming the patient. However, the patient may feel better. Hot fluids must be given only when the patient is fully alert and oriented without any signs of confusion. Patients with moderate and severe hypothermia have a very high risk of vomiting and fluids must not be given to these patients.

6. Do not massage the extremities or the trunk.

7. Do not put the patient in a warm bath or shower.

8. The application of hot packs is very controversial. Patients with moderate to severe hypothermia treated in this way have a higher mortality rate than those treated without hot packs, etc. Furthermore, hot-water bottles or hot pads have the potential to burn the patient. Patients with mild hypothermia may benefit from the careful application of warm pads or hot-water bottles behind the patient's neck (unless a cervical spine injury is suspected), in the groin and the armpit.

Management of Moderate and Severe Hypothermia

Patients with moderate and severe hypothermia by definition have abnormalities of their level of consciousness and variable changes in the heart and respiratory rate. The Attendant's first priority is correction of the ABCs and a careful search for other injuries. Patients with a decreased level of consciousness, with a history of a fall will require immobilization of the cervical spine.

1. As with any other seriously ill patient, the Attendant must clear and stabilize the airway, maintain adequate ventilation and support the circulation.

2. All patients with moderate or severe hypothermia fall into the Rapid Transport Category.

3. Heated, humidified oxygen, if available, should be provided by mask.

4. If assisted ventilation is required, the patient must not be hyperventilated. The Attendant should assist the

patient's own breathing and interpose ventilations to a total of 10-12 breaths per minute. If heated, humidified oxygen is unavailable and assisted ventilation is required, a pocket mask is preferable to a bag-valve mask device because the Attendant can provide warm air with oxygen to the patient.

5. **CPR must be initiated if and only if the Attendant makes a careful and lengthy (up to one minute) search for evidence of a pulse or respirations. Inappropriate use of CPR may precipitate cardiac arrest.**

6. Handle the patient gently. Extricate the patient on a stretcher. The patient may be inappropriately violent or try to walk. The patient may have to be restrained. Rough handling may precipitate a cardiac arrest.

7. *Do not* suppress shivering even if it appears violent. This is the most effective way that the body has to generate heat. Calmly reassure the patient.

8. Remove all wet clothes and replace with dry coverings if available. Wrap the patient in warm blankets and/or a sleeping bag.

9. It is not necessary to have someone undress and rewarm the patient with body contact.

10. Move the patient to a warm environment as soon as possible while awaiting transport to hospital or during transport. Turn the heat up in the first aid room. Turn the heater on high in the ambulance or transport vehicle.

11. *Do not* give the patient any stimulants (coffee, tea) or alcohol.

12. *Do not* give the patient anything by mouth, even warm fluids. Patients with moderate or severe hypothermia are at high risk of vomiting.

13. *Do not* massage the extremities or the trunk. This may precipitate cardiac arrest.

14. *Do not* put the patient in a warm bath or shower.

15. *Do not* apply hot packs or hot-water bottles to patients with moderate or severe hypothermia. Studies have shown that this increases the mortality rate. It is best to let the patient rewarm unassisted until arrival at hospital.

16. Patients with moderate and severe hypothermia must be frequently reassessed. The Attendant must look for changes in the cardiovascular status as well as looking for evidence of other injuries that were not apparent initially.

Part XI, Section C
Burns

Excessive external heat causes damage to the skin and possibly the underlying structures. It may be dry heat, such as fire, friction from a rapidly moving rope, electricity or a scald from hot liquids or vapours. Soft tissue injury from heat is directly related to the duration and intensity of the heat. The extent of damage from a burn depends on the size of the area affected and the depth of tissue involved. The larger and/or the deeper the area involved, the greater the effect on the body as a whole.

CLASSIFICATION OF BURNS

Burns are classified on the basis of the depth of the burn into first, second and third degree. A burn injury may include combinations of first, second and third degree burns.

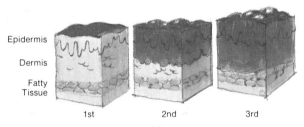

Epidermis

Dermis

Fatty Tissue

1st   2nd   3rd

Depth of Burns

First Degree Burns

First degree burns are those that affect only the outer layer of the skin. A first degree, or superficial, burn usually results in reddening of the skin and pain, such as with mild sunburn or a minor scald. The burn is usually painful initially, then heals in about a week with possible peeling of the outer skin layer.

Second Degree Burns

Second degree burns usually involve the superficial part of the dermis layer of the skin. They are sometimes described as partial thickness burns.

Damage to capillaries causes fluid (plasma) to seep into the damaged tissue, raising the top layer of skin and causing blisters. Severe pain is usually present since nerve endings are irritated and sensitive.

Blisters may not appear for several hours after the injury and the skin may only appear red and mottled (discoloured in patches).

Extensive second degree burns can cause a marked loss of fluid into the blisters and underlying tissues. The effect on the body will depend on the amount of fluid lost. If the loss is excessive, shock may occur. Excessive fluid loss can occur if more than **10%** of the body surface is burned.

Third Degree Burns

Third degree burns involve damage to the full thickness of the dermis layer of the skin and underlying fat. Muscles, bones and deeper structures may be damaged in third degree burns (full thickness burns).

Third degree burns damage the nerve endings so that pain is not a prominent symptom. The burn area may appear charred or may be dry and pale. It may also appear hard, thick and leathery and it may be either black, dark brown or white. In spite of the dry appearance, burn patients may lose a considerable amount of fluid from the burn into the tissue spaces of the area about the burn. Shock due to this fluid loss may be a major complication if the burn involves more than 10% of the body surface.

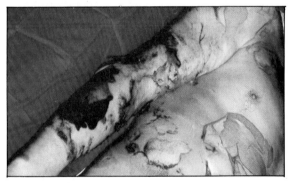

Third degree burn

DETERMINING THE EXTENT OF BURNS

Knowing the exact extent of body surface burned is important for subsequent medical treatment. For initial first aid management and transportation of the patient, the Attendant need only make a quick estimate of the total extent of burn injuries. This information is important so the Attendant can determine if swift transport to hospital is necessary, i.e. Rapid Transport Category.

The fastest and easiest method of estimating the percentages of body surface that is burned is the RULE OF NINES.

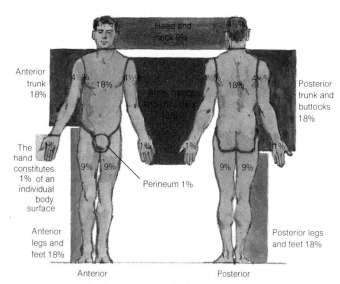

Figure XI-1 The "rule of nines"

The body is divided into multiples of nine (see Figure XI-1). Each upper extremity counts 9%, head and neck together 9%, each lower extremity 18%, the anterior and posterior surfaces of the trunk each 18% and the perineum and genitalia together 1%.

Burns that are considered serious and requiring medical attention at a hospital:

Rapid Transport Category
• any burn with associated smoke inhalation injury
• any burn associated with a decreased level of consciousness
• burns (regardless of type) to more than 10% of the body surface
• significant burns involving the face or eyes
• electrical burns
• burns encircling a limb
• major burns to hands, feet or genitalia
• any third degree burn greater than 2% body surface

Patients who have any of the conditions listed here have serious burns, and they should be transported according to the above guidelines. Although those burns fall into the Rapid Transport Category, some may appear to be of a minor nature; however, if there is any doubt, the Attendant is encouraged to contact the treating physician regarding transport protocol.

MECHANISM OF BURNS

The history of a burn injury is very important to the physician. If the patient was involved with a sudden flash or scalding liquid, most likely there will be first and/or second degree burns. If the patient's clothing caught fire, there may be third degree burns. If the person was burned in an enclosed space, the result may be respiratory burns or smoke inhalation and lung damage. If there was an explosion, there may be other associated injuries.

PRIORITY ACTION APPROACH FOR SERIOUS BURNS

First aid management of the burn patient begins at the scene of injury. The Attendant should follow the Priority Action Approach as outlined in Part III, page 20. The following special considerations must be addressed when assessing the patient with a major burn injury.

1. **Put out the fire.**

   Remove the patient from the heat or the heat from the patient — PUT OUT THE FIRE. Some patients have arrived at hospitals with clothes still smouldering under dressings and bandages. If the clothing is on fire, the patient must be laid down and the flames smothered by rolling him or her in a blanket or by dousing with large quantities of water. Remove all clothing that is still smouldering or retaining heat.

2. **Airway and Respiration**

   The single most important initial consideration is the patient's airway. Is the patient breathing and, if so, is the breathing adequate?
   RESPIRATORY PROBLEMS MUST BE ANTICIPATED IF:
   • the patient has or had a decreased level of consciousness;
   • the patient was burned indoors (closed space);
   • there are facial burns;
   • the patient has been exposed to smoke or hot gases.
   Inspect the face and neck for early signs of swelling. Inspect the nose and lips for burned or singed nasal hairs, lip blisters and soot in the mouth. Have the victim cough and look for soot in the sputum.

Hoarseness, stridor, cough, difficulty swallowing, shortness of breath and retraction of the skin around the lower neck all suggest a smoke inhalation injury. All patients with major burns require supplemental oxygen by face mask at 10 Lpm. For patients with complete or partial airway obstruction, refer to flow chart (Part IV, Section B, page 45). If the patient is having difficulty taking a breath, insert an oral airway. If the patient is not breathing, assisted ventilation is required with a bag-valve mask (or pocket mask) and a high concentration of oxygen.

3. Circulation

Burns do not bleed. However, hypovolemic shock often develops from: 1) fluid loss through burned tissues; or 2) other associated injuries. Rescuers often overlook underlying injuries in patients who have major burns. For all burn victims, the Attendant should follow the Priority Action Approach as outlined in Part III, page 20.

Major Burn Wound Management

1. Cooling. Cooling may limit the depth of the burn for some first and second degree burns (e.g. propane flash or scald). Cooling is soothing and provides some pain relief for all types of burns. Flame burns are usually third degree (full thickness); cooling will soothe but not decrease the depth of injury.

   Cooling should start within 5 minutes of the burn and be applied for a maximum of 10 minutes. Cooling should be limited to **20%** of the body surface. COOLING OF A GREATER PORTION OF THE BODY SURFACE CAN CAUSE HYPOTHERMIA. NEVER APPLY ICE. Any available source of water may be used (e.g. tap water from a kitchen sink or a garden hose). Sterile water or saline solution is neither superior to tap water nor necessary.

   If water is used to put out the fire, the victim's entire body may have to be covered. This is done to put out the fire but should not be prolonged. In these circumstances, once the fire is out, all wet and burned clothing should be removed.

   DO NOT COOL MORE THAN 20% OF THE BODY SURFACE EXCEPT TO EXTINGUISH FLAMES.

2. Remove burned clothing to ensure all smouldering or melting fabric is no longer in contact with the skin.
3. Remove rings, wristwatches and boots, if possible.
4. Elevate burned extremities, if possible. This may decrease fluid loss and tissue swelling. **Do not** splint burned limbs unless there is an obvious dislocation.
5. **Do not** break blisters.
6. **Do not** apply creams, ointments or topical anesthetics to burns.
7. Apply wet dressings to burns less than 20% body surface. Any burn in excess of 20% can be covered with dry dressings or clean sheets. **Do not** apply tight circumferential dressings.
8. After burns are dressed, keep patient comfortable and cover with blankets if necessary.
9. Monitor ABCs frequently en route to the hospital.

MINOR BURN CARE

First Degree Burns

Unless a first degree burn has involved a very large area (i.e. 40-50%) of the body surface, a patient usually does not require hospitalization.

The principal problem in first degree burns is pain which can be relieved by cold water compresses. These should be applied only to a maximum 20% of the body surface. Cold towels are usually effective for burns of the trunk or face.

Second Degree Burns

The principal problems with second degree burns are infection, pain, shock caused by loss of fluid into blisters and infection. Treatment is similar to that of a first degree burn. Cooling applied within five minutes of burn may limit the depth of this type of burn and reduce pain. The first aid treatment is discussed below.

DO NOT DELIBERATELY BREAK BLISTERS BECAUSE THIS MAY LEAD TO SECONDARY INFECTION.

If blisters do spontaneously rupture, allow fluid to drain and treat as outlined below.

The following second degree burns must be treated in a hospital:
- more than 10% of the body surface;
- hands, face, feet or genitals;
- a smoke inhalation injury.

Third Degree Burns

All third degree burns, regardless of size, should be referred to medical attention as soon as possible.

First Aid Treatment for Burns

The Attendant is often confronted with burns that are small but serious. If medical aid is close, these patients should be referred to a doctor.

When distance and transportation problems make it impossible for the patient to receive medical attention within 2-3 hours, these procedures should be followed:

1. Cover the burn with a sterile gauze pad.
2. Clean the skin around the burn.
3. Remove the original gauze pad.
4. Clean burns gently with clean water or saline to remove foreign material. Tap water is satisfactory. DO NOT DELIBERATELY BREAK BLISTERS BECAUSE THIS MAY LEAD TO SECONDARY INFECTION.
5. Apply a topical burn preparation, if available.
6. Cover the area with several layers of sterile gauze.
7. Hold the dressings in place with a conforming gauze bandage. The bandage must be snug enough to keep the dressing from falling off but not tight enough to break blisters or obstruct circulation.
8. Instruct patient to keep burned hands and feet elevated. A patient with burns to the feet should be treated in bed with the feet elevated. **Do not** splint burned extremities.
9. For minor burns that do not require medical attention, the dressing should be changed every two days, or more often if the dressing becomes soiled or wet.
10. If a burn appears infected (usually after 12-24 hours or more), the patient should be seen by a physician.

CHEMICAL BURNS

Chemical burns result from contact with corrosive or caustic substances, usually strong acids or alkalis.

A chemical will continue to burn as long as the substance remains in contact with the skin. Early removal of the chemical is of great importance.

The type of tissue injury varies with the chemical properties of the substance involved. The Attendant should be familiar with the substances used in his/her particular workplace. (See Poisons, Part XII, Section A, page 309, re WHMIS.)

There are three primary factors determining severity of an injury:
- properties of the chemical;
- concentration of the chemical;
- length of exposure to the chemical.

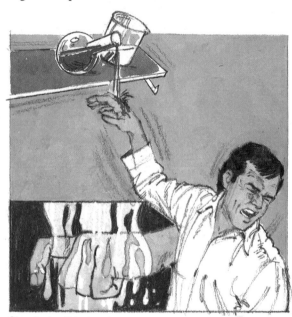

Chemical spill to hand

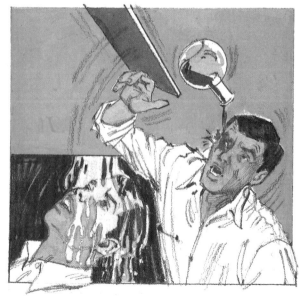

Chemical spill to eyes

Treatment of Chemical Burns

The treatment of chemical burns follows the Priority Action Approach with special emphasis on the following:

1. Immediately dilute and remove the chemical by copious flushing with water. SPEED IS ESSENTIAL.

    Begin flushing immediately, preferably with a hose or shower. Select a comfortable temperature if possible. When it is known that the burn has been caused by an acid or alkali, flush it vigorously with water for 60 consecutive minutes (by the clock).

    When the chemical is known not to be water soluble or the substance causing the burn is unknown and not dissolving in the water irrigations, mineral oil should be liberally applied to the burn site for one minute. Immediately following the mineral oil application, continue to flush with water for 60 minutes.

    The use of buffer irrigating solutions has been considered for years. The purpose of the buffer or neutralizing agent is to neutralize the substance. The idea is logical, but impractical. Neutralizing agents are rarely as available as water and some create heat during the neutralizing process, harming the patient. Water irrigation is safe and practical.

    Dry powder chemicals should be brushed from the skin before flushing is started, unless large quantities of water are immediately available.

2. Remove any of the patient's clothing that is soiled with the chemical. Continue flushing until the burning stops. The Attendant should be careful not to come into contact with the substance.

3. Estimate the degree and extent of the burn using the Rule of Nines, as with a heat burn.

4. Continue flushing or use saline-soaked dressings, reapplied every 30 minutes, if possible.

5. Transport to medical aid, constantly monitoring and recording the patient's condition. It may be necessary to continue flushing the area during transportation.

6. Chemical burns should be irrigated at the scene unless a life-threatening condition develops (e.g. airway obstruction, shortness of breath, shock or decreased level of consciousness).

    If such a life-threatening condition develops, the patient should be upgraded to the Rapid Transport Category and the irrigation continued en route, if possible.

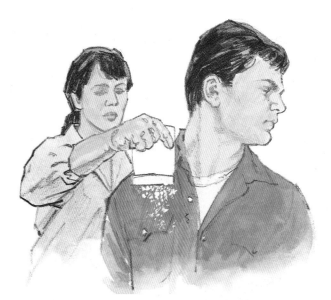

Brush dry chemicals off before flushing

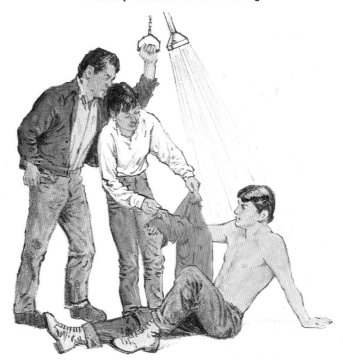

For severe contamination place patient in a shower

TAR BURNS

Burns from molten tar require special consideration. Molten tar adheres to the skin and, as long as it remains hot, it will continue to burn the patient. The tar must be cooled as soon as possible with water. Immersion of the part in, or application of, cool water should be continued for 10-15 minutes.

If the burned area exceeds 20% of the body surface, prolonged cooling should be avoided because it can cause hypothermia. Five to ten minutes is sufficient. Once the tar is cool, it is not necessary to remove it from the skin immediately, unless the nose or mouth is obstructed and breathing is difficult. If the patient's trip to medical treatment is lengthy or delayed, mineral oil on gauze dressings may be applied and left on. The tar will gradually come off as it softens during the next 6-48 hours.

ELECTRICAL BURNS

Electrical contact with the skin and the body can produce devastating effects. The actual burn that the electrical contact produces may appear quite small. The major damage can occur inside the body and the burn is often only visible as entrance and exit wounds. The internal tissues along the pathway of the current may be heated for a moment at 2,500 to 3,000 degrees C and, in effect, cooked.

Harmful Effects of Electrical Burns

- Contact Burns — usually appear as entrance and exit burns, with the appearance of charred or grey, dry tissue. The extent of injury is difficult to assess.
- Flash Burns — these are caused by an electrical flash and can appear as first or second degree surface burns.
- Thermal Burns — clothing can catch fire causing thermal flame burns as described earlier.
- Arcing Burns — these occur when the current jumps from the current source to the victim or from one part of a body surface to another. Arcing can cause contact burns or ignition and burning of clothing.
- Alternating current (AC) may cause muscle spasms. Consequently, if the victim has grasped the current source it may be difficult for the victim to let go.
- The victim may be thrown, or fall, if working at a height (e.g. on a hydro pole). Associated fractures, internal injuries and spinal injuries can occur.
- Electric shock may cause respiratory arrest and/or cardiac arrest. (See Electrical Injuries, Section D, page 293.)

Management of the Electrical Burn Patient

1. CAREFULLY remove the source of contact or the contact from the patient without endangering the rescuer.
2. Institute Priority Action Approach protocols:
   A — Establish an open airway.
   B — Check and maintain breathing.
   C — Check and maintain circulation.
3. Immediate assisted ventilation and/or cardiopulmonary resuscitation (CPR) may be necessary.
   If the electrical shock victim is conscious and breathing, reassure and keep the patient at rest.
4. Because these patients fall into the Rapid Transport Category, any burn or other injury management should be done en route to hospital and monitored closely.

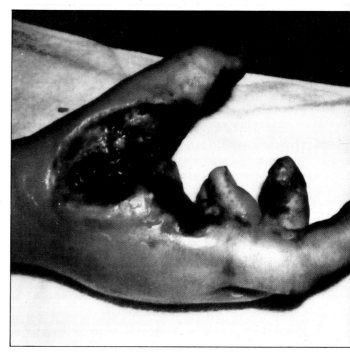

Electrical burn

Part XI, Section D
Electrical Injuries

INTRODUCTION

Electrical injury is a descriptive term for all trauma caused by contact with electrical energy. A wide variety of possible injuries can involve most organ systems. Of importance is the presence of associated injuries due to falls from a height. The electrical charge may result from human activity or a natural cause (i.e. lightning); it may be high or low voltage and it may be direct or alternating current.

The incidence of death due to electrical injury in Canada is seven per million of the population. Approximately one quarter of all electrical injuries are work related, the majority occurring in the industrial environment. Approximately three percent of all burn admissions to hospital result from electrical injury.

TYPE OF ELECTRICAL INJURIES

Electrical injury classifications:
- Electrical flash burns;
- Flame burns caused by the ignition of clothing;
- True electrical injuries, which occur when the current actually passes through the victim;
- Lightning injury.

ELECTRICAL FLASH BURNS

Electrical flash burns are caused by heat released when an arc is formed between the electrical source and a ground. In this case, the arc does not pass through the body. The intense heat of the arc (many thousand degrees) may cause first degree through third degree thermal burns of any part of the victim exposed to the arc. These burns should be managed the same as thermal burns, described in Section C, page 289.

FLAME BURNS

Flame burns caused by the ignition of clothing are common, if associated with high-voltage exposure (e.g. greater than 500 volts). These burns may also be first degree through third degree and are managed as described for thermal burns in Section C, page 289.

TRUE ELECTRICAL INJURIES

The disorders caused in the body by true electrical injuries are complex and poorly understood. Some concepts are clear. The resistance of the skin varies with the moisture content. Therefore, damp skin with perspiration or oil will much more readily conduct electricity into the body. As the electric current travels through various tissues, it generates heat. It is this release of heat that damages the tissues. As the current passes into the body and out, it usually creates an entrance and exit wound. The wounds are often small, irregular, indented and of a whitish-yellow hue. On occasion, the margins may be charred. The entrance and exit wounds may appear quite minor but extensive damage to nerves, vessels, muscles and organs may have taken place as the current passed through the body.

The current always passes through some portion of the body as it seeks ground. In a typical hand-to-hand pathway, both the upper limbs and the organs of the thorax may be injured. As the heart is often affected, the incidence of death is highest with this route. In head-to-foot or head-to-hand pathways, the brain or spinal cord may be injured.

Skeletal muscle is especially vulnerable to repeated stimulation by alternating current. Profound muscle contractions may occur when a victim contacts electrical current. The consequent muscle spasms may prevent a victim from releasing his/her grip, thus extending exposure to the current. Fractures and dislocations may occur as a consequence of these profound muscle contractions or may occur secondarily from falls.

Skeletal muscle, nerves and blood vessels may be irreparably damaged in a high-tension, high-voltage wound. It is estimated that, as a result of these severe injuries, amputation has been necessary in up to 50% of cases. Early aggressive management of these patients in a burn centre will reduce such complications.

Damage to the heart is frequently seen in electrical injury. Even household alternating current frequently precipitates ventricular fibrillation. Complete heart stoppage (asystole) is the major cardiac effect of a direct current electrical injury. Both states cause cardiac arrest and are fatal unless treatment is initiated immediately. Electrical current through the heart can also cause an irregular heart beat or a heart attack, with all of its complications. Please see Part V, Section E, page 117.

Damage to the nervous system is frequently seen. Mild injuries include: anxiety, confusion, headache, dizziness, impaired memory or difficulty concentrating. Much more

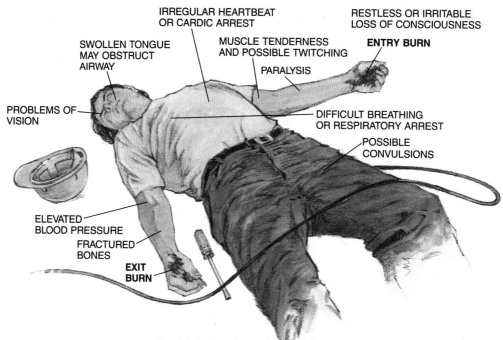

IRREGULAR HEARTBEAT
OR CARDIC ARREST

RESTLESS OR IRRITABLE
LOSS OF CONSCIOUSNESS

SWOLLEN TONGUE
MAY OBSTRUCT
AIRWAY

MUSCLE TENDERNESS
AND POSSIBLE TWITCHING

ENTRY BURN

PARALYSIS

PROBLEMS OF
VISION

DIFFICULT BREATHING
OR RESPIRATORY ARREST

POSSIBLE
CONVULSIONS

ELEVATED
BLOOD PRESSURE

FRACTURED
BONES

**EXIT
BURN**

Possible findings in an electrical injury

serious injuries include: respiratory or cardiac arrest due to direct brain stem injury. Others include: seizures, spinal cord injury with paralysis, and permanent damage to peripheral nerves in the limbs. Eye injuries include immediate burns to the eyes, as well as the subsequent development of cataracts.

The abdomen and its contents may receive serious injury, particularly if the electrical current travels through the torso. The victim may complain of abdominal pain, nausea and vomiting. The abdomen may be tender, distended or rigid. As with blunt trauma, injury to the abdominal organs is more frequent than expected.

Signs and Symptoms of Electrical Injury

The victim of an electrical injury may have any of the following signs or symptoms.
- Respiratory arrest or breathing difficulty.
- Cardiac arrest, irregular heart beat or heart-related chest pain.
- The victim may be unresponsive, have a decreased level of consciousness, be paralyzed or seizing.
- The victim may be restless, irritable, anxious or confused.

- There may be signs and symptoms of shock present.
- The victim may complain of visual difficulties.
- The victim may exhibit entrance or exit burns or associated thermal burns (flame burns are caused by the ignition of clothing).
- There may be fractures and/or dislocations from profound muscle spasm or an associated fall.
- The victim may complain of abdominal pain, nausea and vomiting, and may exhibit abdominal tenderness or rigidity.

Management of Electrical Injuries

The evaluation and management of the injured worker with an electrical injury follows the Priority Action Approach as outlined in Part III, page 20.
1. Extreme *CAUTION* is urged when the Attendant approaches the scene of a victim injured by electricity. Such locations are often very hazardous. If the electrical source is still active or the Attendant is unsure, NO ATTEMPT MUST BE MADE TO RESCUE THE VICTIM unless the Attendant has been trained to do so and all the necessary personnel and equip-

ment are available. The specific protocols for accessing a victim at the site of an electrical accident are beyond the scope of this manual. The Attendant who works in an environment where there is a potential for electrical injuries should obtain appropriate training in those protocols.

2. Perform a primary survey.
3. Ensure an open airway with cervical spine control.
4. Expose the chest to assess for adequate breathing and determine the respiratory rate.
5. Administer high-flow oxygen by mask at 10 Lpm. If necessary, provide assisted ventilation with bag-valve mask and supplemental oxygen.
6. Assess the patient's circulation by feeling for a radial pulse and, if the radial pulse is not found, assess the carotid.
7. Control any obvious major hemorrhage.
8. If the victim has sustained a significant electrical injury, as evidenced by a decreased level of consciousness, signs or symptoms of shock, a serious burn, or injury to the nervous system, heart or abdomen, then the victim should be placed in the Rapid Transport Category.

LIGHTNING

Lightning injuries are frequently mistaken for other conditions. They cause coma, confusion or seizures. Often, a history of a thunderstorm or witness to the lightning strike may be absent, especially if the victim was alone at the time of the strike.

The injury from a lightning strike is distinctly different from other high-voltage electrical accidents because the duration of the strike is so brief. Even though the average voltage may be 10 to 20 million volts, the duration of the current flow is so short that often little energy is delivered to the body. Consequently, the current does not have time to break down the skin or cause internal tissue damage. The lightning primarily splashes over the outside of the individual and does not cause significant burns or tissue damage. The major effects are cardiac and respiratory arrest. An overactivation of the sympathetic nerves to the vessels of the extremities may also occur. This causes diminished peripheral circulation, as evidenced by blue, mottled, cold, pulseless limbs. Other nervous system changes may occur as previously described under electrical injuries. NOTE: The Attendant must carefully examine the victim to rule out injuries which may have been caused by blunt trauma associated with a fall at the time of the lightning strike.

There is a significant incidence of lightning-related deaths and injuries. The most commonly affected groups of people are construction workers, campers and sportsmen.

Lightning strikes may involve more than one victim, as the ground current may spread throughout a small area where individuals may seek shelter from the elements.

It is estimated that lightning strikes are fatal approximately 30% of the time. The major cause of death is cardiorespiratory arrest. The lightning delivers a massive direct current shock to the heart, causing it to stop in asystole. It also shocks the brain stem, causing an arrest of respiration. CPR should be started immediately in those victims without pulse or respiration. In the absence of cardiopulmonary arrest, victims are unlikely to die of any other cause.

Victims of lightning strikes fall into the Rapid Transport Category and should be managed as outlined for electrical injuries on page 294.

Part XI, Section E
Bites and Stings

Bites and stings are sometimes overlooked as life-threatening. Unfortunately, they can, on occasion, become life-threatening very quickly.

BITES

Bites may cause a local and systemic injection of poison into a wound and may also cause a local and systemic invasion of bacteria.

Bites should be managed like any other soft tissue injury: with thorough cleansing, appropriate dressings and referral to medical aid.

STINGS

Stings may be managed at the first aid level except when the patient exhibits a systemic allergic reaction to venom. In these cases there may be considerable danger to the patient. Severe allergic reaction necessitates rapid transportation to a medical facility.

Stings around the mouth or throat and multiple stings are potentially dangerous. They may cause constriction of the airways and a sudden loss of consciousness (coma) and should be treated as a high-priority emergency.

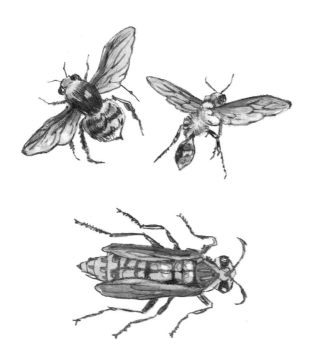

Typical stinging insects

MANAGEMENT OF LOCAL REACTIONS

Some stinging insects leave their sting and poison sacs embedded in the skin. The stinger should be removed under magnification, without squeezing the bag of venom. A sterile needle is used to remove the stinger.

Most people stung by insects have a localized reaction. The stinger and venom cause a local or generalized release of histamine. This substance does not normally circulate but causes localized redness, itchiness and swelling. Commercially available antihistamines are useful for this condition. Strict attention must be paid to recommended dosages. Several antihistamine preparations cause drowsiness. This should be taken into consideration before the patient returns to work.

The local application of ice tends to limit swelling, but stings that occur in the mouth and throat should be treated as potential emergencies.

The wound or local inflammation should be managed in much the same way as most soft tissue injuries. After initial cleansing, application of a preparation containing an aluminum salt (e.g. Burrow's Solution, BuroSol® or an antiperspirant) may provide relief of pain and swelling by inactivating the venom. This should be followed by application of an ice pack.

ALLERGIC REACTION

Most people who have a hypersensitivity to insect stings carry a special antidote kit. Available from most pharmacists, the kit contains a pre-loaded syringe of adrenalin, which has two measured doses, and antihistamine tablets. If stung, these patients will inject themselves. The Attendant should be ready to assist them if necessary. The Attendant must ensure that the instructions provided with the kit are followed.

The symptoms of a systemic allergic reaction may include:
- tightness of throat or upper airway;
- breathing difficulty;
- weakness;
- generalized itching;
- numbness and tingling;
- skin weals (blotchy areas of raised reddish pink swelling);

• anxiety;
• abdominal cramps, diarrhea or vomiting.

The patient may show severe shock symptoms, and may die if the reaction is extreme.

Management of Allergic Reaction

Treatment is supportive and, after initial first aid is rendered, the Attendant should treat the symptoms that are present.

• Maintain an open airway.
• Maintain respiration, artificially if necessary.
• Maintain circulation.
• Give oxygen therapy.
• Transport the patient promptly to the nearest medical facility. This is essential, as these patients require drug therapy to counteract the injected poison.

The condition should be assessed on the patient's reaction to the sting, rather than on the number of stings. If an allergic reaction is noted, the patient needs transport to medical aid. If a special anti-allergy kit is available, it should be used immediately upon medical advice.

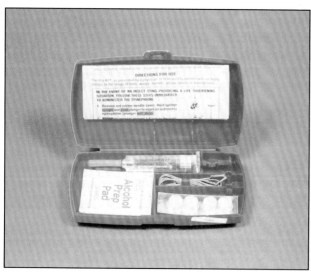

Typical Bee Sting Kit

SNAKEBITES

In BC, poisonous snakebites most commonly occur from rattlesnakes in the interior dry belt of the province. A person can be bitten by a rattlesnake without being poisoned. About 20% of people bitten by poisonous snakes are not injected with venom.

A wide variety of home-remedy snakebite cures have been reported to be successful. Fortunately most of those patients had not actually received venom. The home remedy would have been useless if there had been any venom in the bite. All home remedies should be avoided.

Owing to greater vascularity, bites on the head and neck are more dangerous than those on the extremities.

Venom is a very complex substance that varies greatly from snake to snake. The venom of the rattlesnake causes almost immediate tissue destruction. Blood and fluid leak into the tissues, causing marked swelling. Bruising occurs rapidly and blisters may appear. The skin may be sloughing and appear grossly damaged. The entire limb may swell in a matter of minutes. Pain is often excruciating.

Systemic signs of rattlesnake poisoning are variable and may include:

• development of shock-like state;
• decreased respiration;
• vomiting, abdominal cramps and diarrhea;
• fluid in the lungs (pulmonary edema, see Part IV, Section D, page 74);
• vascular collapse.

Identification of Snakes

Poisonous Snake

1. Snake has eyes with slit-like or elliptical pupils.
2. The mouth has two well-developed fangs hinged to the upper jaw.
3. The rattlesnake has rattles on its tail.

Non-poisonous Snake

1. Round pupils.
2. No developed fangs, but small teeth arranged in rows.

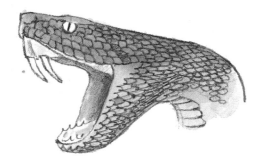

Typical poisonous snake

Identification of Snakebites

Poisonous

1. One or two fang marks with typical puncture wound appearance.
2. If venom is injected, there will be almost instantaneous excruciating pain with associated swelling around the puncture wounds.

Non-poisonous

1. Numerous tiny scratches
2. Little local swelling
3. Usually only slight discomfort and itching

General Management

IT IS IMPERATIVE TO GET A SNAKE-BITTEN PATIENT TO A MEDICAL FACILITY *AS QUICKLY AS POSSIBLE* SO SPECIFIC ANTIVENIN TREATMENT CAN BE STARTED. SUCH PATIENTS FALL INTO THE RAPID TRANSPORT CATEGORY. PERFORM A SECONDARY SURVEY AND TREATMENT EN ROUTE.

If possible, advance notification of the type of snakebite will allow medical personnel to arrange to have the antivenin sent to the facility from a central depot.

Treatment

1. Lay the patient down and keep him/her quiet. Reassure and keep comfortably warm. Do not allow the patient to have any alcoholic beverages.
2. Immediately cleanse the wound with soap and water. Do **not** apply ice. (Use of ice has been associated with an increased incidence of amputation.) Cover the wound with sterile dressings.
3. Do **not** apply a tourniquet or restrictive bandages; it may increase risk of local tissue destruction.
4. Do **not** excise area or perform suction. Such measures have contributed to mutilated extremities.
5. Loosely immobilize affected limb with a splint. Do not elevate affected limb.
6. Apply the general principles of shock management.
7. If possible, the snake should be killed and taken to the hospital for identification.

When working in an area where poisonous snakes may be encountered, the Attendant should establish a protocol with the local hospital. The Attendant should know if:

• antivenin is available at that hospital;
• the patient should be transported to another hospital if antivenin is not available;
• a heli-pad is available (if a helicopter is used).

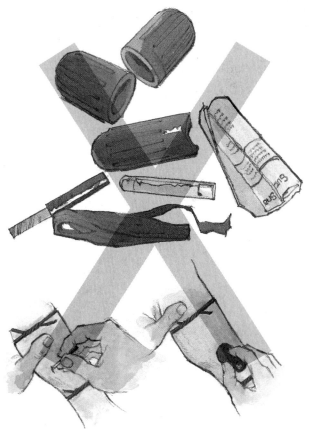

Do not excise area.

WOOD TICKS

Ticks are found throughout British Columbia and become a special hazard during late spring through early summer. Ticks burrow into the skin with their heads, then clamp on firmly with curved teeth, secreting a cement-like substance.

A tick's attachment is so strong that its body is often pulled free from the head.

Ticks carry infectious diseases. Rocky Mountain spotted fever and Lyme Disease are two of the most severe infectious diseases. Early medical treatment usually brings recovery.

Tick paralysis may develop from a tick's bite, especially if it occurs in the neck or spine area. The paralysis begins in the legs, then moves upward. Paralysis slowly improves on total removal of the tick.

It is important to remove a tick as soon as it is found.

The longer an embedded tick remains, the greater the risk of paralysis. The aim is to extract the entire tick, including the head and mouth.

These are methods of removing ticks.

- The Attendant should try to twist the tick out with gentle traction using tweezers.
- Putting some gasoline or kerosene on a cotton ball and taping it loosely over the tick, for 15 to 20 minutes, may cause the tick to loosen its attachment.
- Heavy oils or greases such as mineral oil or petroleum jelly will close off the respiratory opening on either side of the tick's body. It may take 20 to 30 minutes for the tick to back off.
- An ice cube held on the tick may induce the tick to release its hold.
- Application of heat, i.e. a heated needle, matches or a lit cigarette are *not recommended*. The danger of these methods is that the patient may be burned. The tick will usually die with the head remaining in the skin.

If the body parts of the tick are separated from the head and the head cannot be removed, the patient should be sent to medical aid for treatment.

After removal, the area of the bite should be washed well with soap and water. The application of cold to the area may help reduce pain.

Should signs of infection or symptoms appear, such as paralysis, severe headaches, fever or rash, the patient should be sent to medical aid.

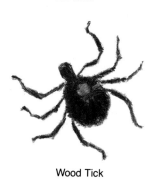

Wood Tick

BITES — ANIMAL AND HUMAN

Because of bacterial contamination, there is a very serious risk of wound infection from animal or human bites. Owing to disease-producing organisms commonly found in the mouths of humans, human bites are usually the most serious. Bites should be treated as a potentially infected major wound. They should be thoroughly cleansed with soap and water, then covered with a sterile dressing and referred to medical attention.

If the patient has an animal bite, try to confine and isolate the animal and contact the closest public health unit.

Rabies

Two of the more serious secondary complications of bites may be rabies and tetanus.

In certain regions, rabies is still common. Rabies is a life-threatening viral illness transmitted by the bite of an infected animal. The possibility of rabies should be considered in the setting of a bite from an unprovoked attack from any animal — wild or domestic. The most common rabid bites are from foxes, bats, raccoons and skunks. In BC, rabies is extremely rare.

Part XI, Section F
Diving Emergencies

NEAR-DROWNING

The term "drowning" means death by suffocation in water or other liquid. "Near-drowning" is the term used for submersion in which an individual survives, at least temporarily.

Mechanisms of Drowning

Low blood oxygen (hypoxemia) is the most important consequence of near-drowning. The degree of hypoxemia depends upon the duration of submersion and whether fluid was aspirated (breathed into the lungs). About 15% of drowning victims do not aspirate water because of either laryngospasm or breath-holding.

Process of Drowning

The panic-stricken person, thrashing about in the water, inhales air in an effort to survive. Starting to sink, he/she tries to take and hold one more deep breath. At that stage, water enters the mouth and nose. The person coughs and swallows, involuntarily inhaling and swallowing quantities of water. As water flows past the epiglottis and enters the trachea, it contacts the larynx and triggers reflex spasm. The laryngospasm seals the airway so effectively that only a small amount of water reaches the lungs. The patient loses consciousness because of a rapid drop in blood oxygen levels. Although the oxygen levels can rapidly decrease to levels incompatible with life, early and vigorous resuscitation can result in rapid and complete recovery. Drowning victims who die with laryngospasm die from true asphyxia — they suffocate from lack of oxygen.

With other victims, the laryngospasm relaxes when the person loses consciousness. Water freely enters the lungs when the spasm relaxes and severe hypoxemia occurs almost immediately. This condition is much more difficult to treat.

There are some theoretical differences between near-drowning in fresh water and in salt water but the net effect of both types of drowning is usually profound pulmonary edema and severe hypoxemia in survivors.

Signs and Symptoms of Near-Drowning

The major signs and symptoms of near-drowning relate to the respiratory and nervous system. The respiratory signs vary considerably in type and severity and may include:
- Absence of breathing
- Wheezing and dyspnea
- Rapid breathing
- Inability to take a deep breath
- Rasping cough
- Expectoration of whitish or pink frothy sputum
- Substernal burning
- Cyanosis

Signs of nervous system impairment may include:
- Restlessness
- Lethargy
- Diminished level of consciousness

Management

Near-drowning victims require prompt and vigorous therapy. Although the mechanism of injury may be somewhat different between fresh and sea water near-drowning victims, the effects and therapy are very similar.

If the victim is responsive but still in the water, a water rescue may be initiated. A swimming rescue is the least satisfactory method of rescue. Many inexperienced individuals have been drowned while attempting a swimming rescue. A life preserver, rope or any floatable object should be thrown to the victim. The basic rule of water rescue is summarized in the lifesaver's motto: "THROW, TOW, ROW, AND ONLY THEN GO."

Unless you are an excellent swimmer, trained in life-saving, DO NOT GO INTO THE WATER TO RESCUE A VICTIM. (Excellent training programs are available through the Royal Life Saving Society of Canada.)

Even if you are a good swimmer, wear a personal flotation device if you are using a boat or attempting a swimming rescue.

The most important immediate action is to restore effective ventilation. Elaborate lung-draining procedures waste valuable time, may induce vomiting and are ineffective. The urgent need is for ventilation, supplemented by high-flow oxygen, if available.

As soon as possible, clear the airway by removing any debris and begin mouth-to-mouth ventilation, even while the patient is still in the water. It may be necessary to blow harder than usual into the mouth of a person who is still in the water because of the water pressure on the chest wall.

When there is no pulse, start CPR as soon as possible.

Administer oxygen at a 10 Lpm when available. Give it in the highest concentration available depending on the type of mask.

Therapy must be continued until the victim recovers or until all resuscitation efforts have been exhausted. The return of consciousness and of spontaneous respiration does not mean the patient is fully recovered. Although ventilatory assistance may no longer be required, it is likely that hypoxemia is present. All patients who have lost consciousness or who have aspirated water fall into the Rapid Transport Category and should be treated with high-flow oxygen and transported to a medical facility.

Such patients must rest, even though they seem to have recovered. Delayed complications such as pulmonary edema are common in near-drowning cases and complex medical procedures may still be required to save the person's life.

Management of the Near-Drowning Victim with Possible Cervical Injuries

It is not uncommon to have cervical spine injuries with many water-related accidents. In fact, there may be injuries anywhere in the spine.

Cervical injury will not be apparent in the comatose victim. Consequently, the Attendant must have a high index of suspicion. If details of the near-drowning are unavailable, the Attendant must assume the victim has a neck injury. That is especially true if there is evidence of head injury.

It is imperative that there is no delay in opening the airway and assisted ventilations, but efforts should be made, if possible, to keep the victim's neck rigid and in a straight line with the body. The use of a modified jaw thrust for opening the airway is recommended. This type of water rescue is demonstrated in Figure XI-2. It requires training and practise in the use of a spine board while in the water. The Attendant who is likely to encounter such situations should practise those techniques. While airway and assisted ventilation should be initiated in the water, effective CPR requires that the victim be out of the water. CPR has not been found to be effective in the water even with the victim on a spine board.

WATER RESCUE – POSSIBLE SPINAL INJURY

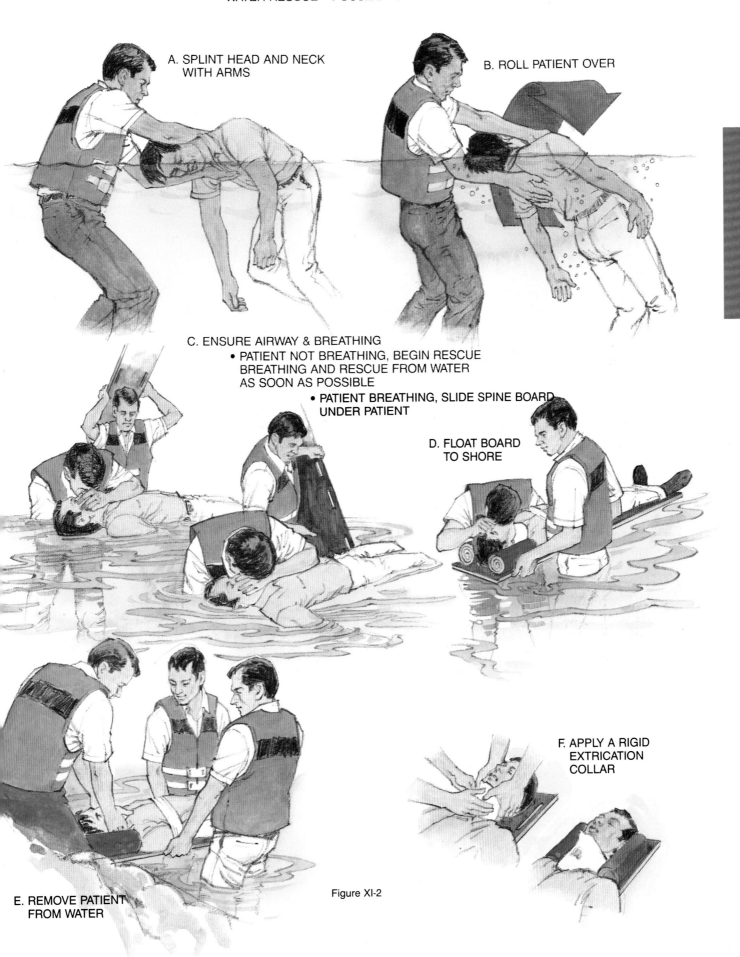

A. SPLINT HEAD AND NECK WITH ARMS

B. ROLL PATIENT OVER

C. ENSURE AIRWAY & BREATHING
- PATIENT NOT BREATHING, BEGIN RESCUE BREATHING AND RESCUE FROM WATER AS SOON AS POSSIBLE
- PATIENT BREATHING, SLIDE SPINE BOARD UNDER PATIENT

D. FLOAT BOARD TO SHORE

E. REMOVE PATIENT FROM WATER

F. APPLY A RIGID EXTRICATION COLLAR

Figure XI-2

EFFECTS OF COLD WATER

Recent studies have shown that a person may survive prolonged submersion in water when the water is colder than 21°C (70°F). That is especially true if the victim is very young. Survival under those conditions occurs as a result of a primitive human response called the dive reflex. The reflex can also be triggered when cold water suddenly hits a person's face. It shuts off the blood flow to most parts of the body, but not the heart, lungs and brain. The cold water temperature also reduces the metabolic rate of the body, reducing the need for oxygen. Whatever oxygen remains in the blood is made available to the brain, where it is most needed.

If person is rescued from cold water:

- Clear the airway quickly and begin artificial ventilation. Provide a high concentration of supplemental O_2 if available.
- Start CPR as soon as possible, if required.
- Prevent further loss of body heat and warm the patient as described in the section on hypothermia.
- Transport to a medical facility quickly, continuing to give resuscitation.

Do not give up on victims who show no sign of life. If the water was cold and the victim young, there is a chance for survival. Successful resuscitations with no disability have been reported in cases where an infant was submerged in cold water for up to one hour.

DIVING EMERGENCIES

Diving accidents may cause a variety of complex medical problems. Immediate and proper attention must be given to the victim at the accident site, but the Attendant must not delay transport to a hyperbaric facility. This will help to minimize residual medical problems after treatment.

Anyone who may have to deal with a diving emergency — instructors, dive supervisors, first aid and rescue personnel — must be able to recognize the signs and symptoms associated with barotrauma, air or gas embolism and/or decompression sickness.

In diving accidents, treatment must be initiated immediately. Treatment includes recognition, maintenance of vital signs, administration of oxygen and arranging immediate evacuation to a hyperbaric facility.

HOW TO RECOGNIZE A DIVING ACCIDENT VICTIM

Barotrauma

Barotrauma may occur in any person who has been breathing air or gas under increased ambient (surrounding) pressure and who surfaces while holding their breath, i.e. under water with SCUBA or even trapped in a submerged vehicle. Lung over-expansion problems may occur from as little as four feet under water and even well-trained divers may have problems on an ascent.

Panic that causes breath-holding or any possible obstructing respiratory problem could result in lung over-expansion during an ascent. With no natural escape routes the expanding air may rupture air spaces in the lungs. This causes lung over-expansion problems (barotrauma) such as pneumothorax, mediastinal emphysema, subcutaneous emphysema and myocardial or cerebral air or gas embolism.

Air/Gas Embolism

Air or gas embolism is the worst of the diving injuries. It is caused by the expanded air or gas with obstructed blood flow. In scuba diving, embolism results from a rapid decrease in the ambient pressure, i.e. breath-holding on ascent for any reason. A major difference between barotrauma and embolism is that the brain may be involved in air/gas embolism.

Immediate History (as described by the diver or witness)

- Rapid or uncontrolled ascent
- Buoyant ascent (ascent with an inflation device)
- Breath-holding on ascent
- A medical history of respiratory problems
- Difficulty in equalizing ears during ascent or descent

Onset of symptoms

Symptoms of air/gas embolism or barotrauma are usually abrupt and dramatic on surfacing.

Signs and Symptoms

- Headache
- Shortness of breath
- Chest pain
- Cessation of breathing
- Decreased level of consciousness
- Collapse or seizures
- Bloody, frothy sputum
- Shock
- Cyanosis
- Visual difficulty
- Nausea/vomiting
- Hearing difficulty
- Speech difficulty
- Lack of balance
- Numbness
- Weakness
- Strange sensations

Management

Barotrauma, Air/Gas Embolism

Conscious Diver

Position the patient supine. The patient's feet should be higher than the head only if:
- the patient's airway will tolerate it
- the feet are raised 6-8 in. higher than the head
- it is done immediately or up to 20 minutes after the incident
- it is maintained for no more than 20 minutes

Treat for shock.
- keep warm
- handle gently

Deliver high percentages of oxygen, i.e. non-rebreathing mask at 10 Lpm.

Transport patient by stretcher.

Diver with a Decreased Level of Consciousness

Breathing and pulse present
- Position patient lateral or supine (for airway management).
- Use oropharyngeal airway.

- Deliver high percentages of oxygen, i.e. non-rebreathing mask at 10 Lpm.
- Assist ventilations as necessary with bag-valve mask with reservoir and oxygen.

Breathing is absent
- Position patient supine.
- Use oropharyngeal airway and sunction if necessary/available.
- Provide ventilation via bag-valve mask with reservoir and oxygen.
- Monitor pulse; deliver CPR as required.

DECOMPRESSION SICKNESS

Decompression sickness can occur in any Scuba diver who dives near or beyond the no-compression limits and/or disregards safe-diving practices when diving deeper than 8 metres (25 ft.) of sea water. Simply stated, decompression sickness may occur if too many inert nitrogen or other inert gas bubbles form in the blood stream or body tissues.

Immediate History (as described by the diver or witness)
- Dives deeper than 8 metres (25 ft.) of sea water
- Violation of dive tables
- Dive monitor (computer) time — depth and/or ascent rate violations
- Hard working dives
- Cold diving conditions
- Dehydration

Onset of symptoms

Decompression sickness has a more gradual onset than barotrauma or air/gas embolism. Symptoms may appear within 15 minutes after surfacing but can be delayed more than 36 hours.

Signs and Symptoms

In the diving industry, decompression sickness (DCS) signs and symptoms are normally separated into two categories:
Type 1: Mild
Type 2: Serious
Type1 may progress to Type 2.

To ensure the proper care by an Attendant for a diver presenting with possible decompression sickness, both

mild and serious symptoms will be covered together.
- Pain, not necessarily localized to a joint, e.g. head, neck, back, abdomen, muscle, extremities
- Skin changes, rash, cyanosis
- Numbness and tingling in the extremities
- Personality change
- Impairment of vision
- Weakness
- Unexplained abnormalities with corresponding DCS history
- Decreased level of consciousness

Management of Decompression Sickness

Both types require assessment at Vancouver General Hospital. The hyperbaric physician may be contacted by calling 875-4111 and stating that there is a "diving accident." The attendant should ask for the hyperbaric physician.

PATIENTS WITH TYPE 1 AND TYPE 2 DCS FALL INTO THE RAPID TRANSPORT CATEGORY.

Conscious Diver
- Place the patient in a position of comfort — at rest.
- Deliver high percentages of oxygen, i.e. non-rebreathing mask at 10 Lpm.
- Transport as a stretcher patient.
- The patient who is able, without compromising the airway, may take oral fluids such as water or juice.

Diver with a Decreased Level of Consciousness

Breathing and pulse present
- Position patient lateral or supine (for airway management)
- Use oropharyngeal airway
- Deliver high percentages of oxygen, i.e. non-rebreathing mask at 10 Lpm.
- Support respirations as necessary with bag-valve mask with reservoir and oxygen.

Breathing is absent
- Position patient supine.
- Use oropharyngeal airway (suction as required).
- Supply ventilation via bag-valve mask with reservoir and oxygen.
- Monitor pulse; deliver CPR as required.

The critical points of field care for an injured diver are:
- Recognition of possible problems based on history and symptoms.
- Non-stop delivery of the highest possible percentage of oxygen, to be continued even if the symptoms seem to pass.
- Appropriate airway management via the use of airways, suctioning and/or patient positioning.
- Constant monitoring of the patient for changes in condition.
- Regardless of how minor the symptoms of decompression sickness may seem it is imperative that the patient does not go back into the water to attempt treatment or to complete omitted decompression stops.
- Patient must be transported directly to a hyperbaric facility. The urgency for transport will depend on the patient's level of consciousness. (The LOC may change.)
- All patients suffering from possible barotrauma, air/gas embolism or decompression sickness, no matter how mild the occurrence, should be seen by a hyperbaric physician.
- Gathering and recording an accurate history in writing for the hyperbaric physician.

Oxygen is an imperative part of the field and medical treatment of diving injuries. When oxygen is breathed, the oxygen tension of the blood is increased. This increased tension helps to rid the blood of nitrogen gas bubbles. The elevated oxygen tension also allows better oxygenation of tissues where the blood supply has been impaired by bubbles.

EMERGENCY EVACUATION

If the patient is a diving accident victim and someone is caring for their immediate medical needs, someone else must be arranging for transportation to a hyperbaric facility. It is necessary then to know how to contact assistance from sea or land.

Communications

1. From the beach (for help that is accessible by land) — contact the provincial ambulance service. Be prepared to provide the following information:
   - Your name and call-back phone number

- Your exact location and any specific information that will help the ambulance crew to locate you quickly
- The patient's condition.

2. From a boat — contact a Coast Guard radio station (Channel 16 marine VHF). Declare an emergency and state "This is a diving emergency." Be prepared to respond with the following information:
   - Your exact location, by marine chart
   - A description of your vessel and status, in danger or not in danger
   - Number of persons on board and their condition
   - The patient's condition in detail.

3. From an isolated location (away from populated centres) — contact the Rescue Co-ordination Centre (RCC) by phone. Be prepared with the following information:
   - Your name and call-back phone number or frequency
   - Your exact location and any information that will help RCC to direct a rescue resource to you.
   - The patient's condition in detail.

Actions

Procedures are in place which ensure that, by making contact with either the ambulance service, a Coast Guard radio station or RCC, an injured diver will be transported, under care, to a British Columbia hyperbaric facility.

Evacuation Preparation

- REMEMBER: OXYGEN DELIVERY MUST NEVER BE DISCONTINUED.
- Diving accident patients are all stretcher patients.
- Ensure that the patient is kept warm (treat for shock).
- Ensure that all responding rescue and ambulance resources understand that this is a diving accident.
- A complete patient history, in writing, should accompany the patient. Describe the events leading up to the accident and treatment actions after the accident. If possible, send the diving buddy with the patient.

If the evacuation is being conducted from a boat at sea by helicopter:

- Try to establish communications with the helicopter to receive their specific directions.
- If communications with the helicopter are not possible:
  - Secure all loose objects on and around the decks.
  - Put all antennae and other movable structures down if they will interfere with the evacuation.

When the helicopter is on the scene:

- Maintain a course into the wind approximately 20 degrees off the bow.
- Maintain a constant speed of 10 to 15 knots. Do not slow down or speed up in an effort to help.
- Allow the lifting device from the helicopter to touch the deck before you touch it. DO NOT TIE IT TO YOUR VESSEL.
- Ensure that your patient is in a life jacket and is secured in the stretcher/lifting device.
- Ensure that all written information is sent with the patient.

Part XII, Section A
Poisons

DEFINITION

A poison is any substance that harms the human body, damaging health or destroying life.

Attendants must know how to deal with hazardous materials and poisonings in the work environment. They must acquaint themselves with all hazardous materials and poisons used at their work sites and the appropriate first aid treatment for each. Employers must comply with Federal Workplace Hazardous Materials Information System (WHMIS) regulations and other applicable occupational safety and health regulations. These regulations require that hazardous and toxicity information be made available to workers who may be exposed to hazardous materials in the workplace. The Material Safety Data Sheets (MSDS) also contain first aid information that is vital to the Attendant. If the information is not available, the Attendant should ask management to obtain it through the manufacturer.

Attendants should use a written procedure for dealing with all poisons and dangerous substances used at their work site. The MSDS are the best source of this information for the Attendant.

The local Poison Control Centre may also be contacted for treatment details. If the local centre cannot provide the information, contact the BC Poison Information Centre at St. Paul's Hospital, Vancouver, at 682-2344, local 2126.

CLASSIFICATION OF POISONS

All poisons can be classified into three general categories:
1. Poisons that are absorbed by inhalation — gases or substances that are breathed in.
2. Poisons that are ingested — substances that are swallowed.
3. Poisons that affect the body through skin contact — substances that come into contact with any body surface (i.e. skin, eye, mouth or other mucous membrane).

GENERAL MECHANISM OF INJURY

Inhaled Poisons

1. Reduction of the oxygen-carrying capacity of the blood, thereby causing tissue hypoxia (e.g. carbon monoxide poisoning).
2. Direct irritation of the lung tissues, which impairs oxygenation of the blood, i.e. chlorine gas.
3. A direct toxic effect on cells; for example, hydrogen sulfide affects brain cells.

Ingested Poisons

Accidental poisoning by ingestion is usually caused by drugs, chemicals and bacterial toxins, such as botulism.

Skin Contact Poisons

Some substances may cause skin destruction or irritation on contact (chemical burn). Other substances may be absorbed when in contact with the skin, eyes or mucous membranes (e.g. pesticides). Some substances can both burn and be absorbed, such as cyanide and phenols.

PRIORITY ACTION APPROACH FOR POISONING

All patients with suspected poisoning should be initially assessed and treated using the Priority Action Approach. The Attendant should follow the step-by-step flow chart. It is also crucial to think ahead and bring all essential equipment to the scene. In general, the following equipment is necessary: long spine board, oxygen, airway equipment and suctioning device if available.

1. Scene Assessment
   Ensure no danger before approaching the patient. If you suspect that the area contains toxic gases or has inadequate oxygen, the proper rescue apparatus must be worn.

   The patient should be extricated to a safe area before initiating your treatment. Do not risk exposing yourself or the patient to further risk.
2. Primary Survey
   Once the patient and Attendant are away from further danger, begin the primary survey.

Airway

Assess the airway and level of consciousness by approaching the patient from the front. Identify yourself briefly: "I am an Industrial First Aid Attendant. I am here to help you. What happened?" The patient's response or lack of response will give immediate information as to the level of consciousness and the the airway. Use the look, listen and feel approach to assess the airway. If an obstructed or partially obstructed airway is suspected, it must be cleared. Refer to the flow chart in Airway Management, Part IV, Section B, page 45. If traumatic injury occurred in addition to the toxic exposure or ingestion (e.g. fall down the stairs or off ladder), remember to immobilize the cervical spine as required.

Breathing

The Attendant assesses the patient's breathing by counting breaths, looking for signs of respiratory distress and noting the depth of the patient's respirations.

If respirations are absent or too slow (less than 10 breaths per minute), assisted ventilation with supplemental oxygen must be initiated immediately. This can be provided with mouth-to-mouth, pocket mask or bag-valve mask device. (Refer to Part IV, Section B, page 51, on Airway Management.) If the patient's breathing is too rapid (greater than 30 per minute), supplemental oxygen by mask, 10 litres per minute, will be required. Assisted ventilation may also have to be provided if the respirations are shallow or laboured.

Circulation

To assess circulation, check the patient's radial, femoral and/or carotid pulses. The pulse is assessed by noting the rate, strength and its regularity. However, for purposes of the primary survey, only the presence or absence of the radial pulse is crucial.

If all pulses are absent, then CPR must be initiated immediately. If only the radial pulse is absent, but the femoral or carotid pulse is palpable, the patient is in circulatory shock and must be transported rapidly to hospital. Supplemental oxygen by mask must be provided.

The primary survey should not take longer than two minutes to complete. By this time, the Attendant should also have noted the patient's level of consciousness. Based on the nature of the ingestion or exposure, the results of the primary survey and the level of consciousness, the Attendant is now able to determine which patient must be transported rapidly to hospital. Outlined below is a list of criteria that place the patient in the Rapid Transport Category.

Rapid Transport Criteria for Poison Victims

1. All patients with a partial or completely obstructed airway.
2. All patients with a respiratory rate less than 10 or greater than 30.
3. All patients with an absent radial pulse.
4. All patients with an altered mental status or decreased level of consciousness.

Finally, if your patient does not initially fall into the Rapid Transport Category, immediate transfer to hospital may still be required. With certain ingestions or exposures, the onset of toxic effects may be delayed. Although the patient may initially appear stable, he or she may deteriorate some time later. Reassess the patient often.

In addition, it is extremely important to identify the suspected poison. After your primary survey has been completed and preparation made for rapid transport as required, the Attendant should always contact Poison Control. Poison Control may advise you to provide additional treatment (e.g. Ipecac, or recommend rapid transport to hospital because of the seriousness of the poisoning). Remember to record the name and the concentration of the suspected poison and send it to the hospital with the patient. If feasible, send the labelled container and the Material Safety Data Sheet (MSDS).

FLOW CHART FOR POISONING

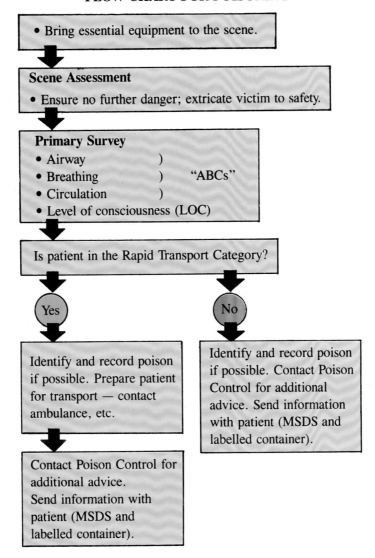

INHALED POISON MANAGEMENT

Oxygen therapy should be given as soon as possible to anyone who may have inhaled a toxic substance. (Moistened oxygen is preferred as it may minimize the irritant effect.)

If the patient is not breathing, give mouth-to-mouth respiration until oxygen can be administered with a bag-valve mask unit or pocket mask. Provided the patient has been extricated to a safe environment, mouth-to-mouth ventilation will not usually pose any health risk to the Attendant. If the patient is breathing, oxygen should be administered through the normal oxygen mask with reservoir at a 10 Lpm.

Keep the patient warm and at complete rest to keep the body's demand for oxygen at a minimum. Any increase in demand for oxygen may cause further hypoxia and increase the toxic effects of the gas throughout the body.

A patient who falls into the Rapid Transport Category must be transported immediately to medical aid. Constantly monitor vital signs en route to hospital.

COMMONLY INHALED INDUSTRIAL POISONS

This section gives an overview of the four commonly encountered poisonous gases. The treatment steps are those outlined previously in the Priority Action Approach.

CARBON MONOXIDE (CO)

Carbon monoxide is especially difficult to detect, being tasteless, colourless, non-irritating and odourless. The hemoglobin in the red blood cells combines chemically with carbon monoxide with an affinity about 250 times greater than that of oxygen. Even a small percentage of carbon monoxide in the inspired air will be quickly taken up by the hemoglobin in the red cells. If sufficient carbon monoxide is absorbed instead of oxygen, the number of red blood cells available to carry oxygen is inadequate. This causes oxygen starvation to the tissues (hypoxia). Smoke inhalation victims often suffer from carbon monoxide poisoning as well as poisoning from other toxic gases.

Signs and Symptoms

Not all patients have every sign and symptom, so it is very important to take a proper history.

The following signs and symptoms are possible with carbon monoxide poisoning:
- headache
- dizziness
- confusion (may appear drunk)
- nausea, vomiting
- drowsiness
- rapid pulse
- dilated pupils
- rapid respirations
- convulsions
- decreased level of consciousness
- death

The cherry-red appearance formerly thought to be associated with all carbon monoxide poisoning is, in fact, rarely seen.

Management

See Inhaled Poison Management.

The critical factor of the management of carbon monoxide poisoning is the speed of which the carbon monoxide may be removed from the body. High-flow oxygen, at the highest concentration available (100% oxygen is preferred; see Oxygen Therapy, Part IV, Section E, page 81), must be provided to speed the elimination of carbon monoxide.

For serious carbon monoxide poisoning that demonstrates a decreased level of consciousness, medical management may necessitate treatment in a hyperbaric unit. Therefore, the receiving physician should be notified that they are receiving a possible carbon monoxide victim.

CHLORINE GAS (Cl)

Chlorine gas has a pungent and disagreeable odour. In large concentrations, it may appear as a greenish-yellow cloud.

Chlorine gas is a respiratory tract irritant. Irritant gases will inflame the lung tissues, causing fluid to accumulate there. This causes the walls of the alveoli to thicken, interfering with the passage of oxygen from the alveoli to the blood. This causes hypoxia.

The inflammatory response to the irritant takes time to develop and its effects are not felt immediately. Never underestimate the seriousness of chlorine gas poisoning because the patient may have little discomfort at first. Even a few breaths of a high concentration may ultimately cause death.

The following signs and symptoms are possible with chlorine gas poisoning and other irritating gases:
- eye irritation
- excessive tearing
- respiratory distress/dyspnea
- coughing
- pain and burning in the throat
- pain and/or discomfort in the chest
- frothy, whitish or pink-tinged sputum
- nausea, vomiting
- cyanosis
- collapse
- death

Management

The crucial point in management is to extricate the victim from further exposure without endangering yourself. Refer to the Priority Action Approach at the beginning of the section.

CYANIDE

Hydrogen cyanide is a colourless gas which has a slight smell of bitter almonds. Not everybody, however, is able to detect this odour. Cyanide is highly poisonous by inhalation, absorption or ingestion. Cyanide — by a direct toxic effect — blocks oxygen use by all cells resulting in immediate toxic death.

Cyanide compounds are widely used as milling reagents and can be generated when any acidic material comes into contact with sodium or potassium cyanide.

Signs and Symptoms

Large doses of cyanide can kill the patient almost instantaneously.

With smaller doses of cyanide, the signs and symptoms can range from mild to severe, depending upon concentration and length of exposure.

The following symptoms are a guide only, as not all patients will have all the signs:
- breath may smell of bitter almonds
- respiratory distress or respiratory arrest
- shock
- possible cardiac arrest
- weakness
- decreased level of consciousness

Management of Cyanide Poisoning

Affected worker who is able to breathe:
- Wrap a single amyl nitrite ampoule in a gauze pad or handkerchief and break it. (The cyanide poisoning antidote kit, which contains the amyl nitrite ampoules, is available only by prescription. The Attendant should periodically check the expiry date of the kit.)
- Hold the ampoule about one inch from the patient's mouth and nostrils for 15 seconds.
- Repeat this procedure at 15 second intervals.
- Break a fresh ampoule every five minutes.
- Administer amyl nitrite until four ampoules are used or medical attention is reached.

Affected worker who is not breathing:
- Administer assisted ventilations immediately.
- When available, a bag-valve mask unit with oxygen should be used.
- Administer CPR if no pulse is present.
- Transport to medical attention. If breathing resumes, apply amyl nitrite as previously outlined.

HYDROGEN SULFIDE (H2S), MERCAPTANS

Hydrogen sulfide is a by-product of many industrial processes.

Hydrogen sulfide is a colourless gas with an odour of rotten eggs. It is heavier than air and collects near the ground. Hydrogen sulfide will burn and will give off sulphur dioxide, which is irritating to the eyes and lungs. Hydrogen sulfide may be explosive when mixed with air.

Hydrogen sulfide can be very dangerous even in small concentrations. It can enter the body through breaks in the skin and by inhalation.

One of the properties of H_2S is that it impairs the sense of smell. This may cause the person to stay in the toxic area without being aware of continuing dangers.

Hydrogen sulfide has a direct toxic effect on the respiratory centre of the brain, causing a person to stop breathing.

Signs and Symptoms

The signs and symptoms of a person exposed to H_2S vary according to the concentration breathed.

Moderate Intoxication

- burning sensation of eyes/throat
- excessive tearing
- loss of sense of smell
- impaired judgment
- loss of balance

Severe Intoxication

- decreased level of consciousness
- collapse
- respiratory arrest
- cardiac arrest

Management

Procedure of H_2S Management same as Cyanide, except do not use the sodium thiosulfate injection.

POISONING BY INGESTION

Poisoning by ingestion in industry is unusual but can occur nonetheless. Several disease conditions look the same as poisoning, such as cerebral hemorrhage, epilepsy, insulin shock, or diabetic coma. Some gastrointestinal conditions, such as acute indigestion or a peptic ulcer, may appear similar to lead poisoning. Therefore, the Attendant must question the patient (specifically ask the patient about possible poisoning, e.g. what, when, how).

Management

The assessment of the patient with suspected accidental poisoning should follow these steps:
1. History.
2. Physical Examination.
3. Treatment.

1. History
   Identify the nature of the poison by chemical name and brand name if possible. Refer to first aid room files, WHMIS or MSDS sheets if necessary.
   * Specifically ask the patient about possible poisoning. What? When? How? Record the details.
   * Keep a sample of the poison and the container or label if possible. Send it with the patient to the hospital if the treatment requires a medical assessment.

2. Physical Examination
   The physical examination should follow the previous guidelines covered in Part III, page 25. However, specific emphasis should be placed on the following physical findings.
   * Look for burns in and around the mouth.
   * Smell the breath for any unusual odours. Note any unusual odours in the immediate area on or about the patient.
   * Ask the patient if he/she is having any difficulty breathing or has a cough and look for any signs of respiratory distress.
   * Evaluate the patient for any signs of a decreased level of consciousness.
   * Ask the patient about any nausea, vomiting or diarrhea. Examine for the presence of abdominal pain.
   * Examine the skin of the extremities and trunk for the presence of rashes, lesions or burns.

3. Treatment
   The first priority is to satisfy the ABCs of patient care.
   A **irway** — is it open and clear?
   B **reathing** — is the patient breathing and, if so, is it adequate?
   C **irculation** — is there a pulse?
   If any of the ABCs are not properly cared for, all other treatment is useless.
   * Identify the ingested poison.
   * Refer to the Material Safety Data Sheets.
   * Phone the Poison Control Centre, either local or provincial (provincial 682-2344, local 2126). If advised by Poison Control, make immediate arrangements for transport of the patient to the nearest hospital.

Conscious and Breathing Patient

1. Non-Corrosive Ingestions
   If the poison is not a corrosive substance or a hydrocarbon, you may receive instructions from Poison Control to induce vomiting by the following methods:
   * For adults, give 30 ml (1 oz. or 2 tablespoonfuls) of Syrup of Ipecac orally. The dose for children under 15 years would be 15 ml (1 tablespoonful).
   * Give the patient one or two glasses of clear fluid 10 minutes after the Ipecac is administered (water or juice).
   * You may receive instructions to provide activated charcoal after the patient has stopped vomiting — the dose would be 50 gm diluted in 8 oz. of water or juice.
   * Poison Control Centre may instruct you to use activated charcoal immediately.

2. Corrosive Ingestions (Acids and Alkalis)
   * Do not make the patient vomit.
   * Do not neutralize.
   * Dilute immediately with 1 to 2 glasses of milk or water.

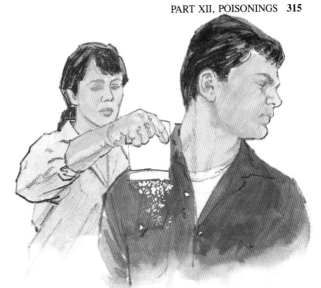

Brush dry chemicals off before flushing.

3. Hydrocarbon Ingestions (Petroleum Products)
Patients with large hydrocarbon ingestions may require Syrup of Ipecac to induce vomiting. However, this should only be administered on advice from the Poison Control Centre. These patients must be observed while vomiting to ensure that no aspiration occurs, because a very serious pneumonia may result if hydrocarbon enters the lungs.

Transport the patient to the nearest medical facility.

DO NOT MAKE THE PATIENT VOMIT IF ANY OF THESE CONDITIONS EXIST:

1. The patient is too drowsy to sit up, has a decreased level consciousness or convulsing.
2. The patient has ingested corrosive acids or alkalis.
3. The patient has ingested a hydrocarbon and the Poison Control Centre has not been consulted.

Breathing Patient with a Decreased Level of Consciousness

Perform primary survey:
1. Assess the scene for hazards.
2. Ensure the patient's airways are clear and unobstructed. If there is any possibility of associated injury, perform airway techniques with C-spine control if possible.
3. The patient who is vomiting or retching must be rolled to the lateral position.
4. Administer oxygen.
5. Be prepared to assist the patient's respiration.
6. Transport to medical aid, carry out secondary survey and further treatment en route, monitoring and recording the patient's vital signs.

DO NOT INDUCE VOMITING IN A PATIENT WHOSE LEVEL OF CONSCIOUSNESS IS DETERIORATING.

DO NOT ADMINISTER CHARCOAL TO A PATIENT WHO CANNOT SWALLOW DUE TO A DECREASED LEVEL OF CONSCIOUSNESS.

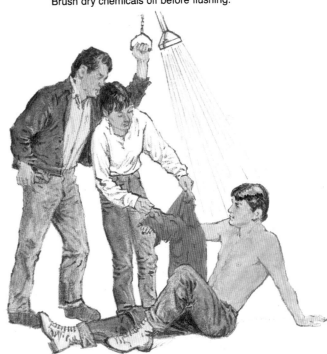

Use a shower for severe spills.

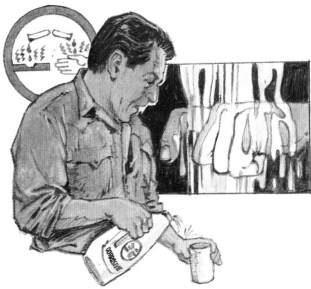

Flush chemicals with large amounts of water.

POISONING BY SKIN CONTACT

It is essential to decontaminate the skin as soon as possible after contact, because as long as the skin is contaminated, some effects may continue. Prolonged contact can result in damage to the skin itself or absorption of the material through the skin. Often the victim is unaware that skin contact has occurred.

Substances that can directly affect the skin or be readily absorbed through it include some insecticides, solvents, cyanides and heavy metals such as mercury, chromium and organic-lead compounds.

Management

Assess the scene for hazards (see page 309).
Priority Action Approach:

A **irway** — is it open and clear?

B **reathing** — is the patient breathing and, if so, is it adequate?

C **irculation** — is there a pulse?

Once the ABCs are assessed and treated, proceed as follows:

- Wash off skin immediately with large amounts of water.
- Remove contaminated clothing.
- The Attendant must take extra precautions to avoid contamination.
- Treat all burned areas as for a dry burn.
- Transport the patient to medical aid.

DO NOT NEUTRALIZE CORROSIVE POISONS WITH ACIDS OR ALKALIS; INSTEAD, FLUSH WITH LOTS OF WATER AND CONTINUE FLUSHING EN ROUTE TO MEDICAL FACILITY IF POSSIBLE.

MANAGEMENT OF CHEMICAL BURNS

(See Burns, Part XI, Section C, page 290.)
Chemical splashes to the eye, see Part VII, Section C, page 172.

HYDROFLUORIC ACID (HF ACID)

Hydrofluoric acid is an extremely corrosive chemical and is one of the strongest inorganic acids. The devastating effects of hydrofluoric acid cannot be overemphasized. Advance planning with a clear, concise treatment procedure must be readily available wherever this chemical is in use.

Signs and Symptoms

Skin Contact

- With solutions less than a 30% concentration of hydrogen fluoride, pain may not be felt for up to 24 hours.
- Solutions of greater than 30% concentration will usually produce immediate pain, which may be excruciating with superficial or deep burns.
- Hydrofluoric acid causes severe burns, slow-healing skin ulcers and may result in loss of fingernails and toenails.

Inhalation

- Possible chemical pneumonitis, pulmonary edema.

Management

- Immediately, flush with copious amounts of running water for at least 60 minutes (by the clock). Patients with associated injuries (i.e. inhalation, severe trauma) will require immediate transport to hospital. Flushing should be initiated at the scene and continued en route to hospital. Do not delay transport.
- Any work site where the potential for hydrofluoric acid injury exists should have a supply of H-F Antidote Gel® (available by prescription only) on site.
- Massage H-F Antidote Gel® onto affected area until pain has ceased. (This could take some time and could be done en route to medical aid.)
- Attendant must use the appropriate glove protection (PVC or neoprene).
- If the gel is not available, soak the affected area with an iced solution of 25% magnesium sulphate (Epsom salts) or iced water.
- If hydrofluoric acid is inhaled, treatment is as for chlorine gas.
- The patient must be transported to medical aid and, if practical, the affected parts should be kept immersed in iced water or solution during transport.

Part XII, Section B
Substance Abuse

INTRODUCTION

Alcohol and other drug abuse is becoming more prevalent in society and in industry. Any person who is under the influence of any foreign substance is a potential hazard to himself as well as his co-workers. Therefore, an Attendant should be aware of the problems associated with drug abuse.

Any substance can be abused. All drugs, legal or illegal, prescription or non-prescription, have the potential to be abused. It is not uncommon for multiple drugs and substances to be abused simultaneously. The purpose of this section is to discuss the most commonly encountered mind-altering drugs and substances.

THE PROBLEM

The WCB Task Force Study on Drug and Alcohol Abuse in the Workplace in 1987 concluded that a typical abuser:

1. is likely to miss work three to five times more often than non-abusers;
2. is up to four times as likely to be involved in an accident;
3. is five times as likely to file a workers' compensation claim;
4. functions at about two-thirds of his or her work potential;
5. requires sick-benefit costs that are three times that of the average employee.

The study also concludes that substance abuse can contribute to serious industrial accidents, as well as hindering the healing process following minor injuries.

TYPES OF ABUSED SUBSTANCES

Commonly abused drugs may be divided into three major groups: depressants, stimulants and hallucinogens.

Central Nervous System Depressants

Common depressants are alcohol, narcotics, barbiturates, tranquilizers and marijuana.

a) Alcohol — the most commonly abused depressant. As it is estimated that five percent of the population are alcoholics, it is likely that the Attendant will encounter alcohol-intoxicated patients in the workplace.

Signs and Symptoms — Alcohol on the breath is a reliable sign that the patient has been drinking. Inappropriate behaviour, bloodshot eyes, loss of coordination and slurred speech may also be present. If excess alcohol has been consumed, the patient may become difficult to arouse. However, the Attendant must not assume that a comatose patient is necessarily intoxicated. The Attendant must be careful not to overlook serious injuries or illnesses in the intoxicated patient. Diabetic coma, serious head injuries or other illnesses may be overlooked in patients considered to be "just drunk".

b) Narcotics — Narcotics are opiates and include opium and its derivatives, morphine, heroin, codeine, Taliven®, Darvon®, etc.

Signs and symptoms of narcotic abuse include pinpoint pupils, shallow, slow respirations, impaired coordination, depressed level of consciousness. These drugs may ultimately cause death from respiratory arrest.

c) Barbiturates and Tranquilizers — Signs and symptoms of intoxication with these drugs are similar to those of alcohol, with drowsiness the predominant symptom.

d) Marijuana and Hashish — can be smoked or ingested. Most common effects are feelings of exhilaration, perceptiveness and self-confidence. The user may demonstrate excessive talking and laughter. With heavy doses, there is generally some perceptual distortion and, with higher doses, hallucinations. Appetite is often stimulated, and there may be a rapid pulse and bloodshot eyes.

Inexperienced users generally report less intense effects. However, if the user is anxious, he/she may become panicky (freak out).

When the effects wear off, a user may feel lethargic and sleepy. The person may suffer from slight nervous irritability or a feeling of sluggishness the next day.

Central Nervous System Stimulants

Common stimulants are cocaine and amphetamines.

a) i) Cocaine — Cocaine is an alkaloid extracted from the leaves of the tropical coca plant. It has two effects: a central nervous system stimulant and a local anesthetic action.

Cocaine is usually available as a white crystalline powder that is inhaled, or "snorted", from spoons or straws. It can also be dissolved and then injected intravenously.

ii) Cocaine Derivatives — In greater demand today are newer, smokable forms of cocaine. These are:

- Freebase: a purified form of cocaine made by applying solvents to ordinary cocaine.
- "Crack": rock-like chunks of processed cocaine.
- Coco Paste: a crude coca preparation, usually smoked on tobacco cigarettes.

Cocaine can cause the following medical emergencies:

i) Cardiac Irregularities: Cocaine, even in small doses, can cause heart attack and cardiac arrest even in otherwise healthy users with no history of heart disease.

ii) Stroke: A cocaine-triggered rise in blood pressure can rupture weakened blood vessels in the brain.

iii) Overdose: Cocaine overdose can produce seizures, coma, respiratory difficulties and/or cardiac arrest.

Common signs of cocaine use are:

- stimulated mental state
- elevated pulse

b) Amphetamines — These drugs have a variety of uses, including offsetting drowsiness and fatigue, appetite suppression and as a decongestant.

The primary effect of amphetamines is hyperstimulation, which is similar to cocaine. Hallucinations may be present. Overdose may have the same effect as cocaine overdose.

Hallucinogens

The common drugs in this group are LSD, mescaline, magic mushrooms, MDA, STP and PCP (angel dust).

The major effects of these drugs are hallucinations. Users may exhibit behavioural changes such as aggressiveness, paranoia and anxiety (i.e. "freaking out"). USERS CAN BE DANGEROUS TO THEMSELVES AND OTHERS AND SHOULD BE WATCHED CLOSELY.

FIRST AID ATTENDANT'S RESPONSIBILITY

The Attendant's main responsibility in cases of drug abuse is to maintain life support while obtaining medical help. The Attendant should be aware that alcohol and drugs may be involved where injuries occur in the workplace. The interpretation of the signs and symptoms may be difficult because of the effects of these substances on the sick or injured worker.

The intent of this section is not to train the Attendant how to deal with the general problem of substance abuse. However, the Attendant may encounter an injured worker where substance abuse has played a significant role. The intent is to heighten the awareness of the Attendant to the possibility of substance abuse when confronted with an injured worker.

If workers with a substance-abuse problem approach the Attendant for help in this general area, they should be referred to the family physician or employee assistance program.

There are a number of support agencies available to assist in the management of a substance-abuse problem. In British Columbia, information, counselling and treatment services can be obtained by calling the toll-free number 1-800-663-1441.

Part XIII
Infectious Diseases

DEFINITION

An infectious disease (communicable disease, contagious disease) is an illness caused by the invasion of a host by organisms such as bacteria, viruses, fungi and parasites. This disease is contagious (transmissible from one person to another) and can be spread by a variety of mechanisms.

ROUTES OF TRANSMISSION

1. Contact
   - Direct physical contact between two individuals
   - Indirect contact where the invading organism is transferred onto a non-living object and from there to another individual
2. Airborne Droplets
   The infective organism is introduced into the air by a cough or sneeze from an infected individual and is contacted by another individual who may inhale it.
3. Vehicle Transmission
   The infecting organism may be ingested from infected food or injected through a blood transfusion or an infected needle.
4. Vector Transmission
   The infectious agent may be harboured in an insect and transmitted to the individual by a bite or sting (e.g. mosquito or wood tick).

TYPES OF INFECTIOUS ORGANISMS

1. Bacterium
   These are microscopic single-cell organisms capable of self-replication (reproduction) (e.g. staphylococcus, tetanus, gonorrhea).
2. Virus
   These are even smaller organisms requiring the presence of host tissue to replicate (e.g. influenza, HIV, hepatitis, herpes).
3. Parasite
   A plant or animal that lives upon or within another living organism and derives a benefit from it, at the expense of the host (e.g. Giardia, tapeworms, lice).
4. Fungus
   Another microscopic simple cellular structure having infectious properties (e.g. yeast, ringworm).

Each of these infectious organisms is capable of causing one or more specific disease entities if introduced to a host under favourable circumstances. That may not occur right away (the incubation period) because time is required for the organisms to become established. The incubation period may be as short as a few hours (e.g. food poisoning) to a few days (e.g. influenza) or as long as several years (e.g. AIDS).

On the other hand, the disease may never develop because of the ability of the host to successfully "fight it off" (the immune response).

It is also possible that the disease will be only partially controlled and a carrier state may develop. Here, the victim would have no symptoms but would nonetheless be capable of spreading the disease to others (e.g. hepatitis B, HIV disease).

RESPONSIBILITY OF THE ATTENDANT

Early recognition of the symptoms of infectious disease is important for two reasons:
1. so that the patient can be referred to medical aid as soon as possible;
2. so that fellow workers can be protected from contracting the disease as early as possible.

In remote areas, it may be necessary to care for the contagious patient for some time. Therefore, special precautions should be taken to protect not only the other workers but also the Attendant.

PREVENTION OF INFECTION

The probability of spreading infection can be reduced by strict adherence to accepted isolation policies and procedures. Protocols for handling infectious — or potentially infectious — materials should also be in place and rigidly followed.

The importance of effective hand washing by the Attendants and all visitors to an isolated patient's room cannot be overemphasized. Vigorous hand washing, even with ordinary soap for 15-30 seconds, is the single most effective measure in infection control. Virtually all transiently acquired microorganisms can be eliminated in this way.

ISOLATION POLICIES AND PROCEDURES

FIRST AID ROOMS SHOULD NOT BE USED AS ISOLATION ROOMS, BECAUSE OTHER PEOPLE MAY REQUIRE THE ROOMS FOR EMERGENCY CARE.

Strict isolation in a non-hospital setting is difficult to maintain but, in the case of a serious, highly communicable disease, every effort should be made to adhere as closely as possible to the ideal protocol, depending upon facilities and equipment available to the Attendant. The less exposure the infectious patient has to other people, the better. Isolation protocols differ somewhat, depending upon the mode of transmission of the specific infectious disease.

Four levels of infection control precautions:
1. Contact
2. Respiratory
3. Enteric
4. Blood/Body Fluids

1. CONTACT PRECAUTIONS

Patients may have infections spread by direct hand contact or by contact with infectious material, such as secretions, pus or contaminated articles. They should be advised to avoid direct contact with others until appropriate medical treatment can be initiated. This is called contact precautions.

The Attendant will have to decide what degree of isolation is necessary in a particular case. Contact precautions would obviously not be indicated for a superficial wound infection or athlete's foot. However, for a large abscess draining pus, contact precautions are appropriate.

- Hand washing — careful hand washing with disinfectant soap before and after contact with the patient.
- Gloves — for direct handling of infected materials.
- Disposal — of contaminated dressings and materials in specially marked double plastic bags.
- Gowns — optional, depending on risk of one's own clothes becoming contaminated.
- To avoid contamination, it is preferable to treat grossly infected wounds in a room other than the first aid room.
- Avoid unnecessary contamination of first aid equipment or furniture.

2. RESPIRATORY PRECAUTIONS

These are for patients whose infections are spread by air droplets that are coughed, sneezed or breathed into the environment. This is rarely indicated except in cases of active TB.
- Mask must be worn by the patient.
- Gloves are necessary if touching the patient is required.
- Hand washing as in "Contact Precautions".
- Disposal of directly infected materials as in "Contact Precautions".
- Keep door closed and patient confined to room.

3. ENTERIC PRECAUTIONS

Enteric precautions should be used to prevent spread of disease transmitted by direct or indirect contact with infected feces and contaminated articles (e.g. hepatitis A).

The patient must be instructed to use good personal hygiene principles, especially careful and thorough hand washing when using toilet facilities or eating. The patient must not share food, drinks or personal belongings (e.g. toothbrush).
- Confinement not necessarily required.
- Hand washing as in "Contact Precautions" — especially important for the patient.
- Gloves — required if handling patient or contaminated materials.
- Disposal of contaminated dressings and materials in specially marked double plastic bags.

4. For complete details, see Universal Precautions, page 325. BLOOD/BODY FLUIDS PRECAUTIONS

BLOOD AND BODY FLUIDS SHOULD BE TREATED AT ALL TIMES AS IF KNOWN TO BE CONTAMINATED. GLOVES ARE MANDATORY. In addition, the following precautions should be taken:
- Masks are recommended for the Attendant when the patient is coughing up blood or other secretions.
- Hand washing and gloves — as in "Contact Precautions".
- Take extra care to prevent needle stick or other puncture wounds.
- Disposal of contaminated dressings and materials in specially marked double plastic bags.

- Blood spills should be cleaned up immediately using a household bleach solution diluted 1:10 with water.
- All first aid equipment should be decontaminated as outlined in Part XI, Section E, page 213.

INFECTIOUS DISEASES

Detailed discussion of the many communicable diseases that might be encountered by the First Aid Attendant does not fall within the scope of this book. However, a few selected diseases will be discussed, with emphasis on the practical aspects of diagnosis and treatment that might be useful to the Attendant.

SCABIES

Scabies is an infestation of the skin caused by a microscopic mite. It can be identified by these characteristics:

- Skin penetration, visible as small pimples and/or blisters. May also be palpable as fine bumps on the skin surface in the early stages, before anything is visible.
- Burrows, visible as linear tracks, are formed by mites under the skin.
- Lesions are most frequently found between the fingers and toes, on the anterior surfaces of the wrists and ankles, in the armpits and folds of the skin and along the belt line. The face and palms are usually spared.
- Itching is usually present with the primary infestation and may be intense. It is usually worse at night.

Mode of Transmission

The infection is spread by direct contact. However, casual contact is not usually sufficient to permit the spread of scabies to another individual. Closer contact, such as sharing the same bed or the same towel, is more likely to result in the communication of this disease to others. Merely examining the scabies victim does not put the Attendant at risk, particularly if proper hand washing techniques are observed following the examination.

Treatment

The treatment of choice is available without a prescription in British Columbia. A lotion and/or a shampoo containing 1% gamma benzene hexachloride is usually used. A shampoo is used on all hair-bearing areas as per label directions. The lotion is applied to all affected areas after a long, hot bath, used according to label directions. The treatment is repeated after 24 hours. Use of these products beyond the manufacturer's recommendations may cause toxic side effects. Normal bathing may be resumed after this time. Clothing and linen should be thoroughly laundered.

LICE (PEDICULOSIS)

Lice are tiny insects that infest the hair, skin and clothing. There are three distinct types:

1. Head Lice
2. Body Lice
3. Pubic Lice (Crabs)

HEAD LICE

Head lice generally prefer the fine hairs on the head, particularly around the ears. They also infest the eyebrows and eyelashes. Adults, larvae and nits (eggs) are all visible. Adults are 3-4mm in length and, if observed closely, can often be seen moving. Nits appear as tiny black specks of sand, usually clinging to a hair.

Their presence can be suspected in situations of overcrowding in dwellings, less than adequate hygiene facilities and when grooming items might be shared (combs and brushes).

Treatment

Shampoo containing 1% gamma benzene hexachloride is used. It should be applied once, then the hair is combed with a fine-tooth comb to remove dead lice and nits. The treatment is usually repeated in four days. Contact precautions should be maintained until the treatment is effective.

The most common mistake made in delousing patients is inadequate application of the shampoo. All scalp and hair surfaces must have the shampoo thoroughly worked in and well rinsed, followed by a comb-out.

BODY LICE

Body lice are not found on the body but, instead, in the clothing. They anchor themselves on the clothing and reach across to suck blood from the infected person. The patient may be covered with scratch marks but have no actual lice found on the body.

Treatment

Shampoo containing 1% gamma benzene hexachloride should be applied to the body, although nearly all the lice are in the clothing. Lice and nits in clothing can be destroyed by laundering in hot water (60°C, 140°F) for 20 minutes. Drycleaning or gas autoclaving will also destroy lice and nits.

PUBIC LICE — "CRABS"

Pubic lice can infest the hairs of the pubic area, armpits, eyelashes and eyebrows. In a hairy person, they may be found over the entire body.

Mode of Transmission

A common mode of transmission is intimate body contact. Pubic lice can also be acquired by sitting on an infested toilet seat. However, other venereal diseases are not transmitted by toilet seats.

Treatment

Shampoo containing 1% gamma benzene hexachloride is usually applied thoroughly to the affected area and the dead nits and lice are removed with a fine-tooth comb. The treatment should be repeated in four days. Crabs do not infest clothing, so no special treatment is necessary for the clothes other than regular laundering.

FUNGAL INFECTIONS

SCALP RINGWORM

This is a fungal infection and, in spite of the name, is not a worm. It almost always occurs in children and appears as round, grey, scaly bald patches on the scalp. The patient should be referred to a physician for treatment and should not use another person's hat or comb.

BODY RINGWORM

This is a fungus causing ringed, scaling, itchy areas on exposed skin surfaces. It is often transmitted from infected household pets. Treatment is the same as for scalp ringworm.

JOCK ITCH

This is also a fungal disease, causing marked itching in the groin and characterized by sharply demarcated, reddish lesions with clear centres. This occurs in athletes and others who perspire excessively. Mild cases can be treated with local drying measures and an antifungal medication.

ATHLETE'S FOOT

Athlete's foot is another fungal disease. It causes itching, burning and scaling between the fingers and toes of the hands and feet, possibly associated with nail destruction. Treatment and prevention is by personal hygiene, including thorough washing and thorough drying of the affected areas. The fungus that causes the condition cannot survive in a dry environment. It is frequently encountered in public showers and changing rooms in and around gymnasiums and swimming pool facilities.

Treatment

There are a variety of commercially available applications, some of which are non-prescription. Patients should be advised to seek medical advice and treatment for these conditions. Incorrect self-diagnosis and treatment can result in unwanted complications or delayed recovery.

GASTROENTERITIS (FOOD POISONING)

Food poisoning is a general term applied to a variety of clinical entities caused by a number of different agents. Most, but not all, food poisoning is the result of "an infection". A few of the causes are:

* viral, bacterial or parasitic infection;
* food intolerance;
* organic poisons (shellfish or mushrooms);
* inorganic chemicals and toxins (nitrites, MSG);
* side effects of some drugs (antibiotics);
* stress.

The Attendant should suspect food poisoning when a group of people develop similar symptoms, all within a short period of time.

Symptoms usually include vomiting and/or diarrhea and/or abdominal cramps, in the absence of fever.

Treatment

The basic principles of treatment for food poisoning are:

1. Restrict solid food intake.
2. Encourage clear fluid intake (e.g. water, juice, soft

drinks or clear soups). Give small amounts frequently rather than a lot at once, and avoid all milk products.
3. Provide medication, such as antinauseants.
4. Ensure adequate rest.

The patient should be referred for medical treatment in the following situations:
- blood in stool;
- vomiting blood;
- fever;
- marked weakness;
- severe abdominal pain;
- dehydration.

The most commonly encountered types of food poisoning are usually mild and self-limiting, and symptoms usually resolve within a few days. In isolated areas with questionable drinking water, consider parasitic infections (Giardia/beaver fever). When there is a history of recent out-of-country travel, consider more serious causes (e.g. hepatitis, typhoid), and refer promptly to medical aid.

HEPATITIS

Hepatitis is an inflammatory disease of the liver which can be caused by a variety of agents, including infectious organisms, toxic chemicals and a few medications.

They may be very difficult to differentiate on the basis of etiology. For purposes of this section, the most commonly encountered types of hepatitis will be discussed — those caused by viral infections.

Types of Viral Hepatitis

- Hepatitis A
- Hepatitis B
- Others (Hepatitis C and D, Mononucleosis Virus, etc.)

The Attendant should have some understanding of how the disease works and have a sound knowledge of safe handling techniques, to avoid putting the Attendant or others at serious risk of contracting the condition.

Signs and Symptoms

All forms of hepatitis have similar signs and symptoms. It is virtually impossible to distinguish the different types of hepatitis on the basis of their clinical presentation, which can be done only by specific laboratory tests. Signs and symptoms may include:

- weakness and fatigue;
- nausea and vomiting;
- diarrhea;
- abdominal pain and tenderness — especially right upper quadrant;
- loss of appetite (anorexia) and weight loss;
- dark-coloured urine and light-coloured stools;
- jaundice — yellow eyes and skin;
- prolonged course — weeks or months.

HEPATITIS A

This type is also known as infectious hepatitis; it is generally acquired through ingestion of contaminated food or water. The virus lives in the bowel of infected persons and escapes into the environment through fecal contamination. It is not spread by blood products.

HEPATITIS B (SERUM HEPATITIS, HBV INFECTION)

Hepatitis B is the most serious form of hepatitis likely to be encountered by the IFA Attendant. It is spread by blood-to-blood contact (needle stick, transfusion), by mucous membrane contact (saliva and other body fluids) and by sexual contact.

It is difficult for the Attendant to identify a patient who may be harbouring HBV, because of the high prevalence of asymptomatic carriers in the general population. Those who do not exhibit the classic signs and symptoms of the disease may be unaware that they can pose a health threat to others.

Adding to the difficulty in identifying such patients is the fact that there is a long incubation period (up to six months) and a very slow onset of the disease, during which time it can be transmitted to others.

The Attendant should also be aware that there are certain high-risk groups where the prevalence of HBV is likely to be higher than in the general population. They include IV drug abusers, homosexuals and people from Asian or African countries.

Of all those who develop serum hepatitis, about 80% will have a full recovery and somewhere between 1% and 15% will die. Importantly, 5%-10% of all those infected with HBV will become lifetime carriers who are asymptomatic, but nonetheless capable of transmitting the disease to others.

Precautions for Hepatitis B Prevention

For complete details, see Universal Precautions, page 325.

- Wear disposable gloves at all times when in contact with blood or saliva. Be extremely cautious if your hands have any open scratches or sores.
- Observe recommended hand washing practises.
- Clean up blood spills promptly with a dilute bleach solution (household bleach diluted 1:10 with water).
- Avoid needle sticks wherever possible.

NOTE: IF INADVERTENTLY EXPOSED TO THE BLOOD OR SALIVA OF A KNOWN CARRIER OR HIGH-RISK INDIVIDUAL, THE ATTENDANT SHOULD SEEK MEDICAL ADVICE IMMEDIATELY REGARDING THE POSSIBILITY OF IMMUNIZATION AGAINST HBV.

OTHER FORMS OF HEPATITIS

A number of other viruses have been known to cause hepatitis (e.g. the virus that causes mononucleosis, hepatitis C, formerly called Non-A, Non-B). They are more rare than HBV and generally pose less of a threat to the IFA Attendant and others.

HIV DISEASE AND AIDS

There has been a great deal of interest and concern in the last few years over the rapidly rising incident of HIV disease (human immunodeficiency virus), ultimately manifesting itself as AIDS (Acquired Immune Deficiency Syndrome). It has been of particular interest to pre-hospital care providers, including the first aid Attendant, because of its prevalence in society today in unsuspecting individuals who are unaware of their potential ability to infect others. Furthermore, there is a strong indication that, even with the best medical technology, the disease, once contracted, is not only incurable but eventually fatal.

A relatively new disease, the human immunodeficiency virus has come into widespread recognition only within the last 10 years.

Formerly confined to a relatively small segment of the community in this part of the world, now it affects virtually all groups in society — old and young, male and female, and all racial and socioeconomic groups.

Certain high-risk sub-groups for this disease still exist.

They include:
- "IV" drug abusers;
- homosexuals, bisexuals;
- hemophiliacs and other recipients of therapeutic blood products;
- people from certain high-prevalence nations (Haiti and certain Central African nations).

The HIV attacks certain blood cells vital to a healthy immune response. The immune system weakens significantly, allowing the victim to become highly susceptible to other infections (opportunistic infections) and certain types of cancer (Kaposi's sarcoma). In the early stages of HIV disease, the sufferer tends to recover from those events but, as time goes on, and the immune system is compromised further, recovery becomes more difficult. In addition to the above, patients with "full-blown" AIDS may exhibit any or all of the following symptoms.

Signs and Symptoms
- Multiple swollen lymph nodes
- Fever and night sweats
- Malaise and fatigue
- Weight loss
- Recurrent diarrhea
- Shortness of breath
- Dementia (loss of intellectual capacity)

Modes of Transmission

HIV is a rather fragile virus outside of the human body. It dies rapidly with drying, changes in temperature and exposure to common disinfectants. It does not survive on dry surfaces (e.g. toilet seats, dry skin, eating utensils). It is not transmitted by casual contact, coughing, sneezing, hand shakes or kissing. Nor is it communicated by sharing of food or drink, mosquito bites, hot tubs or swimming pools, nor by toothbrushes.

There is no direct current evidence that HIV disease is transmittable through human tears, saliva, stool or urine. The HIV virus is transmitted from an infected person ONLY through:
1. blood-to-blood contact;
2. sexual contact.

Diagnosis and Outcome

Blood testing is the only confirmatory test for the presence of the HIV virus. Seropositivity or seroconversion will occur in 94%-97% of victims within three months of acquiring the virus. It is believed that all seropositive patients will eventually develop AIDS. It is also thought that 50% of all victims will show some form of the disease within 10 years of testing positive for the HIV virus. It is still believed that AIDS will eventually prove to be fatal 100% of the time.

Statistics

To put things in perspective: in Canada to date (1990), not one case of work-acquired AIDS has been reported among all health care workers. Furthermore, there have been only 34 such confirmed cases world-wide.

It is estimated that, on an international basis, perhaps one to two health care workers will die of AIDS annually. This compares to about 300 workers who will die each year from work-acquired hepatitis B.

It should also be remembered that the vast majority of these serious infections have arisen following needle-stick type injuries. Of course, that type of injury would be exceedingly rare in the industrial first aid setting.

As of May 1990, British Columbia had recorded 734 cases of AIDS since 1981. Approximately half of those people have died.

UNIVERSAL BLOOD, BODY FLUID PRECAUTIONS (HIV/AIDS Precautions)

Largely because of increasing concern over the rising incidence of AIDS, in 1985 the Centre for Disease Control in the USA was asked to devise a set of precautions for the health care setting, in an effort to limit its spread. Guidelines subsequently developed are known as "Universal Precautions".

The following section is an excerpt from the MMWR (Morbidity and Mortality Weekly Report), Volume 38/No. S-6, February 1989 — U.S. Dept. of Health and Human Services, Public Health Service Centre for Disease Control, Atlanta, Georgia.

Disinfection, Decontamination and Disposal

The only documented occupational risks of HIV and HBV infection are associated with parenteral (including open wound) and mucous membrane exposure to blood and other potentially infectious body fluids. Nevertheless, the precautions described below should be routinely followed.

1. Needle and Sharps Disposal
   All workers should take precautions to prevent injuries caused by needles, scalpel blades and other sharp instruments or devices during procedures; when cleaning used instruments; during disposal of used needles; and when handling sharp instruments after procedures. To prevent needle-stick injuries, needles should not be recapped, purposely bent or broken by hand, removed from disposable syringes or otherwise manipulated by hand. After they are used, disposable syringes and needles, scalpel blades and other sharp items should be placed in puncture-resistant containers for disposal; the puncture-resistant containers should be located as close as practical to the use area (e.g. in the ambulance or, if sharps are carried to the scene of victim assistance from the ambulance, a small puncture-resistant container should be carried to the scene as well). Reusable needles should be left on the syringe body and placed in a puncture-resistant container for transport to the reprocessing area.

2. Hand Washing
   Hands and other skin surfaces should be washed immediately and thoroughly if contaminated with blood, other body fluids to which universal precautions apply or potentially contaminated articles. Hands should always be washed after gloves are removed, even if the gloves appear to be intact. Hand washing should be completed using the appropriate facilities, such as utility or restroom sinks. Waterless antiseptic hand cleanser should be provided on responding units to use when hand-washing facilities are not available. When hand-washing facilities are available, wash hands with warm water and soap. When hand-washing facilities are not available, use a waterless antiseptic hand cleanser. The manufacturer's recommendations for the product should be followed.

3. Cleaning, Disinfecting and Sterilizing
   The methods and applications for cleaning, disinfecting and sterilizing equipment and surfaces in the prehospital setting have already been discussed in "First Aid Room Techniques". These methods also apply to housekeeping and other cleaning tasks.

4. Cleaning and Decontaminating Spills of Blood
All spills of blood and blood-contaminated fluids should be promptly cleaned up using an EPA-approved germicide or a 1:10 solution of household bleach in the following manner WHILE WEARING GLOVES. Visible material should first be removed with disposable towels or other appropriate means that will ensure against direct contact with blood. If splashing is anticipated, protective eyewear should be worn along with an impervious gown or apron which provides an effective barrier to splashes. The area should then be decontaminated with an appropriate germicide. Hands should be washed following removal of gloves. Soiled cleaning equipment should be cleaned and decontaminated or placed in an appropriate container and disposed of according to agency policy. Plastic bags should be available for removal of contaminated items from the site of the spill.

Shoes and boots can become contaminated with blood in certain instances. Where there is massive blood contamination on floors, the use of disposable impervious shoe coverings should be considered. Protective gloves should be worn to remove contaminated shoe coverings. The coverings and gloves should be disposed of in plastic bags. A plastic bag should be included in the first aid kit or the car which is to be used for the disposal of contaminated items. Extra plastic bags should be stored in the police cruiser or emergency vehicle.

5. Laundry
Although soiled linen may be contaminated with pathogenic microorganisms, the risk of actual disease transmission is negligible. Rather than rigid procedures and specifications, hygienic storage and processing of clean and soiled linen are recommended. Laundry facilities and/or services should be made routinely available by the employer. Soiled linen should be handled as little as possible and with minimum agitation to prevent gross microbial contamination of the air and of persons handling the linen. All soiled linen should be bagged at the location where it was used. Linen soiled with blood should be placed and transported in bags that prevent leakage. Normal laundry cycles should be used according to

the washer and detergent manufacturers' recommendations.

6. Decontamination and Laundering of Protective Clothing
Protective work clothing contaminated with blood or other body fluids to which universal precautions apply should be placed and transported in bags or containers that prevent leakage. Personnel involved in the bagging, transport and laundering of contaminated clothing should wear gloves. Protective clothing and station and work uniforms should be washed and dried according to the manufacturer's instructions. Boots and leather goods may be brush-scrubbed with soap and hot water to remove contamination.

7. Infective Waste
The selection of procedures for disposal of infective waste is determined by the relative risk of disease transmission and application of local regulations, which vary widely. IN ALL CASES, LOCAL REGULATIONS SHOULD BE CONSULTED PRIOR TO DISPOSAL PROCEDURES AND FOLLOWED. Infective waste, in general, should either be incinerated or should be decontaminated before disposal in a sanitary landfill. Bulk blood, suctioned fluids, excretions and secretions may be carefully poured down a drain connected to a sanitary sewer, where permitted. Sanitary sewers may also be used to dispose of other infectious wastes capable of being ground and flushed into the sewer, where permitted. Sharp items should be placed in puncture-proof containers and other blood-contaminated items should be placed in leak-proof plastic bags for transport to an appropriate disposal location.

Prior to the removal of protective equipment, personnel remaining on the scene after the patient has been cared for should carefully search for and remove contaminated materials. Debris should be disposed of as noted above.

Fire and Emergency Medical Services

The guidelines that appear in this section apply to fire and emergency medical services. This includes structural fire fighters, paramedics, emergency medical technicians and advanced life support personnel. Fire fighters often provide emergency medical services and therefore encounter the exposures common to paramedics and emergency medical technicians. Job duties are often performed in uncontrolled environments, which, due to a lack of time and other factors, do not allow for application of a complex decision-making process to the emergency at hand.

The general principles presented here have been developed from existing principles of occupational safety and health in conjunction with data from studies of health care workers in hospital settings. The basic premise is that workers must be protected from exposure to blood and other potentially infectious body fluids in the course of their work activities. There is a paucity of data concerning the risks these worker groups face, however, which complicates development of control principles. Thus, the guidelines presented below are based on principles of prudent public health practise.

Fire and emergency medical service personnel are engaged in delivery of medical care in the prehospital setting. The following guidelines are intended to assist these personnel in making decisions concerning use of personal protective equipment and resuscitation equipment, as well as for decontamination, disinfection and disposal procedures.

Personal Protective Equipment

Appropriate personal protective equipment should be made available routinely by the employer to reduce the risk of exposure as defined above. For many situations, the chance that the rescuer will be exposed to blood and other body fluids to which universal precautions apply can be determined in advance. Therefore, if the chances of being exposed to blood is high (e.g. CPR, IV insertion, trauma, delivering babies), the worker should put on protective attire before beginning patient care. Table XIII-b sets forth examples of recommendations for personal protective equipment in the prehospital setting; the list is not intended to be all-inclusive.

1. Gloves

   Disposable gloves should be a standard component of emergency response equipment, and should be donned by all personnel prior to initiating any emergency patient care tasks involving exposure to blood or other body fluids to which universal precautions apply. Extra pairs should always be available. Considerations in the choice of disposable gloves should include dexterity, durability, fit and the task being performed. Thus, there is no single type or thickness of glove appropriate for protection in all situations. For situations where large amounts of blood are likely to be encountered, it is important that gloves fit tightly at the wrist to prevent blood contamination of hands around the cuff. For multiple trauma victims, gloves should be changed between patient contacts, if the emergency situation allows.

   Greater personal protective equipment measures are indicated for situations where broken glass and sharp edges are likely to be encountered, such as extricating a person from an automobile wreck. Structural fire-fighting gloves that meet the Federal OSHA requirements for fire fighters' gloves (as contained in 29 CFR 1910.156 or National Fire Protection Association Standard 1973, Gloves for Structural Fire Fighters) should be worn in any situation where sharp or rough surfaces are likely to be encountered.

   While wearing gloves, avoid handling personal items, such as combs and pens, that could become soiled or contaminated. Gloves that have become contaminated with blood or other body fluids to which universal precautions apply should be removed as soon as possible, taking care to avoid skin contact with the exterior surface. Contaminated gloves should be placed and transported in bags that prevent leakage and should be disposed of or, in the case of reusable gloves, cleaned and disinfected properly.

2. Masks, Eyewear and Gowns

   Masks, eyewear and gowns should be present on all emergency vehicles that respond or potentially respond to medical emergencies or victim rescues. These protective barriers should be used in accordance with the level of exposure encountered. Minor lacerations or small amounts of blood do not merit the same extent of barrier use as required for exsanguinating victims or massive arterial bleeding. Management of the patient who is not bleeding, and who has no bloody body fluids present, should not routinely require use of barrier precautions. Masks and eyewear (e.g. safety glasses) should be worn together, or a face shield should be used by all personnel prior to any situation where splashes of blood or other body fluids to which universal precautions apply are likely to occur. Gowns or aprons should be worn to protect clothing from splashes with blood. If large splashes or quantities of blood are present or anticipated, impervious gowns or aprons should be worn. An extra change of work clothing should be available at all times.

3. Resuscitation Equipment

No transmission of HBV or HIV infection during mouth-to-mouth resuscitation has been documented. However, because of the risk of salivary transmission of other infectious diseases (e.g. herpes simplex and Neisseria meningitidis) and the theoretical risk of HIV and HBV transmission during artificial ventilation of trauma victims, disposable airway equipment or resuscitation bags should be used. Disposable resuscitation equipment and devices should be used once and disposed of or, if reusable, thoroughly cleaned and disinfected after each use according to the manufacturer's recommendations.

Mechanical respiratory assist devices (e.g. bag-valve masks) should be available on all emergency vehicles and to all emergency response personnel that respond or potentially respond to medical emergencies or victim rescues.

Pocket mouth-to-mouth resuscitation masks designed to isolate emergency response personnel (i.e. double lumen systems) from contact with victims' blood and blood-contaminated saliva, respiratory secretions and vomitus should be provided to all personnel who provide or potentially provide emergency treatment.

TABLE XIII-a
SUMMARY OF TASK CATEGORIZATION AND
IMPLICATIONS FOR PERSONAL PROTECTIVE EQUIPMENT

Joint Advisory Notice Category[1]	Nature of Task/Activity	Personal protective equipment should be:	
		Available?	Worn?
I.	Direct contact with blood or other body fluids to which universal precautions apply	Yes	Yes
II.	Activity performed without blood exposure but exposure may occur in emergency	Yes	No
III.	Task/activity does not entail predictable or unpredictable exposure to blood	No	No

[1] US Department of Labor, US Department of Health and Human Services. Joint advisory notice: protection against occupational exposure to hepatitis B virus (HBV) and human immunodeficiency virus (HIV). Washington, DC: US Department of Labor, US Department of Health and Human Services, 1987.

TABLE XIII-b
EXAMPLES OF RECOMMENDED PERSONAL PROTECTIVE
EQUIPMENT FOR WORKER PROTECTION AGAINST HIV
AND HBV TRANSMISSION[1] IN PREHOSPITAL[2] SETTINGS

Task or Activity	Disposable Gloves	Gown	Mask[3]	Protective Eyewear
Bleeding control with spurting blood	Yes	Yes	Yes	Yes
Bleeding control with minimal bleeding	Yes	No	No	No
Emergency childbirth	Yes	Yes	Yes, if splashing is likely	Yes, if splashing is likely
Blood drawing	at certain times	No	No	No
Starting an intravenous (IV) line	Yes	No	No	No
Endotracheal intubation, esophageal obturator use	Yes	No	No, unless splashing is likely	No, unless splashing is likely
Oral/nasal suctioning, manually cleaning airway	Yes[4]	No	No, unless splashing is likely	No, unless splashing is likely
Handling and cleaning instruments with microbial contamination	Yes	No, unless soiling is likely	No	No
Measuring blood pressure	No	No	No	No
Measuring temperature	No	No	No	No
Giving an injection	No	No	No	No

[1] The examples provided in this table are based on application of universal precautions. Universal precautions are intended to supplement rather than replace recommendations for routine infection control, such as hand washing and using gloves to prevent gross microbial contamination of hands (e.g. contact with urine or feces).

[2] Defined as setting where delivery of emergency health care takes place away from a hospital or other health care facility.

[3] Refers to protective masks to prevent exposure of mucous membranes to blood or other potentially contaminated body fluids. The use of resuscitation devices, some of which are also referred to as "masks", is discussed on page 327.

[4] While not clearly necessary to prevent HIV or HBV transmission unless blood is present, gloves are recommended to prevent transmission of other agents (e.g. herpes simplex).

LEGAL ASPECTS

From a legal perspective, the IFA Attendant has a responsibility to treat all patients promptly and effectively regardless of their "HIV status". To refuse to do so would be not only unethical but could be deemed discriminatory and negligent in a court of law. By following the recommended precautions and safety procedures in caring for patients — even those known or suspected of being HIV positive — the Attendant need have no fear for his/her own personal health and safety.

Part XIV, Section A
Stroke (Cerebrovascular Accident–CVA)

INTRODUCTION

The brain cells require a constant supply of oxygen and nutrients in order to perform their vital functions. Consequently, there are four major arteries feeding the brain: the two carotid arteries anteriorly and the two vertebral arteries posteriorly. Any interruption in the arterial blood flow to any part of the brain beyond four minutes will result in permanent damage to that part of the brain.

A STROKE is the layman's term for a cerebrovascular accident (CVA) and is the term for the brain damage caused by the sudden blockage or rupture of a cerebral artery. Strokes result in permanent damage to brain tissue and the victim is left with some degree of permanent disability. Strokes are one of the most common causes of serious disability in adults. They are the third leading cause of death in North America. Males and females are affected equally. Although most strokes occur in the elderly, they can occur in young, apparently healthy adults.

TYPES OF STROKES

There are two main types of strokes:
- Ischemic strokes
- Hemorrhagic strokes

Ischemic Strokes

Ischemic strokes are caused by the blockage or narrowing of a cerebral artery. The term "ischemia" means a local deficiency of blood flow. Ischemic strokes account for the majority of strokes (approximately 75%).

There are two major types of ischemic strokes:
- Cerebral thrombosis
- Cerebral embolism

A cerebral thrombosis develops in the same way as coronary artery disease. See Part V, Section E, page 115. Atherosclerosis develops in the arteries of the brain, causing the vessel walls to narrow and also causing a roughened inner surface. A thrombus (blood clot) can then form on the roughened area, obstructing the blood flow to the brain tissue beyond the blockage. The same risk factors that promote coronary artery atherosclerosis similarly affect the brain's arteries.

A cerebral embolus is a stroke caused by the obstruction of a cerebral artery by a clot that formed elsewhere in the body (usually the heart) and travelled to the brain. Patients with heart disease in the form of a myocardial infarction or with irregular heart beat are at higher risk for cerebral embolus. An embolism is not always clotted blood. It may be any foreign material or gas (see Diving Emergencies, Part XI, Section F, page 304), which can obstruct the flow of blood to brain cells.

Hemorrhagic Strokes

A hemorrhagic stroke is caused by the rupture of a cerebral artery. Brain damage results from the bleeding into the surrounding brain tissue as well as the impaired circulation caused by the ruptured vessel. The hemorrhage usually occurs at weakened dilated regions of the wall of the blood vessel (aneurysm). This weakness is primarily caused by atherosclerotic damage. However, occasionally, an aneurysm may be a developmental abnormality that the victim is born with. The rupture of congenital aneurysms is one of the major causes of stroke in young, previously healthy adults.

SIGNS AND SYMPTOMS OF STROKE

The following three different events can interrupt blood flow to the brain. These can cause three different groups of signs and symptoms.

1. Cerebral Thrombosis — The clot formation with blockage of the cerebral arteries causes specific losses of body functions (e.g. partial paralysis, partial numbness, loss of speech, etc.) BUT generally without pain, headache or seizures.
2. Cerebral Embolism — This problem may cause a sudden convulsion, coma and/or paralysis.
3. Arterial Rupture — This disorder is frequently accompanied by a sudden severe headache, "the worst headache the patient has ever had", a fainting episode or a decreasing level of consciousness, and often profound nausea and vomiting. The patient may not have any specific loss of body function (i.e. may not have any local paralysis).

Regardless of the different initial presentations, the signs and symptoms of stroke are variable, depending upon the location in the brain that is affected and the extent of damage to the brain tissue.

General Signs and Symptoms of Stroke That May be Present

1. Mental Function
   - Decreased level of consciousness

- Confusion
- Trouble communicating (e.g. understanding or having garbled speech)
- Dizziness
- Seizures

2. Motor Function
   - Inability to speak or slurred speech
   - Facial weakness with a one-sided droop of the mouth and/or drooling
   - Sudden clumsiness or weakness of an arm or leg
   - Paralysis on one (most common) or both sides of the body
   - Decerebrate or decorticate posturing (see Part III, page 27)
   - Difficulty swallowing

3. Change in Vital Signs
   - Pupils may be unequal in size or may be dilated
   - May have rapid or very slow, strong pulse
   - May demonstrate irregular respirations

4. Complaints
   - There may be a loss of feeling (numbness) or "pins and needles" sensation in one side of the body
   - Severe headache
   - Nausea and/or vomiting
   - Amnesia
   - Visual difficulties (e.g. partial blindness)

Prior to a stroke, some patients may experience warning symptoms in the form of a transient episode with symptoms that resemble a stroke but spontaneously resolve after seconds, minutes or hours. Such an episode is called a *Transient Ischemic Attack*. It is caused by a temporary blockage of a cerebral artery. Such patients should be treated as though they had a stroke and should be managed as described below. They must definitely see a physician. With appropriate medical care, a complete stroke may be prevented.

MANAGEMENT OF THE STROKE VICTIM

The evaluation and management of the worker with a suspected stroke follows the Priority Action Approach outlined in Part III, page 20. Stroke victims with a diminished level of consciousness will often have airway and respiratory problems. Workers with a suspected stroke should be transported to hospital rapidly once they have been evaluated.

1. Assess the scene.
2. Determine the level of consciousness and assess the airway. Ensure that there is an adequate airway, ruling out a C-spine injury and position the patient appropriately.
3. Ensure that breathing is adequate by assessing rate and chest movement. Assist ventilations with supplemental oxygen, if necessary.
4. Apply high-flow oxygen at 10 Lpm but do not leave the comatose stroke victim unattended with a mask affixed to the face, as the patient may aspirate if he or she vomits.
5. Assess the patient's circulation by feeling the radial pulse. If it is not present, check the carotid artery.
6. Control any major hemorrhage.
7. Conduct a rapid body survey.
8. Insert an oral pharyngeal airway if the patient has a diminished level of consciousness.
9. Suction as needed and if necessary.
10. The Attendant should prepare the patient for rapid transportation to a medical facility. Patients who have a diminished level of consciousness should be transported in the lateral or ¾ prone position. The ¾ prone position is acceptable for non-traumatic emergencies, providing there is no concern for spinal injury. If they are conscious, transport with the head and shoulders elevated.
11. Obtain history. When obtaining the history, in the presence of an apparent stroke, the Attendant should ask the patient or co-workers if there are any medical problems (e.g. past heart disease, high blood pressure, diabetes, etc.) and whether the patient has experienced any symptoms of a transient ischemic attack in the past.
12. Perform a secondary survey, including a neurological exam. The Attendant should assess the level of consciousness using the Glasgow Coma scale. Pupil response should be noted and recorded. The Attendant should then test for arm and hand as well as leg and foot strength and sensation on both sides of the body.
13. En route to the hospital, the Attendant must be alert

for changes suggestive of increasing intracranial pressure, which may be due to either intracranial hemorrhage or swelling of the brain. Danger signs include:

- a decreasing level of consciousness over time;
- profound vomiting, which is persistent;
- a slowing and strengthening of the pulse into the 40-50 beats per minute range;
- increasing pupil size or inequality of the pupils.

14. Remember the patient with a CVA may be unable to speak. Nevertheless, they most probably will be able to hear what is going on about them, as well as understanding what is being said. Invariably, they will be upset or frightened and it is important that the Attendant use a reassuring manner and be careful of statements made in front of the patient.

Part XIV, Section B
Seizures

INTRODUCTION

In this section, the assessment and treatment of seizures is reviewed. Different types and cause of seizures must be kept in mind by the Attendant when assessing the patient with a suspected seizure disorder. A Priority Action Approach to seizure management is presented. The important role of the Attendant in determining the seizure history is emphasized. Most seizures, although frightening and dramatic, are self-limiting. By using an organized approach to assessment and treatment, the Attendant will usually prevent any life-threatening complications. Most seizures can ultimately be controlled and these patients can usually lead healthy lives.

Seizures are the manifestation of a massive discharge of electrical impulses from the brain cells. Most people consider the term "seizure" to mean generalized uncoordinated muscular activity associated with loss of consciousness. In fact, there are many different types of seizures.

TYPES OF SEIZURES

Seizures may be classified as generalized or focal, depending on whether or not the entire brain is involved.

Generalized seizures are of two types:
- Grand mal
- Petit mal
  Focal seizures are also of two types:
- Focal motor
- Temporal lobe seizures (formerly called psychomotor seizures; also called complex partial seizures)

Generalized Grand Mal Type Seizures

These seizures are the most common type. They follow a classical pattern. Initially, the patient may have a sensation (aura) that something is about to happen. The patient may cry out. The sensation takes many forms — a sound, a feeling of dizziness or anxiety, a characteristic smell — but for the patient it is always the same and serves as a warning that a seizure is about to occur. This sensation is called the AURA and lasts only a few seconds.

The patient then develops a convulsion. It is characterized by a loss of consciousness (coma). The patient usually falls to the ground. There is a generalized contraction of all muscles associated with rigid extension of the body. The extremities and trunk are stiff not limp. The patient also develops rapid jerking activity of the extremities associated with tight jaw muscles and clenched teeth. The latter may lead to biting the tongue. The patient often turns blue; the breathing often becomes loud and gurgling. The patient often appears to be in danger of respiratory arrest. Loss of bladder control is also common and involuntary urination may occur. This convulsion is referred to as the ictal phase of the seizure. It may last from one to several minutes but rarely longer.

The convulsion is followed by a period of decreased consciousness, which represents the recovery phase (postictal phase) of the seizure. During the postictal period, the patient's level of consciousness gradually improves from unresponsiveness to confusion. Slowly, over a period of 10 to 30 minutes, the patient usually regains full consciousness. In the postictal period, the patient's extremities are limp and flaccid as opposed to the rigid and jerking activity seen in the convulsive or ictal period. Initially, there may be no response to any stimuli. The patient may also appear apneic and cyanotic. Assisted ventilation may be required. Patients usually begin breathing on their own. Regaining consciousness, the patient is usually confused, with no memory of the seizure. The patient may also be combative during this time. Ultimately, the patient regains previous normal status.

Generalized Petit Mal Type Seizures

Petit mal type seizures are very brief (less than one minute) and usually occur in children. This type of seizure often goes unnoticed. The patient characteristically stares into space and does not respond to questions. The patient is unable to speak. Characteristically, the patient does not fall to the ground or exhibit convulsive activity as in the grand mal type seizures. The patient's eyes may remain open and the eyelids may flutter. After the seizure, the patient returns to the previous state and resumes full activity. The briefness of the seizure and the lack of convulsive activity is the reason why these seizures are often unnoticed. Such seizures usually disappear by adulthood.

Focal Motor Seizures

Focal motor seizures involve only the part of the brain that controls motor activity. Typically, only one part of the body is affected by twitching or shaking (e.g. twitching of one side of the face, jerking movement of one arm or one leg). A focal motor seizure may progress to a generalized grand mal type seizure. Focal motor seizures may last for several minutes and may recur frequently.

It may be difficult to differentiate a focal motor seizure from a generalized grand mal type seizure. The key is whether or not the patient is unresponsive. The patient who is conscious and responds to verbal stimuli is not having a generalized grand mal type seizure.

Temporal Lobe Seizures (Psychomotor Seizures, Complex Partial Seizures)

These seizures are primarily characterized by altered behaviour and are not associated with a decrease in the level of consciousness or convulsive activity. They often start with a period of dizziness or a strange metallic taste in the mouth. This is similar to the aura associated with generalized grand mal type seizures. The seizure itself is characterized by an altered mental status and a display of automatic behaviour. The changes in the mental status are quite variable, ranging from mild confusion to uncontrollable anger. The patient may walk about aimlessly, resist any assistance and seem unresponsive. Hallucinations and disturbances of memory have also been recorded. The patient may also exhibit incessant automatic behaviour such as chewing, grimacing or fumbling with clothes. The absence of the characteristic coma and convulsive activity makes these types of seizures very difficult to diagnose. Often, they are unrecognized for some time or are mistaken for other diseases that cause behavioural disorders.

EPILEPSY AND STATUS EPILEPTICUS

Seizures may occur only once in a lifetime from a specific cause (e.g. hypoxic episode, electrical injury). When seizures become chronic (i.e. recur at intervals), the patient is classified as having epilepsy. Epileptics (patients with epilepsy) are usually aware of their condition, are usually on regular medication to prevent or lessen the frequency of seizures and often carry medic alert bracelets to identify their condition. Therefore, the Attendant must understand the following:

• Patients with their first-time seizure do not necessarily have epilepsy.

• Patients with epilepsy may still have seizures despite being on medication.

Occasionally, a patient may have a prolonged seizure where the convulsive activity lasts for 20 minutes or more. Other patients may have two or more successive seizures without regaining full consciousness in between. These situations define status epilepticus. Status epilepticus is a life-threatening medical emergency requiring rapid transport to hospital.

Status Epilepticus

• Prolonged seizure with convulsive activity lasting longer than 20 minutes.

• Two or more successive seizures without regaining consciousness in between.

CAUSES OF SEIZURES

Patients with epilepsy may have started their seizures at an early age. It is important to differentiate patients with epilepsy from those patients who are having their first-time seizure. The first onset of the seizure is potentially more serious and life threatening when compared to patients with established epilepsy who happen to have a seizure.

Seizures may be caused by a variety of conditions, including the following.

1. Not taking prescribed anti-convulsive medication
2. Alcohol intoxication and/or alcohol withdrawal
3. Drug abuse or overdose
4. Hypoglycemia in diabetic patients on medications or insulin
5. Stroke
6. Head injury
7. Meningitis or other infections of the brain
8. High fever, especially in infants
9. Severe hypoxia
10. Cardiac arrhythmias
11. Hypertension, especially in the latter months of pregnancy

The Attendant should attempt to identify and, if possible, treat the underlying cause.

HISTORY

There are many other movement disorders that may resemble a seizure. For example, a simple faint associated with trembling of the extremities may be mistaken for a seizure. It is obviously very important to differentiate between true seizures and other disorders that may resemble a seizure. The only reliable method is based on obtaining factual data from the patient and witnesses. It is not the Attendant's responsibility to make the exact diagnosis, but obtaining the history is extremely important. The Attendant therefore plays a crucial role in patient assessment in such cases. The Attendant should obtain the following information from the patient or witnesses on all cases of a suspected seizure.

- Determine and record, if possible, the name and phone number of a direct witness (someone who actually witnessed the event).
- Was the patient comatose at anytime? Was the patient unresponsive during the event?
- What was the patient doing prior to the attack?
- Was there an aura?
- Where did the seizure begin (i.e. in an arm or face) and did it progress to a generalized seizure?
- When did the seizure start and how long did the convulsion last?
- In what direction were the eyes pointed or were they closed?
- During the convulsion, were the extremities limp or rigid?
- What was the patient's colour (cyanotic or pale)?
- Did the patient bite his/her tongue? The Attendant should examine the tongue closely.
- Was the patient incontinent of urine?
- Did the patient have a postictal phase of confusion or unresponsiveness and, if so, how long did it last?
- Has the patient had seizures before?
- Is the patient on any anti-convulsive medication (common anti-convulsive medications are Dilantin, Phenobarbital, Tegretol, Valproic Acid)? Bring all the patient's medication to hospital, if possible.
- Does the patient have any other neurological, respiratory or cardiac illnesses?

PRIORITY ACTION APPROACH TO THE PATIENT WITH A SEIZURE

The cornerstone of first aid treatment of seizures consists of maintaining an adequate airway and protecting the patient from injury. There is little that the Attendant can do during the convulsive phase of the seizure.

1. The patient should be lying down in the lateral or ¾ prone position to maintain the airway. If a cervical spine injury is suspected (e.g. the patient has suffered a head injury or a fall), the cervical spine will have to be manually stabilized as well as possible during the seizure.

2. Clothing around the neck should be loosened.

3. DO NOT TRY TO FORCE AN ORAL AIRWAY OR BITE STICK INTO THE MOUTH OF A CONVULSING PATIENT. This can cause injury and bleeding within the oral cavity, further compromising the patient's airway. The Attendant should wait until the convulsive activity has ceased. In the postictal phase, the patient is usually flaccid and comatose. Clearing the airway (finger sweep or suction) is then easier and more effective. An oral airway may be inserted at this time. Suctioning, if available, is extremely useful in the immediate postictal period.

4. Supplemental high-flow oxygen by mask should be provided to all seizing and postictal patients. During the convulsions, the patient is usually deeply cyanotic and respiratory arrest seems imminent. It is extremely difficult to provide assisted ventilation to these seizing patients whose teeth are clenched and chest muscles are tense. The Attendant should provide oxygen at 10 Lpm by mask and wait until the convulsion has stopped. Then, assisted ventilation may have to be provided until the patient is breathing adequately.

5. It can be extremely difficult to assess the pulses in a patient who is actively seizing. The Attendant may be able to feel only the femoral or carotid pulses. Occasionally, the patient may have to stop seizing before a pulse can be adequately detected.

6. At the end of the convulsion, the patient is often unresponsive. The postictal phase may be variable (i.e. 10-30 minutes). Special attention to the airway

and ventilation must be provided by the Attendant. A thorough examination for injuries sustained before or during the seizure must be made. They should be treated accordingly.

7. After treating the ABCs, the Attendant must obtain a complete history of events that surrounded the seizure. As the patient is usually unable to recall the exact sequence of events, bystanders may be able to provide useful information.

8. All patients who have experienced a seizure must be transported to hospital for further medical evaluation. If possible, their medication should be brought with them. Patients with a first-time seizure are potentially more serious than those with established epilepsy.

9. Patients with status epilepticus fall into the Rapid Transport Category. They may have to be transported while still convulsing. In this situation, it is imperative that they be adequately secured in the lateral or ¾ prone position to prevent injury to themselves during transport.

10. Some patients may be partly aware of their surroundings and, consequently, statements should be made with care around them. It should also be remembered that patients with seizure disorders are self-conscious of their condition and therefore all patients should be handled with sensitivity.

Part XIV, Section C
Diabetes

Diabetes is a systemic disease that affects many different organs of the body. Diabetics have an increased risk of heart disease, atherosclerosis of the blood vessels, stroke and kidney damage. The main disorder in diabetes is the body's inability to regulate the level of blood sugar (glucose). The severe long-term complications of diabetes are directly related to the patient's inability to control the blood sugar by diet, medications or insulin injections.

THE ROLE OF INSULIN AND BLOOD SUGAR

Glucose is a cell's primary source of fuel. From glucose, the body's cells obtain the necessary energy to perform their vital functions. Without glucose, the cells' energy stores become depleted and they begin to malfunction. Certain cells, such as brain cells, are more dependent than others on adequate glucose levels in order to maintain normal function. Therefore, the signs and symptoms of low levels of blood sugar (hypoglycemia) usually involve the nervous system.

Insulin is a hormone produced by specialized cells in the pancreas, an organ within the abdominal cavity. Insulin's specific function is to transport glucose into the body's cells. Without insulin, the body's cells are unable to take up glucose, and cell dysfunction ensues. Given the presence of high blood sugar levels, in the absence of insulin, the body's cells are unable to utilize it.

TYPES OF DIABETES

There are two types of diabetes:

1. *Type I or juvenile onset diabetes.* These patients usually develop diabetes in childhood or adolescence. Their diabetes is caused by a total lack of insulin. All these patients require supplemental insulin to control their disease. These diabetic patients are therefore insulin-dependent and take injections of insulin to control their blood sugar levels.

2. *Type II or adult onset diabetes.* This is a milder form of the disease. The body is still able to make insulin but it is insufficient to provide the necessary control of blood sugar. In many of these cases, the body requires higher than normal levels of insulin to control its blood sugar levels. The pancreas is unable to keep up with the demand. Many of these patients can control their diabetes by diet alone; however, others require specific medication to stimulate the production of insulin by the pancreas. In the most severe case of type II diabetes, patients may be insulin-dependent and require insulin injections to control their disease.

Diabetes is essentially incurable but the disease can be controlled by following a careful diet and using medication (insulin or specific pills) where necessary. Diabetics may monitor their blood sugar levels by checking their urine for blood sugar. When the level of blood sugar exceeds a certain amount, it spills over into the urine. Therefore, the high level of blood sugar can be detected by testing the urine for sugar. Other diabetics may actually monitor their blood levels of glucose by testing blood samples obtained from a finger prick. These patients have special portable machines called glucometers, which analyze the level of glucose in the blood sample.

EMERGENCIES IN DIABETIC PATIENTS

Diabetics may develop complications of the disease which may present as a medical emergency. Two emergencies that the Attendant will most commonly treat are:
- hypoglycemia (low blood sugar)
- hyperglycemia (high blood sugar)

HYPOGLYCEMIA

Hypoglycemia is a potentially life-threatening emergency because of the brain's dependency on adequate levels of glucose. Hypoglycemia is also called insulin shock or insulin reaction. However, the Attendant must realize that patients do not necessarily have to be on insulin in order to develop hypoglycemia. Adult diabetics who are taking pills to control their blood sugar are also at risk for hypoglycemia. Non-diabetic patients who are heavily intoxicated with alcohol may develop hypoglycemia. Diabetic patients who drink alcohol excessively are at very high risk of developing hypoglycemia.

The major causes of hypoglycemia are:
- diabetics on hypoglycemic pills or insulin with insufficient food intake;
- diabetics on hypoglycemic pills or insulin who have worked or exercised strenuously and used up all their available glucose;
- diabetics who have taken too much insulin or extra doses of their hypoglycemic medications.

Signs and Symptoms of Hypoglycemia

The Attendant must suspect hypoglycemia whenever a diabetic patient becomes confused or behaves irrationally. Because of the brain's dependency on adequate levels of glucose, failure to quickly recognize and treat hypoglycemia will result in deterioration of the patient into coma and possibly death.

The earliest signs of hypoglycemia are:
- hunger;
- pale, clammy skin;
- dizziness, trembling, weakness;
- confusion, restlessness, irrational behaviour.

As hypoglycemia progresses, the patient may develop slurred speech or collapse, or lapse into a coma. Seizures are also quite common. The patient's respirations and pulse may increase somewhat but, characteristically, they often remain normal despite the changes to the patient's level of consciousness.

It is not uncommon for an Attendant to mistakenly diagnose the diabetic patient with hypoglycemia as alcohol intoxication. The signs and symptoms of alcohol intoxication are quite similar to hypoglycemia. Certainly, diabetics and alcohol intoxication can co-exist in any one patient. Failure to promptly treat hypoglycemia may result in permanent brain damage or death.

The responsible Attendant will identify co-workers who are diabetics, especially those on insulin or hypoglycemic medication, and suspect hypoglycemia whenever they become ill.

Treatment of Hypoglycemia

The basic principle of treatment is to provide glucose in any form. If the patient is conscious, any sugar-containing substance will suffice — honey, syrup, sugar and water, fruit juice, soft drinks (not diet drinks) or candy. The Attendant should not be concerned about giving too much sugar. Sips of juice or small amounts of candy are insufficient. A full glass of juice with sugar added or a whole candy bar is usually required. All these patients, even if they regain their normal status, should be referred for medical evaluation by a physician.

If the patient is found comatose, or is too confused to be able to take anything by mouth, the Attendant has limited options. In the past, it has been recommended to place a small amount of sugar under the patient's tongue.

In other cases, a concentrated glucose jelly or glucose tablets that are commercially available have been recommended. The risk of choking or aspirating liquid is very high in these patients, even if the patient is placed ³/₄ prone or suction equipment is available. The only effective way to give sugar to these patients is intravenously. Therefore, all comatose, severely confused or stuporous diabetic patients must be transported rapidly to hospital. After conducting the primary survey and treating any other life-threatening conditions, the Attendant should still attempt to place a teaspoon of sugar or concentrated sugar solution (honey, syrup, etc.) under the patient's tongue while awaiting transport or en route. The patient should be in the lateral or ³/₄ prone position. The Attendant must take care not to place the sugar at the back of the throat because it may cause the patient to choke or aspirate. Special attention must be devoted to maintaining the airway of the comatose patient. Assisted ventilation may be required if breathing is inadequate. All comatose, stuporous or confused patients also require supplemental high-flow (10 Lpm) oxygen by mask.

HYPERGLYCEMIA

When a diabetic's blood sugar rises to high levels, a chain of events is triggered in the body's metabolism. In the absence of adequate amounts of insulin, the body's cells are unable to use the glucose and they begin to malfunction. High levels of blood glucose cause excessive urination, which in turn causes severe dehydration and thirst. The changes to the body's metabolism result in acid waste products accumulating in the blood. This causes a loss of appetite, nausea, vomiting and deep, rapid breathing. The breath has a characteristic fruity odour, caused by the accumulation of these acid waste products.

This sequence of events develops gradually, usually over the course of a few days. However, it can progress to coma and, ultimately, death if not adequately treated. At this extreme, hyperglycemia becomes a true emergency.

Causes of Hyperglycemia

As mentioned previously, diabetes can only be controlled by following a strict diet and taking medications as prescribed. The most common causes of hyperglycemia are:

- not following diet, i.e. too many calories or sugar;
- excessive alcohol intake;
- not taking prescribed medications or insulin correctly;
- infection (e.g. the flu, pneumonia, gastroenteritis).

Signs and Symptoms of Hyperglycemia

The earliest signs of hyperglycemia are:
- thirst;
- excessive urination;
- loss of appetite;
- weakness, dizziness.

As the hyperglycemia progresses and the other derangements in the body's metabolism appear, the following signs and symptoms develop:
- nausea, vomiting;
- deep, rapid breathing;
- dry mouth;
- breath has a characteristic fruity odour;
- weak, rapid pulses;
- warm and dry skin;
- decreased level of consciousness, coma.

When faced with a stuporous or comatose diabetic patient, it can be often difficult to determine if the patient is suffering from hypoglycemia or hyperglycemia.

It is important to note that diabetics are not immune to head injury, stroke, seizure or any of the other causes of coma (see Part VI, Section B, page 127). The Attendant must consider all of the possible causes of coma when assessing a comatose patient who happens to be a diabetic.

The differences between hyperglycemia and hypoglycemia are shown in Table XIV-a.

TABLE XIV-a

HYPOGLYCEMIA HYPERGLYCEMIA

	HYPOGLYCEMIA	HYPERGLYCEMIA
History		
Food intake	Insufficient	Excessive
Insulin or medications	Excessive relative to food intake	Insufficient
Onset of symptoms	Rapid	Gradual
Symptoms		
Thirst	Absent	Present
Hunger	Present	Absent
Vomiting	Uncommon	Common
Urination	Normal	Excessive
Physical Signs		
Odour of breath	Normal	Fruity, sweet
Breathing	Normal	Rapid
Pulse	Normal, maybe increased slightly, strong pulse	Rapid, weak
Skin	Pale, clammy, wet	Warm, dry
Seizures	Common	Uncommon
Response to Treatment with Sugar		
	Rapid improvement	No change

Despite the differences noted in the above table, it may still be unclear. Failure to treat hypoglycemia risks permanent brain damage and possibly death to the patient. Providing additional sugar to the hyperglycemic patient in coma will not cause any additional harm. The Attendant must administer sugar to all diabetic patients with a decreased level of consciousness unless the history, signs and symptoms *clearly* indicate hyperglycemia or other causes of coma.

Treatment of Hyperglycemia

There is little that the Attendant can do to treat hyperglycemia. These patients require prompt treatment in hospital with intravenous fluids and insulin. The Attendant must complete the primary survey and stabilize, as best as possible, the ABCs. The comatose patient requires special attention to the airway. Assisted ventilation may be required. All comatose patients require supplemental high-flow oxygen (10 Lpm) by mask.

Part XV
Psychiatric Emergencies

COMMUNICATION AND PERSONAL INTERACTION SKILLS

How the Attendant communicates and interacts with the patient, bystanders, the patient's co-workers or relatives may have a great impact on the effectiveness of first aid. Communication is the act of having one's thoughts understood by another person. It is a two-way process. Appropriate personal interaction is the manner of communicating calmly and reassuringly with the patient: alternately speaking and carefully listening so the patient feels emotionally supported. Effective personal interaction involves both verbal and non-verbal skills. Non-verbal communication involves body language, such as posture, touching and eye contact.

When an individual experiences an injury or illness, it is usually also emotionally stressful. The stress arises from response to the body disorder but also from feelings that the patient is in a situation over which self-control has been lost. Similarly, bystanders or relatives may also be stressed, as they feel unable to help. Both the patient and bystanders may feel they are in crisis. Whether the crisis is real or imagined, it must be managed. By practising good communication and personal interaction skills, the Attendant will provide emotional support, lessen emotional stress and initiate appropriate crisis management.

SIGNS AND SYMPTOMS OF EMOTIONAL STRESS REACTION IN THE PATIENT

1. Anxiety
   - One of the most common responses
   - May arise from specific fears (e.g. fear of pain, permanent disability or even death)
   - May be generalized fear (e.g. fear of loss of control over the situation)
2. Depression
   - May be sad as a consequence of loss of normal body function
3. Anger
   - May be demanding, resentful and hostile to the Attendant or others around them
4. Denial
   - The reaction by which the patient minimizes the injury or illness
   - Commonly seen with the onset of symptoms of a heart attack and with victims of violence

SIGNS OF EMOTIONAL STRESS REACTION IN CO-WORKERS, BYSTANDERS OR FAMILY

Those at the scene with the patient may exhibit a number of responses to the stress of the injury or illness. They may exhibit all of the emotional responses described for the patient. More commonly, however, there is often a feeling of guilt in co-workers who may feel in part responsible for the patient's injuries, or amongst family members. This particular emotion may cause them to be very aggressive in their demands for action. They may question the Attendant's competency and demand that the patient be sent to hospital before appropriate assessments and interventions have taken place.

A cool, unflustered manner, with a persistent use of communication and personal interaction skills will greatly alleviate fear and stress in the patient and others at the scene and put the Attendant in control. The Attendant must try not to become angry or upset with people displaying inappropriate behaviour, by remembering that this only reflects their fear and feelings of inadequacy.

GOOD COMMUNICATION AND PERSONAL INTERACTION SKILLS

- Be calm and reassuring — tell the patient you are a trained First Aid Attendant, there to help.
- Use the patient's name and establish personal interaction by looking at him/her "straight in the eye".
- Use language that the patient can understand and always speak clearly and slowly. Explain what you are going to do and reassure the patient as you carry out each procedure — do this even if the patient is confused or comatose.
- Providing there is no immediate life-threatening condition, allow enough time for the patient to respond to your questions. Injuries or illness or consequent emotional stress can cloud the patient's thinking, requiring more time to respond, even to simple questions.
- Tell the truth. Otherwise, you will destroy the patient's trust in you. You may not tell the patient everything but, generally, a direct, specific question deserves a direct, specific answer, given to the best of your ability and training.
- Use appropriate body language. This includes good

eye contact and a non-threatening posture. A reassuring pat on the hand or shoulder will often go a long way to calming the anxious patient.
- Avoid being coldly detached or becoming angry or irritated with the patient — keep your own emotions under control.

EMOTIONALLY DISTURBED PATIENTS

The various emotional reactions displayed by an injured or ill patient, which have been described as *emotional stress reactions,* are quite common and might be encountered by the Attendant. In most cases, appropriate communication and personal interaction skills will reassure the patient.

At times, patients may not behave as expected and their emotional response interferes with your assessment and treatment. These patients still respond to people around them and are not apparently dangerous to themselves or others. They may be very anxious or fearful and do not calm down as care is initiated. As such, these patients are experiencing an EMOTIONAL EMERGENCY. This reaction may represent an underlying psychiatric disturbance but it may just result from the stress of the immediate injury or illness. Avoid labelling such a patient as a "psycho" or "mental case".

These patients may require more time and understanding and reassurance in order to cope with the stress of the injury or illness. Continue to use the skills outlined above. If there are no critical interventions required, spend more time conversing with these patients, listening calmly to them and providing more reassurance.

DISRUPTIVE PATIENTS AND PSYCHIATRIC EMERGENCIES

Disruptive patients behave in a manner that presents danger to themselves and others or causes a delay in treatment. The standard skills for good communications and personal interaction outlined earlier may be ineffective with such patients but should still be tried.

Behaviour which should no longer be considered to be a stress reaction or an emotional emergency but more likely a psychiatric emergency includes:
- Take no action to help themselves and do not allow others to care for them.
- Continue to be enraged or very hostile or threatening.

- Try to hurt others or the surroundings.
- Try to harm themselves.
- Withdraw and no longer respond to others or the surroundings.
- Are very depressed, with symptoms of hopelessness, helplessness, unworthiness or guilt.
- Behave irrationally and inappropriately.

If, at the scene, a patient is displaying inappropriate behaviour, the Attendant may not be able to rule out an illness or an injury. The Attendant may assume that the patient is exhibiting signs of a *psychiatric emergency.* The psychiatric emergency may have a medical or physical problem as its cause.

IT IS IMPORTANT THAT THE ATTENDANT ATTEMPT TO RULE OUT PHYSICAL OR MEDICAL CONDITIONS THAT MAY BE THE CAUSE OF THE DISRUPTIVE BEHAVIOUR.

The major medical and physical causes of disruptive behaviour include:
- Alcohol and other drug abuse (e.g. stimulants, cocaine, diet pills, psychedelics or narcotics). THIS IS THE MOST COMMON CAUSE OF DISRUPTIVE BEHAVIOUR. THE ATTENDANT MUST ALWAYS SUSPECT UNDERLYING ASSOCIATED CONDITIONS (e.g. head injury).
- Diabetes, especially insulin reactions causing hypoglycemia. Hyperglycemia from diabetes may also cause disruptive behaviour.
- Seizures.
- Head injuries.
- Severe infections and/or very high fever.
- Organic brain syndrome — neurological disorders (e.g. minor strokes). These are primarily seen in the elderly.

Clues which may point to a physical or medical basis for the disruptive behaviour include:
- Sudden onset of symptoms — psychiatric illness usually develops over weeks or months.
- Unusual odour on the breath (e.g. alcohol or fruity odour).
- Impaired memory — with most psychiatric disorders, the memory is intact and the patient is oriented to time, person and place.
- The patient may be incontinent.
- Hallucinations are more likely visual. In psychiatric

disorders, hallucinations are usually auditory (e.g. the patient hears voices).

Psychiatric Illness

There are many psychiatric disorders which may cause a wide variety of abnormal behaviour. Conditions that may be encountered include:

- Suicidal act — the patient may have made a suicide attempt or may be threatening suicide.
- Manic behaviour — the patient is often very agitated, speaking rapidly and may not complete sentences. May exhibit pacing and have an expanded perception of personal importance or capability (grandiose).
- Depression — the patient is usually sad and withdrawn, with low self-esteem.
- Paranoia — the patient may believe that others (including the Attendant) are trying to harm or even kill him/her.

Patients exhibiting true psychiatric emergencies may be very volatile and may exhibit a great variety of behaviour in a short period. They may appear calm one minute, then become violent the next.

Management of the Disruptive Patient

The greatest concern is the aggressive or violent patient. Effective evaluation and treatment of the violent patient requires the Attendant to follow a Priority Action Approach.

The first priority is the *protection* of the Attendant and others at the scene, then adequate control of the patient. This may require physical restraint. The second priority then becomes the assessment of the patient and prompt transport to hospital.

Whether the patient exhibits violent behaviour, has been observed to be violent, has threatened to be violent or is considered potentially violent, the Attendant's first obligation is self-protection and others. ADEQUATE PROTECTION REQUIRES THE SUMMONING OF ADEQUATE FORCE. At least five able-bodied individuals will be needed to physically restrain the patient. The police should be summoned urgently in order to assist the control of the patient and to authorize the application of restraints and transportation to hospital against the patient's wishes. Often, just the presence of the police in uniform will help subdue the violent individual.

PROCEDURES TO BE FOLLOWED WHEN INTERVIEWING THE UNRESTRAINED VIOLENT OR POTENTIALLY VIOLENT PERSON

- Think of your own safety! Do not isolate yourself from other sources of help.
- Always be alert for weapons or indication that the patient will use physical force. Immediately withdraw and stay in a safe area until the police can control the scene. DO NOT TRY TO GRAB AWAY A WEAPON.
- Do not put yourself in danger by action that may be considered threatening by the patient.
- Always ensure that you have an escape route.
- Maintain an open exit — do not sit or stand in a location that blocks the patient's exit, and the door should remain open. If the patient bolts out of the room, do not try to intervene. The patient's recapture and restraint should be left to the police.
- Maintain adequate distance. The Attendant should not try to shake hands or reach towards the patient. Stand at least eight feet away. Maintain adequate distance, to avoid pressuring the violent patient.
- Listen and sympathize. That will allow the patient to ventilate anger and frustration verbally instead of physically.
- Promise anything — if the patient becomes more violent before adequate force arrives, then promise anything. It may distract the patient or defuse the situation temporarily until adequate force arrives. It may buy time.
- Avoid eye contact. The usual benefits of good eye contact can have the opposite effect with a violent patient. Looking at another person directly in the eye may represent a personal challenge or threat and precipitate further violence.
- Maintain a submissive posture. Since the violent patient is likely to respond violently to a challenge, the Attendant who adopts a rather submissive posture may reduce this perceived challenge. A slightly slouched posture turned somewhat away from the patient may be effective.
- Be decisive. Decisive and swift action is appropriate when adequate numbers of helpers are available to bring the situation under control. Violent patients are

best managed with swift restraint and rapid transport to a medical facility for evaluation.

If a patient has been successfully restrained by others prior to the Attendant's arrival, those restraints should not be removed until the patient has been assessed in a hospital setting. With appropriate help, the restraints may need to be replaced so that they cannot injure the patient. If the patient becomes violent in the presence of the Attendant, sufficient numbers of helpers must be summoned and a plan made for restraint by a coordinated team of helpers. The worst mistake the Attendant can commit is to try to physically subdue the patient single-handedly or with inadequate force. Such ineffective measures always make the situation more unstable. Anxiety and belligerence increase because the patient recognizes that he/she is out of control and unmanageable. In such a state, the patient may harm the Attendant or other bystanders.

Physical restraint of a violent patient should be swift and certain but not brutal. Adequate restraint requires the patient be subdued with an overwhelming and coordinated force. The most widely recommended tactic requires one helper to be available for each limb. Police officers or helpers should be assigned to a limb in advance and, at a given time, all grab and immobilize the designated limbs at the major joint (knee or elbow) simultaneously. The team then manoeuvres the patient to a stretcher for further restraint.

A show of force with at least four persons and one additional team leader may be enough to subdue a violent patient. The team should be spaced apart and standing about 20 feet away from the patient when possible. The effective means of restraining the patient is for each member to grab one limb at the major joint; this four-point restraint generally immobilizes the patient. Under certain circumstances, a chest restraint may be used or, under other circumstances, the patient should be restrained in a prone or side position.

Prior to restraining the patient, the leader should speak calmly and inform the patient that violent behaviour is inappropriate and will not be tolerated. If the patient remains violent, the team can approach from all sides; each team member grabbing the previously assigned limb at the major joint, with the leader remaining in control.

An alternative method, useful when the patient has a knife or club, requires the use of a mattress as a shield for four or five helpers. To disarm the patient, gradually advance with the mattress, forcing the patient against the wall. Two mattresses held at each end work equally well to sandwich a menacing patient in the middle. The show of adequate force may be sufficient to quiet the violent individual and permit the Attendant to conduct an evaluation before proceeding.

If violent behaviour is expected but has not been observed, the Attendant should summon sufficient force in advance to stand by as the patient is evaluated. That group should be nearby but out of sight.

Physical restraint involves some risk to the patient and a small probability that the restraint will increase the patient's anxiety and belligerence. In most cases, however, the patient will become calmer after restraint. The patient knows that someone else is in charge and that he/she does not need to fear these uncontrolled impulses. Four-point restraints that leave the patient "spread eagle" on a stretcher carry the risk of aspiration if the patient should lose consciousness or vomit. Restraining the patient on his/her side or in a prone position reduces the risk, but the only sure protective mechanism is to place the restrained patient under continuous supervision. This precaution has the added advantage that someone is able to talk to the patient. Restraints made of sheets or blankets or wide bandages are the safest and most effective if leather restraints are not available. An additional form of belt restraint across the chest may be needed; however, the Attendant must ensure that the restraint does not seriously impair respiration.

Following restraint, the patient may plead for release, promising to be calm if the restraints are removed. The patient must be informed that the restraints need to be left in place until an adequate medical evaluation can be conducted.

The restrained patient must be searched for weapons. Knives and other weapons must be removed and kept away from the patient.

If you help a police officer or physician to restrain a patient, make certain that the restraints used will not cause soft tissue damage (i.e. handcuffs). Soft restraints for the wrists and ankles can be made from triangular bandages. Most provincial ambulances carry leather restraints, which are the most effective. Handcuffs should not be removed until soft restraints are well secured and all concerned are certain that the patient will not be able to escape. Once the appropriate restraints are placed on the patient, they should not be removed, even if the patient appears to be acting rationally. The removal of the restraints is the responsibility of the attending physician or the police.

GUIDELINES FOR MANAGING DISRUPTIVE PATIENTS WHO ARE NON-VIOLENT

- Use the communication and personal interaction skills recommended at the beginning of this section.
- Remain as calm as possible. Remain well mannered and show respect to the patient.
- Do not be judgmental. The patient may be convinced his/her thoughts are valid no matter how ridiculous they seem.
- Do not force the patient to make decisions if that ability has been lost. The Attendant should make all the decisions. Be persuasive and supportive. However, if it seems important for the patient to maintain some control, allow the patient to participate in non-essential decisions.
- Try to obtain as much history from bystanders or co-workers regarding any past history of psychiatric disturbance or medications for same.
- Consider all patients with psychiatric symptoms at risk for escape. Have someone stay with the patient at all times.

- If any weapons are found in the course of assessment or treatment, they should be confiscated. Patients especially likely to have concealed weapons are patients with suicidal thoughts, paranoid thoughts or severely disturbed individuals. If the Attendant is concerned about the possibility of concealed weapons, ask the police to check the patient for them.
- Ask specific questions requiring more of an answer than a simple yes or no, in order to help determine whether the patient has lost contact with reality. Encourage the patient to explain his/her feelings or situation.
- Do not be uncomfortable if there are lapses or silent periods in the patient's speech. Remain attentive but relaxed.
- Once the Attendant has an understanding of the patient's problem, explain it to the patient. The Attendant should emphasize the need for medical care and the steps to be taken to get the patient to hospital.
- If the scene is very noisy or busy, the Attendant may wish to take the patient to a quieter area to conduct the interview or assessment. Be sure that help is readily available and do not become trapped between the patient and the exit.

Part XVI, Section A
Lifts, Carries, Stretchers

This section outlines the basic techniques of lifts, carries and stretchers.

To avoid injury, every Attendant needs a thorough knowledge of the biomechanics of lifting. Back injury from poor lifting technique is the most common cause of disability amongst pre-hospital emergency-care providers.

BIOMECHANICS OF LIFTING

- Be aware of your physical capabilities and don't try to handle too heavy or awkward a load. When in doubt, seek help.
- Position your feet shoulder width for balance and to maintain a firm footing.

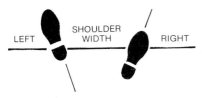

Feet at shoulder width

- Bend the knees.
- While lifting or holding, keep the back straight and rely on leg and shoulder muscles. Tighten the muscles of the buttocks and abdomen to brace the back (pelvic tilt).

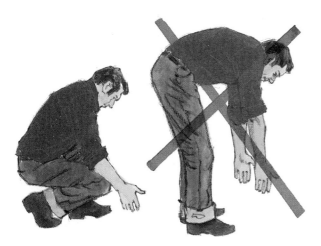

Use the legs to lift.

- Keep the patient close to your body.
- Do not twist your back while lifting, but pivot with the feet.
- Carry out all lifts and carries slowly, smoothly and in unison with helpers.
- Whenever possible, try to slide or roll a heavy patient, rather than lifting.

Following this procedure will ensure proper patient handling and lifting:

1. Inform the patient.
2. Prepare the patient for transport.
3. Lift and carry the patient to a lifting device.
4. Place and secure the patient on the spine board and/ or stretcher.
5. Lift and load the stretcher into the transportation vehicle.

INFORMING THE PATIENT

Prior to any movement, the Attendant should always inform the patient of the manoeuvres to be carried out. This communication allows the patient to understand and assist if he or she is able. It also helps to dispel any fears the patient may have about being lifted and placed on a carrying device.

The Attendant must reassure the patient during the lift. He or she may have a fear of being dropped. By providing calm reassurance during any manoeuvre, the Attendant assures the patient's cooperation and comfort. This should be done regardless of the patient's level of consciousness.

PREPARING THE PATIENT FOR ROUTINE TRANSPORT

Prior to performing a lift, the Attendant should follow these steps:

- Place a blanket between the patient's legs.
- Secure the legs at the mid-thighs, knees, mid-tibia/ fibula and ankles, using wide triangular bandages.

LIFTING AND CARRYING THE PATIENT TO A LIFTING DEVICE

When performing lifts, the Attendant is responsible for instructing and coordinating helpers. THE ATTENDANT MUST ASSUME THE BEST POSITION TO CARE FOR THE PRIORITY INJURY SITE. In the case of multiple injuries, the airway and/or cervical spine control are the highest priority.

For low-priority patients where rapid transport is not indicated, it is helpful to do a "dry run". A person of about the same size and build as the injured worker should be used. This will not only bolster the helpers' confidence but may avoid injuries.

There are many methods of lifting and transferring patients to a lifting device, each with particular advantages. The location, availability of help and the nature of injury will dictate the best method. Practising the various methods of lifting patients ahead of time will be helpful in preparation for an actual emergency. The Attendant may wish to train designated stretcher teams for emergency responses at the work site.

Two-Person Fore-and-Aft Lift

- The Attendant is on one side of the patient and lifts the patient's shoulders.
- The helper is positioned at the patient's head, supporting the head and lifting the back of the patient.
- As the patient reaches a sitting position, the helper at the head drops to one knee and supports the patient against the helper's leg.
- This helper then passes his or her arms around the patient and grasps the patient's wrists; the right hand grasps the right wrist.
- The Attendant then passes his or her arms under the patient — one under the thighs and the other under the calves.
- The Attendant and the helper squat. The head-end helper has the patient's back on his or her chest and the Attendant's knees are on either side of the patient.
- On a signal from the helper at the patient's head, both rise simultaneously and place the patient on a stretcher.

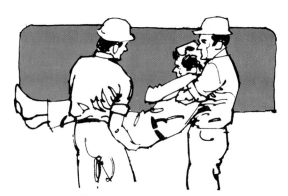

Two-person, Fore-and-Aft lift

Two-Person Lift, Patient Supine (Figure XVI-1)

This method should be used with caution because of the strain it places on the lifters' backs.

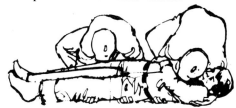

1. Preparing to do a two-person lift

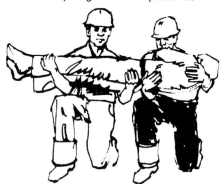

2. Patient curled into the chest

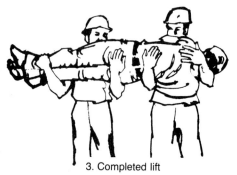

3. Completed lift

Figure XVI-1

- The Attendant and the helper should position themselves beside the patient, both on the same side and down on one knee. Both should be on the same knee.
- Instruct the patient to place the arms across the chest and to remain still, preferably with the legs straight.
- The person closest to the patient's head places his or her arm under the patient's neck, cupping the opposite shoulder of the patient, with the patient's head cradled in the elbow. This helper slips his or her other arm under the small of the patient's back.
- The foot-end Attendant lifts the patient's hips slightly and slides one arm under the patient's pelvic area. The other arm is slid under the patient's calves.
- The patient is lifted as a unit and curled into the lifters' chests.
- Lifting with their legs, the Attendants stand upright.
- The Attendants then move to the stretcher and gently lower the patient with a slight roll.

Multi-Person Direct Lift (Figure XVI-2)

Ideally, there should be six people to do this lift, although it is also possible with five, depending on the size of the patient.

If trained stretcher teams are not available, the Attendant should do two or three practise lifts at the scene, using a volunteer. Practise lifts should not be done for patients who fall into the Rapid Transport Category because it wastes time. The Attendant must take charge of the lift and direct the co-workers. The Attendant must always be at the priority injury site.

- One person kneels at the patient's head and one at the feet. The head and neck are manually stabilized by grabbing the muscles at the base of the neck (trapezius muscles) with one hand and the head with the other hand. The patient's head is supported between the forearm and hand.
- The remaining four people will be beside the patient. Three will be on one side and the other will be opposite them. All these people will kneel on one knee, preferably the same knee, and with their raised knees lined up at about the same level. The Attendant will take the position closest to the priority injury site. The heaviest part of a person's body is between the neck and the hips, so the strongest lifters should be at these areas.

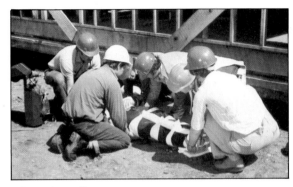

1. Preparing to lift

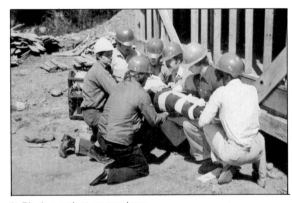

2. Placing patient on one knee

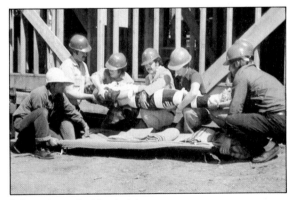

3. Lowering patient to stretcher

Figure XVI-2 Multi-person direct lift

- The two centre helpers slide their hands towards each other, palms up, until their fingertips touch. The other two helpers on the side also slide their hands under the patient, palms up, as far under the patient's body as possible.

- On a signal from the Attendant, the patient is raised and placed on the raised knees of the three helpers. The patient must be lifted as a complete unit and supported in alignment.
- The single helper on the far side of the patient puts the stretcher or spine board where the patient was lying. The helper then slides his or her hands back under the patient.

The Log-Roll

Another way to get a patient on a spine board is to roll instead of lift. This may be necessary if the footing is difficult or obstructions make lifting a problem. The procedure can be difficult when the patient is found in an awkward position.

- The Attendant should position the helpers as for the multi-person direct lift, with the Attendant at the priority injury site.
- The helpers at the feet and head of the patient must steady and support these parts of the body.
- The helpers at the side of the patient should be positioned at the chest, waist and knees. These helpers should place one hand on each side of the patient's body. Those at the chest and waist should place their hands outside the patient's arms.
- On a signal from the Attendant, the helpers along the patient's side apply pressure inwards to maintain rigidity and support.
- At the Attendant's signal, the three helpers roll the patient toward themselves, as if they were rolling a log. The patient must roll as a unit, with the head and neck in alignment to the rest of the body.
- Another helper places the spine board beside the patient, opposite the three helpers.
- The spine board should be placed behind the patient. The Attendant signals to roll the patient back onto the board again, as a unit without twisting the body.

Single-Person Log-Roll

When the patient's airway must be quickly drained of vomitus or blood, the Attendant may have to perform a log-roll to the lateral position without help.

- The Attendant must kneel beside the patient, level with the patient's abdomen.

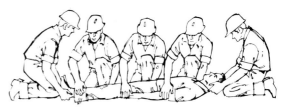

Position helpers.

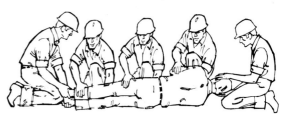

Roll patient.

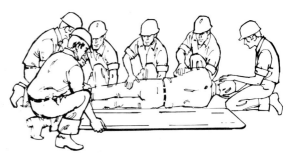

Place spine board.

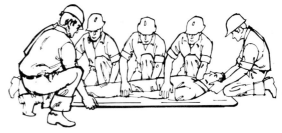

Roll patient onto spine board.

- The Attendant should place the patient's closest arm above the patient's shoulder.
- The Attendant then puts one hand at the side of the patient's head and neck.
- With the other hand, the Attendant reaches across and grasps the patient's clothing just below the waist.
- With one smooth motion, the patient is rolled against the Attendant. THE ATTENDANT MUST CRADLE THE HEAD AND NECK AND TRY TO KEEP THEM IN LINE WITH THE REST OF THE PATIENT'S BODY.

- The Attendant positions the patient's leg to prevent rolling fully prone.
- The patient's head should be positioned in line with the C-spine.

Alternative methods of lifting patients may have to be used by the Attendant. They should be used only when the health and safety of the patient or Attendant are in question. These are the alternative methods:

- Two-handed seat
- Four-handed seat
- Chair carry
- Drag carry

Two-Handed Seat (Figure XVI-3)

- Two Attendants kneel on the knee on either side of the patient. Each Attendant must pass one arm around the patient's back, grasping the clothing.
- The Attendants pass their other arms under the patient's thighs and grip hands, either with a hook grip or wrist lock. The arms of the patient are placed around the Attendants' shoulders.
- On a given signal, both Attendants rise.
- The Attendants should keep their backs straight and lift with their legs.

Four-Handed Seat (Figure XVI-4)

- The two Attendants kneel on one knee on either side of the patient and each Attendant should grasp his/her own left wrist.
- The Attendants now grasp each other's free wrist.
- The patient's arms are placed around the Attendants' necks and rises so the Attendants can place their four-handed seat in position.
- At a given signal, the Attendants should rise, keeping their backs straight and lifting with their legs.

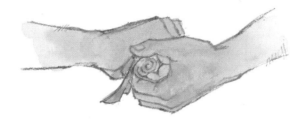

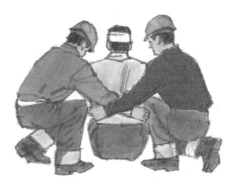

Figure XVI-3 Two-handed seat

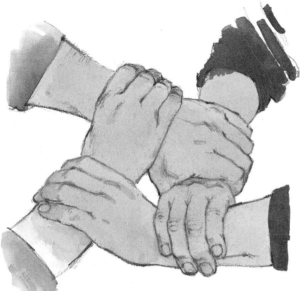

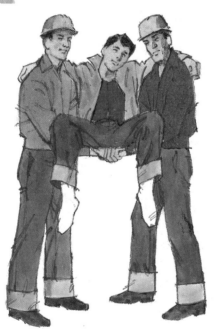

Figure XVI-4 Four-handed seat

Chair Carry

The chair carry is used by two Attendants to carry a conscious patient through narrow passages and down narrow stairs.

- The chair must be sturdy and have a straight back.
- Place the chair beside the patient and with the fore-and-aft lift, place the patient on the chair. Alternatively, if the injuries permit, raise the patient's legs and attempt to carefully slide the back of the chair under the buttocks and back.
- One Attendant is at the feet, facing the patient. The other Attendant stands at the patient's head.
- The patient is instructed to grasp the sides of the chair.
- The head-end Attendant grips the top or side of the chair back and carefully tilts it backwards, using the feet and bracing the legs of the chair.
- The foot-end Attendant grasps the front legs of the chair as close to the floor as possible.
- On a signal from the head-end Attendant, they lift the chair.

Drag Carry

The drag carry is used to move a patient who cannot move voluntarily, and must be rescued quickly from hazards such as fire, smoke or gases. This method keeps the Attendant and patient low, where the air is freshest. It is also used in confined spaces where the Attendant cannot stand up.

- With the patient on the back, quickly tie the wrists together.
- The Attendant straddles the patient facing the head and places his/her own head through the patient's arms. The Attendant then raises the patient slightly with his/her neck.
- The Attendant crawls on hands and knees, dragging the patient.
  When going down stairs, the Attendant should reverse the position and crawl backwards, supporting the patient's head.

SECURING THE PATIENT

STRETCHERS AND LIFTING DEVICES

There are many kinds of stretchers and lifting devices. The more common types are:

- Canvas army-type (Furley stretcher)
- Wheeled cot (multi-level)
- Basket stretcher
- Robertson orthopedic
- Helicopter stretcher
- Spine board

All these devices will carry the patient's entire body.

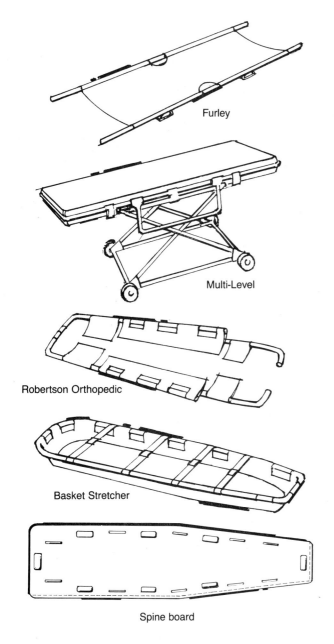

Furley

Multi-Level

Robertson Orthopedic

Basket Stretcher

Spine board

Spine Boards

Most spine boards are made of rigid plywood. They should have bevelled edges on one side and one end for sliding under the patient. Most boards are approximately 1.8 metres long. If spine boards are used in conjunction with basket stretchers, the board must fit within the stretcher. Spine boards should have holes for patient securing straps and hand holes for lifting.

If the spine board is to be used in helicopters:

- The back of the board should not have any runners attached to it.
- There must be two 1.5cm bolts on the head of the board, 20.5cm apart, to lock the board to the back seat of the helicopter.

General Principles for Securing Patient for Routine Transport

The patient must be secured to the spine board so that it may be lifted, rotated, or even raised vertically without significant patient movement. For example, the patient should be adequately secured to the board so that it can be turned onto its side to facilitate drainage of blood or vomitus when the patient's airway becomes compromised.

FOR LONG TRANSPORTS, ESPECIALLY OVER ROUGH TERRAIN, THE SPINE BOARD MUST BE WELL PADDED.

Securing ties should hold the patient's arms to the body rather than to the device, in case intravenous therapy is needed.

The securing ties should be high enough on the chest and low enough on the abdomen to allow the patient to breathe with minimal restriction and discomfort. The ties should provide security without constriction. All buckles or knots should be padded so they do not press against the patient.

Before loading for transportation, a patient with suspected cervical spine injuries must have the neck immobilized with a hard cervical collar. The head must also be immobilized between two 4.5 kg sandbags or other supports such as rolled blankets. The head must be secured to the board with tape, a triangular bandage or Velcro® straps across the forehead and around the board. Preferably, straps or triangular bandages should be used to secure the patient. Rolled blankets should also be placed on each side of the patient to prevent movement. See Figure XVI-5. The Attendant must remember that the *objective is to immobilize;* the position of the securing ties may have to be altered because of injuries.

Whenever a patient is secured to a spine board, the Attendant should remember the following guidelines:

- The patient's arms are left free for physicians or

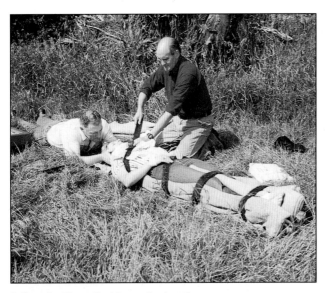

A. Securing the patient to a spine board

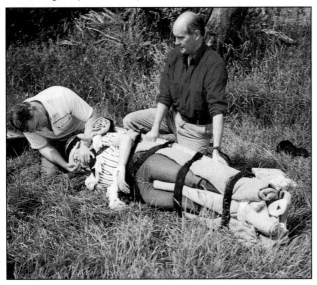

B. Turning the spine board to facilitate drainage
Figure XVI-5

qualified emergency personnel to start intravenous therapy.

- The patient's arms are also left free for checking and monitoring of the pulse.
- The patient is securely immobilized onto the spine board so that he/she can be turned onto the side or raised vertically without any significant movement should the need arise during extrication.
- The chest is easily accessible to the physician by

simply undoing the ties or straps on the patient's chest.

- The lower chest and the upper abdomen are left free of restrictive ties or straps to allow the patient to breathe with minimal restriction and/or discomfort. If the patient complains about the top tie or strap, loosen it as soon as a stable environment has been reached.
- All body hollows (as well as body parts that contact the board) must be padded for patient comfort.

Patient Immobilization and Packaging for Rapid Transport

From the time the Attendant has determined that the patient's condition warrants rapid transport to hospital, it is imperative that aside from attending to life-threatening situations involving AIRWAY, BREATHING and CIR-CULATION, all efforts should be directed to "packaging" the patient for safe transport as rapidly as possible.

This means that if, during the primary survey, the Attendant reaches the decision that the patient falls into the Rapid Transport Category, the Attendant should only:
- complete the primary survey;
- carry out critical interventions relating to compromised airway, breathing and circulation;
- conduct a rapid body survey.

THE PRIMARY SURVEY, CRITICAL INTERVENTIONS AND PATIENT SECURING SHOULD NOT TAKE LONGER THAN 15 MINUTES.

The Attendant should then immediately proceed to "package" the patient and direct others to arrange for the appropriate transportation. The vital signs and secondary survey should be conducted AFTER the patient is packaged and en route to hospital or while the patient is waiting for the transport vehicle.

These recommended techniques are used for patient packaging for rapid transport. This way the patient is thoroughly immobilized and secured to a padded long spine board or stretcher. As the long spine board is the universal transport device available throughout industry, it is used in the following examples.

The term "patient packaging" is used so that the Attendant will think of the patient as a fragile, priceless article that must be shipped some distance and may be exposed to inadvertent rough handling and/or moved through all manner of positions. For example, in transit, the patient may be exposed to the shaking and thumping of a rough logging road or to air turbulence in an air evacuation. Alternatively, the patient may have to be turned rapidly as a unit into the lateral position to protect the airway if vomiting occurs, or the stretcher may have to be put on its side to get it into an aircraft. For the multiple trauma patient with suspected C-spine injury, it is imperative that the patient be firmly secured with appropriate padding to the spine board or stretcher, so that the patient does not move and associated injuries are protected and not aggravated.

THE TECHNIQUES USED FOR PATIENT IMMOBILIZATION AND PACKAGING FOR RAPID TRANSPORT SUPERSEDE AND REPLACE ALL OTHER IMMOBILIZATION AND SPLINTING TECHNIQUES TAUGHT IN THIS COURSE ONCE THE PATIENT FALLS INTO THE RAPID TRANSPORT CATEGORY.

Summary of Advantages of Rapid Transport Patient Packaging

- Patient is rapidly prepared for transport.
- The airway can be more easily managed while protecting the cervical spine.
- The method affords some chest wall stabilization for associated chest injuries.
- There is effective immobilization of other injuries, reducing their aggravation (e.g. spine injuries, pelvic fractures or lower limb fractures).
- The patient is protected from further injury en route.
- Have effective control of the delirious patient.

Equipment Required

1. A hard cervical collar of appropriate size.
2. Long spine board.
3. At least seven 2 meters x 5 cm (6' x 2") heavy Velcro® straps or, alternatively, safety-belt-type straps with quick-release buckles. These are the preferred straps. However, triangular bandages and/or 5 cm (2″) tape may be used.
   - one to secure the head;
   - two to cross the upper chest. Each strap passes under the axilla on one side and over the opposite shoulder;
   - two to crisscross the pelvis;

- one to secure the knees;
- one to secure the ankles.
4. Six regular blankets or comparable padding:
   - one to fold and place on the spine board for padding;
   - one folded to fit between the legs;
   - two folded longways to run from the axilla to below the ankles on each side;
   - one folded as a horseshoe or cut in half and rolled to secure the head and neck; (NOTE: Acceptable alternative padding and support for the head and neck include 4.5 kg sandbags or large foam blocks.)
   - one to cover the patient if necessary, depending on the weather.
5. A triangular bandage to secure the feet and ankles with a figure-of-eight tie.

Procedure for Packaging of Patients in the Supine Position

The patient should be moved into the supine position according to the protocols outlined in the section on spinal injuries and their management (Part VI, Section D, page 149).

THE HEAD AND NECK SHOULD BE SECURED LAST! THE HEAD AND NECK SHOULD BE MAINTAINED IN THE ANATOMICAL POSITION MANUALLY OR WITH SANDBAGS WHILE THE REST OF THE PACKAGING IS APPLIED.

Industrial First Aid Attendants should follow the steps outlined pictorially (see Figure XVI-6). However, the sequence of strap application may have to be varied depending on the circumstances. THE ONLY FIRM RULE IS TO APPLY THE STRAPPING TO THE HEAD LAST.

While packaging is being carried out, it is imperative that the patient's condition, especially relating to the airway, breathing and circulation, be regularly reassessed. If necessary, the Attendant may have to delegate the packaging procedures to others while attending critical interventions (e.g. airway management, assisted ventilation, control of major hemorrhage, etc.). In this instance, the Attendant would supervise others from the head and then check all the strapping and padding once the critical interventions have been concluded.

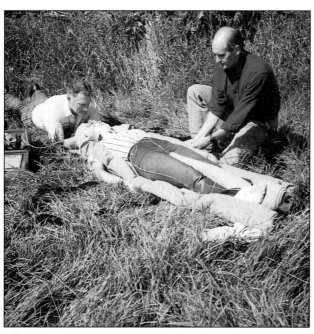

1. Manually stabilizing the neck while padding the patient and spine board

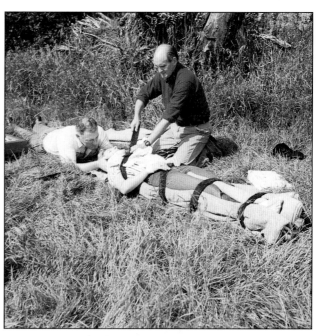

2. Securing the patient to the spine board

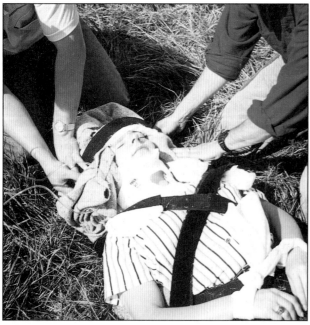

3. Securing the head to the spine board last

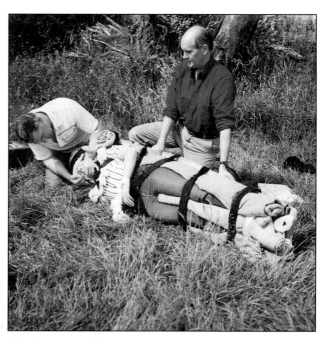

4. Packaging complete

Figure XVI-6

All strapping should line up with the other side and should cross over the midline anteriorly to allow rapid access to the patient for further assessment. It should be firmly secured so that the patient will not move on the stretcher during transportation. If Velcro® straps are used, it is recommended that the tapes overlap one another at least 25 to 30 cm (10-12") in order to ensure a solid contact. It is important that the Velcro® straps be applied fuzzy side towards the patient. When they are pulled through the slots in the spine board, they should be twisted 180°, cinched-up firmly and applied to themselves, fuzzy to hooked side.

The situation may arise when the Attendant must delegate some critical interventions (i.e. assisted ventilations with bag-valve mask) to previously trained assistants. In such cases, it is imperative that the Attendant recheck the effectiveness of the treatment rendered by the other helper frequently and not become so distracted with packaging or other activities that the patient's condition deteriorates without the Attendant's knowledge and the appropriate intervention.

Although it is important to try to reduce patient discomfort and the aggravation of injuries, it may sometimes be necessary to roll the patient onto an injured part (e.g. fractured pelvis). The need may arise because of airway and C-spine concerns, which take precedence over other injuries. The Attendant must focus on treatment procedures that maintain the airway, breathing and circulation, and expedite the patient's rapid transport.

Such a situation might arise (for instance) if the Attendant is concerned for a patient's airway. The patient may have to be rolled onto a fractured pelvis, or possibly a fractured femur on that side, in order to manage the airway efficiently. Though this is perhaps less than ideal from the point of view of the fracture, the airway problem, being potentially life-threatening, takes precedence!

Procedure for Packaging of Patients in the Lateral Position

The patient should be moved into the lateral position according to the protocols in the section on spinal injuries and their management (see Part VI, Section D, page 157).

The major indications for transporting the patient with suspected cervical injury in the lateral position are:
- facial injuries with active bleeding in the nasal or oral airway;
- active vomiting;
- patients with a decreased level of consciousness who cannot be continuously monitored by the Attendant;
- stretcher limitations, i.e. inability to rotate the spine board or stretcher should the patient vomit;
- helicopter evacuations; if the stretcher is suspended below the helicopter during rescue operations, the patient cannot be monitored effectively so the lateral position is required.

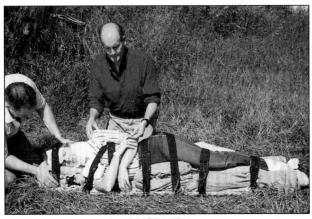
ANTERIOR VIEW
Securing the patient in the lateral position for rapid transport

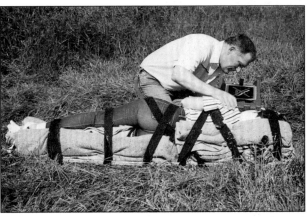
POSTERIOR VIEW
Note the padding to maintain the lateral position

THE HEAD AND NECK SHOULD BE SECURED LAST! The head and neck should be maintained in a neutral position manually, with sandbags, or with padding, while the rest of the packaging is applied.

The Attendant should follow the same steps as outlined pictorially for the supine patient. However, the sequence of strap application may have to be varied depending on the circumstances. THE ONLY FIRM RULE IS TO APPLY THE STRAPPING TO THE HEAD LAST.

IT IS IMPORTANT TO CAREFULLY PAD THE SPINE BOARD AND ALL PARTS OF THE PATIENT THAT CONTACT THE BOARD IF TRANSPORTING THE PATIENT IN THE LATERAL POSITION.

More attention must be paid to filling in hollows and spaces, both anteriorly and posteriorly, not only for the comfort of the patient but also to ensure the patient will not move around during transport.

Please review again all the instructions for packaging the supine patient as they are, for the most part, equally applicable to packaging the patient in the lateral position.

Canvas Stretcher (Furley Stretcher)

Furley stretchers consist of two wooden poles and a canvas stretcher. The canvas must be checked regularly for rotting and tearing. If soiled, it can be washed with soap and water.

- Undo the straps and open the stretcher.
- Lock the spreading bars by pushing them with your feet.
- Secure the centre hinge of the bars with a triangular bandage or tape.
- Check the canvas before placing the patient on it, to be sure it will not fold up under the patient's weight or tear away from its anchor points on the side rails.
- Be sure the patient is well secured before carrying.

Robertson Orthopedic Stretcher (Clamshell)

The clamshell stretcher is an aluminum lifting device which adjusts in length and separates into two halves. THIS STRETCHER IS A LIFTING DEVICE AND IS NOT FOR CARRYING PATIENTS.

- Place the stretcher alongside the patient and adjust the length. The ends should extend two inches past

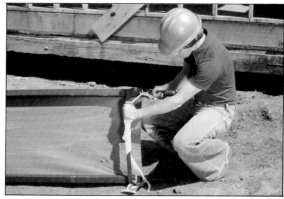
Securing spreader bars

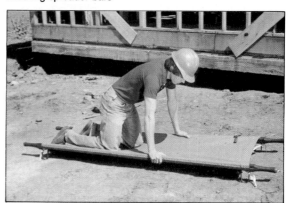
Checking canvas

the patient's head and feet.
- Remove the head support and release the Velcro® attachments.
- Separate the two halves by undoing the releases at the head and foot.
- Place one half on each side of the patient.
- Slide the two halves under the patient, one at a time. Roll the patient slightly if necessary.
- Hold the foot section securely and slowly. Latch the head end, being careful not to pinch the patient's buttocks with the two halves.
- Place the head support under the patient's head, Velcro® attachments upright. Support the head.
- Secure the Velcro® attachments, being careful not to snag the patient's hair.

- Secure the Velcro® attachments on the head support firmly by pinching them together.
- Place the clamshell on a stretcher or spine board and remove it from under the patient.

Two people can lift a spinal trauma patient with a clamshell if he/she weighs under 90 kilograms. If the patient is between 90 and 113 kilograms, four people can do the lift, one at each end of the device and one each side at the middle. This will prevent sagging. A heavier patient cannot be lifted with a clamshell; therefore, another method must be found.

Basket Stretcher

There are various types of basket stretchers, made of metal or fibreglass:
- Blankets should be placed under the patient for comfort.
- A spine or litter board at the bottom makes loading and unloading easier.
- The fibreglass basket stretcher will accommodate the clamshell stretcher.
- The patient must be secured if the stretcher is to be carried over a long distance or uneven ground.

Roll Cot or Multi-Level Stretcher

The multi-level stretcher weighs approximately 30 kg and has an elevating head. The stretcher can be raised or lowered, using the end or side release. When raising or lowering the stretcher, listen for a click that indicates that the release is in place.

The stretcher has two safety bars ("D" bars), and should have straps to secure the patient. The stretcher must never be lifted by the "D" bars. The stretcher has a footrest to keep the patient from sliding off. The footrest and handle may be placed upright and the covers wrapped over the handle to remove pressure from the patient's feet.

The multi-level stretcher has a few disadvantages. It is very unstable when fully extended because of the high centre of gravity and it may tip over, especially if all the wheels are facing in one direction. The patient is usually most comfortable when the head of the stretcher is raised slightly.

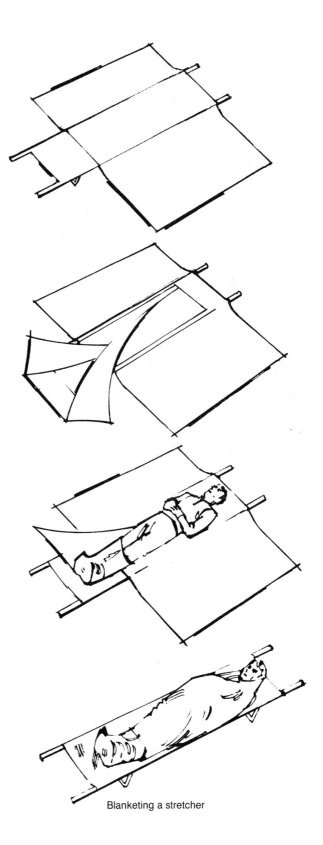

Blanketing a stretcher

Carrying the Multi-Level Stretcher

The multi-level stretcher is most suitable for use on smooth surfaces.

- Wheeling a stretcher when it is set low can cause back problems, so it should be raised to a comfortable height and lowered when it must be carried across rough ground.
- Reduce patient discomfort by making turns slowly and lifting the stretcher over obstacles.
- When carrying the stretcher on an incline, always carry it so that the patient's head is higher than the feet. Instruct the patient to keep his/her head on the pillow, legs straight and arms folded across the chest.
- Use a side-carry to load any stretcher.
- When loading the stretcher into a vehicle, first lower the stretcher, then, keeping the back straight, lift with the legs.
- NEVER lift with the backrest, footrest or "D" bars.

When unloading the multi-level stretcher, lower it to the ground before extending the undercarriage.

Most roll-cot stretchers can be positioned so that the patient is semi-sitting, or with the knees flexed. The Attendant should take advantage of these facilities.

Helicopter Stretcher

The helicopter stretcher is a flat, aluminum spine board. The helicopter is equipped with these stretchers and the pilots usually know how to use them. The helicopter stretcher is hinged in the middle and folds in half for easy storage. The Attendant must ensure that the stretcher is opened and laid with the correct surface up, so it will not accidentally fold in half during use. *If the Attendant is unsure that the company spine board will fit the helicopter, the pilot should be asked to bring one.*

LIFTING AND LOADING A CARRYING DEVICE

When lifting a patient on a carrying device, the Attendant uses the same body mechanics as lifting a patient. The objective of each lift is to complete it as safely and as efficiently as possible.

When loading a stretcher, the Attendant should:
- Use proper lifting techniques. Use enough helpers.
- Carry the patient feet first. If stretcher bumps into anything, the head won't take the force of the blow.

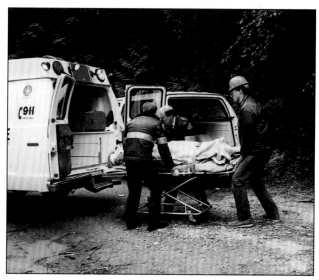
Loading a patient into the ambulance

- Carry the patient feet first down stairs or steep inclines as well (keeps abdominal organs away from diaphragm).
- When the stretcher is placed in the ambulance, the patient's head should be at the front.
- Never run with a stretcher. A quick orderly walk accomplishes the same objective without danger of tripping and falling.
- Ensure that the appropriate securing devices are in place.
- Use padding under a basket stretcher if the road is going to be rough (a partially filled inner-tube or a piece of 6″ thick foam the size of the stretcher may be used).
- Secure the stretcher to ensure that it doesn't move during transport.

SUMMARY

Patient lifts and carries are skills learned and perfected through training and practise. The only way an Attendant can be sure of using the best technique for a specific situation is to continually practise the skills outlined in this section.

The Attendant should remember that there is NEVER an excuse for a patient falling off a stretcher. Only negligence allows this to happen.

Part XVI, Section B

Multiple Casualties, Disasters and Triage

The ultimate challenge to the Attendant is an accident or disaster involving multiple casualties. The situation requires maximal use of all the Attendant's skills and judgment, often in a setting of mass panic and ongoing hazards.

A disaster situation may be defined as any emergency that overwhelms the available medical resources. A disaster cannot be defined simply by the number of injured. Treating two injured patients in a wilderness setting can be much more challenging than ten patients in a multi-vehicle accident with a multitude of bystanders, police officers, firefighters and ambulance attendants available to assist.

There is no substitute for disaster planning. Forming a rescue team among co-workers and practicing periodically will ensure that, when the emergency arises, the team will be fully prepared.

As an Attendant, your first responsibility is to CALL FOR HELP. You cannot do it all by yourself. Call for the rescue team and get help from other workers or bystanders.

It should be apparent from the nature of the disaster whether or not transport to hospital will be required. Usually, transport to hospital is required. The Attendant must call early for emergency assistance involving multiple casualties.

The Attendant must be able to provide as much of the following information as possible to the dispatcher when calling for emergency assistance:

1. Location of the disaster:
   - exact address;
   - specific location of that address — especially if it's a large plant or multi-storey building;
   - useful landmarks if in a rural or wilderness setting.
2. Attendant's telephone number and extension — enabling the dispatcher to call back if further information is required.
3. Type of accident or disaster.
4. Estimated number of victims (however, a precise count of victims should be performed as soon as possible).
5. Estimated type and extent of injuries as soon as can be determined.
6. Hazards at the scene:
   - fire;
   - downed wires;
   - hazardous materials (e.g. chemicals, explosives);
   - landslide, avalanche, unstable debris.
7. Access to the scene:
   - is the road open or blocked by the accident;
   - remote area (e.g. accessible only by helicopter);
   - water access only.
8. Special situations:
   - boating accidents — divers required;
   - severe weather conditions (e.g. hypothermia);
   - special extrication equipment required.

On the basis of the initial information, the dispatcher will be able to determine the number of ambulances and the need for other services (e.g. fire, police, coast guard, etc.). If the Attendant can only provide limited information, delay in mobilizing the appropriate personnel and equipment will occur. It is better for the Attendant to overestimate the number of victims and extent of injuries, rather than come up shorthanded on vehicles and personnel.

The First Aid Attendant and other rescuers must not blindly rush into a hazardous environment to extricate and treat victims. It is important to remember that dead or injured heroes cannot save lives. **Be careful!**

When faced with multiple patients in a disaster situation, the Attendant must prioritize the patients for treatment and transport, determining which patients are critically ill and require rapid transport to hospital. **The process of sorting out and prioritizing patients is called triage.**

The first rule of triage is to DO THE GREATEST GOOD FOR THE GREATEST NUMBER. Sorting and prioritizing injuries and allocating the limited resources require skill, judgment and experience. The Attendant must initiate a triage process, but responsibility for triage should be handed over to a more experienced person as soon as possible. That person may be an ambulance attendant, nurse or, ideally, a physician.

At the same time, the Attendant must select an appropriate triage area — where patients can be safely assessed, treated and transported.

The triage area must be established using the following guidelines:

1. The triage area should be large, well lit and preferably protected from the environment.
2. The triage area should be located at a safe distance from any known hazards.
3. The triage area should also be situated so that the entire disaster site can be seen.
4. The triage area should be located between the accident scene and the evacuation vehicles so that orderly patient flow — i.e. triage — assessment — treatment — transport — can be maintained. The Attendant should not take more than 10 seconds to choose the triage area.

The Attendant must delegate one or two assistants to bring all necessary medical supplies, equipment, stretchers, spine boards, etc. to the triage area. Once the area has been selected and assistants delegated to obtain all necessary equipment, the Attendant initiates the triage process.

TRIAGE OF VICTIMS

Using the primary survey and the Rapid Transport Criteria, the Attendant moves rapidly from one victim to another, identifying those who require immediate treatment and prioritizing patients for transport to hospital. The following rules of triage apply:

1. Only immediate life-threatening conditions are identified and treated in the initial triage round, i.e. airway obstruction, open chest injuries or major external hemorrhage.
2. Salvage of life takes precedence over salvage of limbs.

The Attendant, as triage officer, should stop only to treat immediate life-threatening conditions. HE/SHE MUST SURVEY ALL THE PATIENTS AS QUICKLY AS POSSIBLE IN ORDER TO DETERMINE THE NUMBER OF VICTIMS AND TO OBTAIN AN OVERALL EVALUATION OF THE DISASTER SCENE. Therefore, the Attendant, as triage officer, completes the primary survey and treats only immediate life-threatening conditions before moving on to the next patient. Triage assessments should not take more than two minutes per patient. Assistants are delegated to provide first aid.

In this initial round of triage, patients who are obviously dead or who are in cardiac arrest are bypassed in favour of those patients who have life-threatening but salvageable conditions. Although this seems cruel and uncaring, in a disaster situation the Attendant must do the greatest good for the greatest number. The limited personnel and resources must be directed to those victims who can be saved. The chance of survival for the victim of a traumatic cardiac arrest is very small. Unless all the other victims have very low priority injuries, the cardiac arrest victim must be bypassed.

Patients with any life-threatening conditions identified on the primary survey are triaged as the highest priority. Examples of patients in this category are those with airway obstruction, open chest injuries and major hemorrhage with shock.

Using the general rules of triage, those patients with any of the other Rapid Transport Criteria are assigned the second priority. Examples of patients in this category are:

*   Patients with flail chest;
*   Patients with penetrating injuries to the head and neck, abdomen or groin;
*   Patients with two or more proximal long-bone fractures;
*   Patients with spinal cord injury;
*   Patients with burns greater than 10% body surface area;
*   Patients with severe head injury;
*   Patients with extremity amputation.

The third priority of patients includes those patients whose treatment and transportation can be delayed temporarily. Examples of such patients include those with moderate burns, spinal injuries without evidence of spinal cord injury, open or displaced fractures, eye injuries.

The low priority group are those patients who may be best described as "the walking wounded". These patients will primarily have soft tissue injuries, sprains, closed simple fractures and other minor injuries.

Once the initial round of triage has been completed and a more accurate assessment of the extent of injuries has been obtained, the dispatcher must be updated. A more accurate estimate of the number of victims, with the extent of their injury, must be provided.

TRIAGE TABLE

PRIORITIZATION OF INJURIES IN MULTIPLE-CASUALTY SITUATIONS

PRIORITY I

1. Airway obstruction
2. Penetrating chest injury
3. Major hemorrhage with shock

PRIORITY II

1. Patients with flail chest
2. Penetrating injury to the head and neck, abdomen or groin
3. Two or more proximal long-bone fractures
4. Spinal cord injury
5. Burns greater than 10% body surface area
6. Severe head injury
7. Extremity amputation

PRIORITY III

1. Moderate burns
2. Spinal injuries without evidence of spinal cord injury
3. Open or displaced fractures
4. Eye injuries
5. Mild head injury (GCS greater than 13)

PRIORITY IV

1. Soft tissue injuries
2. Sprains
3. Closed simple fractures
4. Other minor injuries

PRIORITY V

Dead, traumatic cardiac arrest*

*NOTE: The patient with a traumatic cardiac arrest can be given a high priority only if all other victims are in a low priority.

After the highest priority patients are identified and treated, and the dispatcher updated, the second round of triage is begun. Trauma patients require reassessment. For example, those patients who are initially stable may deteriorate. The triage process must be repeated to reassess the patients' changing clinical status. During this round of triage, more definitive first aid can be provided to the patients with second or third priority injuries.

The process is repeated until all the patients have been treated and transported. In most instances, more experienced medical personnel (e.g. ambulance attendants, nurses or a physician) may arrive and take over the role of primary triage from the Attendant. The triage person is responsible for delegating assignments and tasks to assistants and bystanders.

DATA COLLECTION AND RECORD KEEPING

If possible, one person at the scene should be assigned the task of identifying and recording the names of all victims. Equally important is an attempt to determine if there are any undiscovered victims. Some victims may be trapped; others may run from the accident scene in a state of shock or panic; some victims may be transported to hospital by other witnesses unbeknownst to the Attendant.

In most disaster situations involving experienced personnel, a tag identification system is attached to each victim, outlining patient information as well as medical history, physical examination treatment provided and priority status.

PRIORITIES FOR EVACUATION OF MULTIPLE CASUALTIES

In most mass-casualty situations, there are usually sufficient vehicles to maintain a steady flow of evacuated patients. By the time patients are extricated, assessed, prioritized and treated, the first ambulances have usually arrived, and assistance is available.

Generally, those patients with the highest priority, who are stabilized first, are evacuated first. In certain instances, there may be room for only one patient at a time in the transport vehicle. The highest priority patient must be evacuated first. In other situations, where there may be room for multiple patients, it is best to evacuate one high priority patient with one or two low priority ("walking wounded") patients. Each situation differs significantly and the optimal solution is best determined at the scene, taking into account all the factors.

All patients, but especially those in Priority I or II, must not be evacuated unattended. Depending on the complexity of the injury and ongoing requirements for treatment, the best qualified individual must go with the patient(s). Patients with minor injuries who require little or no treatment may be evacuated with almost anybody who is available. High priority patients who require constant attention to their airway, for example, will require a qualified person to attend en route to hospital. Once again, the optimal choice should be made at the scene, taking into account the needs of the patient to be evacuated, as well as the needs of those patients awaiting transport.

Finally, as each vehicle leaves the disaster scene, the dispatcher must be notified as to the number of victims en route, the extent of their injuries and an estimated time of arrival. It is also important that the dispatcher be asked to notify the hospital with all the pertinent information.

SUMMARY

This section has reviewed the approach and management of multiple casualties in a disaster situation. Above all, the Attendant must try to take command of the situation with as much self-assurance and efficiency as possible. At the same time, the Attendant must recognize his or her own limitations.

Part XVI, Section C
Transportation

The Attendant's responsibilities are not necessarily completed after the patient assessment and first aid treatment have been provided at the scene. Preparing the patient for transport and ensuring optimal transportation to the hospital is also the Attendant's responsibility.

The Industrial First Aid Regulations of the WCB of British Columbia state: "Every employer shall, at his own expense, furnish to any worker injured in his employment, when necessary, immediate conveyance and transportation to a hospital or physician or qualified practitioner for initial treatment." As the First Aid Attendant is usually the employer's representative, he or she is usually responsible for ensuring compliance with the regulations.

The First Aid Regulations also state: "Before commencing operations, the employer shall have written procedures for transporting injured workers to medical aid." First Aid Attendants must learn the existing procedures for transporting injured workers, preferably before the need to use them arises. The Attendant may have to recommend changes or institute new procedures as necessary. As differences exist between job sites, no one transport protocol can be devised that would be applicable in all situations. Procedures for transporting injured workers must address all the following concerns and needs:

- Type of terrain over which the patient must be transported
- Location of the patient
- Distance to the nearest hospital and surface travel time
- Availability of an industrial ambulance or other properly equipped transport vehicle
- Response time to the work site by the ambulance service
- Maintenance procedures and equipment needs for the ambulance or transport vehicle
- Equipment and manpower requirements to assist with patient transport
- Special needs for remote work sites — helicopters, fixed-wing aircraft or marine vessels may be required for patient transportation
- Communications with ambulance dispatch, hospital and other transportation agencies

- Backup procedures in case of equipment failure or weather conditions

It is usually impossible to predict all the different types of problems that can arise when transporting patients, especially from remote work sites. Practise drills at different locations on the work site are the best method of evaluating the transportation procedures.

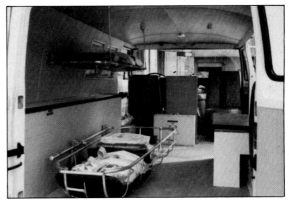

Industrial ambulance

INDUSTRIAL AMBULANCES AND EMERGENCY TRANSPORTATION VEHICLES

Some industries are required to have an emergency transportation vehicle (ETV) at the work site. Other industries must maintain an industrial ambulance at a location central to their various work sites. If the surface travel time from the work site to the hospital is greater than 20 minutes, consideration should be given to maintaining an ETV. In some areas, the ambulance service's response time may differ significantly between day, evening, night or weekend times. It may be necessary to develop different transportation procedures for emergencies when ambulance personnel are "on call".

National standards exist for ambulance design. Industrial First Aid Regulations already establish the minimum standard equipment required for the vehicle. The following guidelines are recommended for selecting and equipping an industrial ambulance or ETV:

1. The vehicle should have a patient compartment that can accommodate two patients on stretchers. The Attendant should be able to communicate directly with the driver. Direct access between the driver and patient compartment is desirable.

2. The patient compartment should be large enough so that there is sufficient room for an Attendant to kneel and perform CPR.

3. There should be sufficient space at the head of the patient to assist ventilation and maintain the patient's airway.

4. There should be no protrusions between the stretchers nor over the head and chest of either stretcher patient.

5. The patient compartment must be well lit, heated if necessary and easily cleaned.

6. All equipment necessary for patient care during transport must be permanently installed, secured or stored in cabinets. On rough roads at high speed, unsecured items can become dangerous missiles.

7. The vehicle should be equipped with two-way radio communication between the Attendant and the job site. It is also desirable to be able to directly communicate with ambulance dispatch and the hospital from the vehicle.

8. The chassis must provide optimal riding performance. Adequate road clearance or four-wheel drive may be necessary in certain locations.

The Attendant should also ensure that the industrial ambulance or ETV is always in good working order. The vehicle and its equipment must be checked on a regular basis.

OPERATION AND TRANSPORTATION GUIDELINES

Throughout this manual, guidelines are given to Industrial First Aid Attendants to assist them in transportation decisions. Whenever a patient falls into the Rapid Transport Category, the Attendant must follow these guidelines:

• The transportation vehicle must be operated in a safe manner at all times, according to local traffic laws and to ensure the safety and comfort of all passengers.

• For industrial ambulances, the Attendant must ensure that the driver is properly licensed to operate the vehicle. This should be done prior to an accident occurring. (In BC, a Class 4 licence is required.)

If the Attendant has any doubts about the operation of emergency vehicles, the local law enforcement agencies or Motor Vehicle Branch should be contacted for direction.

PATIENT CHECKLIST PRIOR TO SURFACE TRANSPORT

1. Position the patient appropriately. The Attendant must think ahead and anticipate problems. Murphy's Law always applies during patient transports ("whatever can go wrong will go wrong").

Individuals are more susceptible to motion sickness when they are ill. Strapped down to a stretcher for a long, bumpy or twisting ride increases the risk of vomiting. The Attendant must anticipate the problem and position the patient accordingly. There are two options:

• Ensure that the patient is secured to a spine board or other lifting device which can then be easily rotated, when necessary, to the lateral position, facing the Attendant.

• Position and secure the patient in the lateral position, facing the Attendant, for transport after completion of the patient assessment and treatment.

The best choice is left to the Attendant's judgment, taking into account the needs of the patient, the length and difficulty of transport and the availability of equipment and assistance.

2. Maximize patient comfort.

For long transports, especially over difficult terrain, the patient must be firmly secured. The Attendant should remember that a hard spine board is very uncomfortable and extra effort should be made to pad the board. Bunched-up clothing, belts and objects in pockets should be removed before securing the patient for transport. The patient with spinal cord injury is particularly at risk for developing pressure sores. If necessary, pre-heat the vehicle to keep the patient warm.

3. Extremity injuries must be splinted to reduce pain and prevent further injury if the patient is to be subjected to a long and rough transport. Even if the patient is in the Rapid Transport Category, extremity injuries must be immobilized and well secured if the patient is to be transported over rough terrain for a long period of time. On the other hand, only limited immobilization may be necessary for Rapid Transport Category patients if the transport time is short or the

ride is relatively smooth. All splints, bandages and stretcher securing straps must be checked before transport.

4. The Attendant must check the equipment. The Attendant must ensure there is a sufficient supply of oxygen. All basic life support equipment must be available and in good working order (e.g. bag-valve mask units, suction device, if available). There should also be plenty of dressings, bandages and blankets. All equipment should be permanently labelled so that it will be easy to retrieve from the hospital or ambulance service.

5. Remember to bring along the patient's medications, if possible. If poisoning is suspected, it is important to bring along the container to assist the physician in treating the patient.

6. Repeat and record the patient's vital signs. These will serve as the baseline for monitoring purposes en route.

7. Reassure the patient. Explain what procedures are to be done. Tell the patient where and how he or she will be transported. Even if the patient has a decreased level of consciousness, it is always important to explain things. When patients have a decreased level of consciousness, it does not necessarily mean they cannot hear or understand what is happening.

8. The Attendant must direct the driver. A slower, smoother ride may be required depending on the patient's condition.

9. The Attendant must enforce the no-smoking rule inside the vehicle. Passengers, assistants and the driver must all comply.

10. Contact the ambulance dispatcher to provide an update on the patient's condition and the estimated time of arrival. If the patient is being transported directly to a hospital, contact the hospital (usually the emergency department). It is very important to report any changes in the patient's condition, especially if there has been a deterioration.

11. The Attendant must bring along the patient evaluation sheet. An extra pad may be useful to record the vital signs en route if there is insufficient space. These notes can be transcribed to the patient evaluation sheet at the final destination.

12. The patient's personal effects should be brought along on the transport. During the initial assessment and treatment, it may be necessary to remove watches, wallets, rings, etc. It is best to ask an assistant to hold onto them initially. The Attendant must remember to bring or send them along with the patient to the hospital.

PATIENT CHECKLIST DURING TRANSPORT

En route, the Attendant must monitor the patient in order to recognize and, if necessary, treat any changes in clinical status. It is important to recognize that the patient's condition may vary with time after injury. Some effects of injury may be delayed in onset and not be apparent initially. These injuries may only manifest themselves during transport and the Attendant must be ever alert to recognize them.

1. The Attendant must pay careful attention to the airway and the risk of vomiting during transport. If the supine patient retches or vomits, he or she must be rotated to the lateral position to prevent aspiration. The airway must be kept clear. Drainage by gravity may not be sufficient and the Attendant must clear the airway using a finger sweep or suction device (if available).

2. Monitor the vital signs. Worsening of the vital signs may represent a deterioration of a recognized injury or the presentation of a previously unsuspected injury. For example, a decrease in the strength of the patient's pulses probably indicates the development of hypotension and impending shock from blood loss. If the Attendant had already suspected an intra-abdominal injury with internal bleeding, the changes in the patient's vital signs probably represent a deterioration in the recognized intra-abdominal injury. On the other hand, if internal bleeding was not previously suspected by the Attendant, the changes in the vital signs indicate the delayed presentation of an unsuspected injury causing blood loss. The most likely sources of internal blood loss are injuries of the chest and abdomen and pelvic fractures.

The vital signs must be reassessed and recorded every 10 minutes on all patients:
- who fall in the Rapid Transport Category;
- who have head, chest or abdominal injuries.

Patients who are not in the Rapid Transport Category should have the vital signs reassessed every 30 minutes. However, if there are any concerns, the Attendant should reassess more frequently.

3. If the patient's condition deteriorates into cardiac arrest, the Attendant must initiate CPR. Continue to transport the patient to hospital. Trauma patients who suffer cardiac arrest have a very small chance of survival and will survive only if they can get to a hospital rapidly.

4. The Attendant must carefully reassess and re-examine known sites of injury. Check dressings and bandages for evidence of ongoing bleeding or impaired circulation. Splints must be reassessed to ensure that there has been no significant change in position. The neurological and circulatory status of injured limbs must be monitored. Patients with head, chest or abdominal injuries must also be closely re-examined to detect any changes. As part of patient monitoring, the Attendant performs a limited physical examination, focussing not only on the injured areas but also looking for evidence of new injuries.

This limited examination must be repeated every 30 minutes during transport. Patients in the Rapid Transport Category may require more frequent reassessments, depending on the status of the vital signs. In general, the sicker the patient, the more frequent the reassessments.

5. Reassure the patient. Keep him or her as comfortable as possible.

6. Recording the vital signs and results of the physical examination during transport is extremely important. The Attendant must document the time of the reassessments and the results clearly on the patient evaluation sheet. During transport, it may be easier to jot the findings and times down on a notepad and rewrite them on arrival at the hospital.

TRANSFER OF PATIENT RESPONSIBILITY

When the ambulance service arrives or the patient reaches the hospital, there is a transfer of patient responsibility from the Industrial First Aid Attendant to the ambulance attendants or medical staff respectively. The Attendant will be requested to provide specific information regarding the patient. If the patient evaluation sheet has been completed, it should be given to the person assuming patient responsibility. The Attendant should provide the following information:

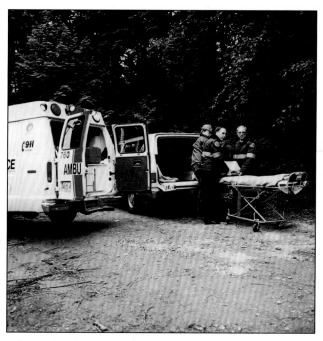

B.C. Ambulance meets ETV en route to hospital

1. Description and time of the injury
2. Mechanism of injury
3. Patient's chief complaint(s)
4. Associated symptoms
5. Patient's past medical history, medications, allergies
6. Initial patient vital signs
7. Initial findings on physical examination
8. Suspected diagnoses
9. Treatment provided
10. Complications or new injuries during transport
11. Last set of vital signs and time
12. Last findings on physical examination and time

The ambulance attendants or hospital medical staff may repeat all your questions to the patient. They may remove your dressings and untie your splints. Although this may appear to be detrimental to patient care and perhaps wasting precious minutes of the "golden hour", it is usually required because the person assuming medical responsibility for the patient must perform a thorough patient assessment. If you are concerned about these delays, you may politely ask the person in charge to explain.

You should also ask if further assistance is required (e.g. in lifting or moving the patient or assisting with any treatment). In certain cases, the First Aid Attendant may be asked to assist with the transport by the ambulance service to the hospital.

After the transfer of care, gather all of your equipment for the return trip. In many cases, equipment such as splints or spine boards may still be required. Arrangements should be made to pick up the items later. This emphasizes why all the Attendant's first aid equipment must be properly labelled. It is easy for equipment to be lost when it becomes mixed up with that of the ambulance service or hospital.

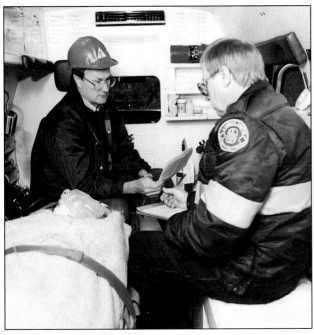

First Aid Attendant provides patient information to B.C. Ambulance attendant

CHECKLIST AFTER TRANSPORT

On completion of the patient transport, the industrial ambulance or ETV must be cleaned and prepared for reuse. The First Aid Attendant's responsibilities include the care and maintenance of the vehicle.

1. Replace or clean soiled linen.
2. Clean all equipment that was used for the patient.
3. Refill all first aid supplies in the vehicle.

4. Replace used oxygen cylinders.
5. Wash the stretcher and floor or other areas of the ambulance as required.
6. Refill the gas tank, check the oil, coolant and tires. Perform any other maintenance checks that may be required.

The Attendant must also clean the equipment and refill the supplies in the first aid kit. Finally, the Attendant must submit the appropriate reports to his or her employer.

LOCAL AMBULANCE SERVICE

In British Columbia, the BC Ambulance Service operates province-wide as the sole agent. In other provinces and countries, there may be a variety of agencies providing ambulance service. It is imperative that the First Aid Attendant know how to access the ambulance service, understand its capabilities and know its response time to the work site.

In BC, the ambulance possesses equipment that may not be available to the First Aid Attendant (e.g. suction device). Most ambulance attendants are specifically trained to handle major trauma patients, especially those who fall into the Rapid Transport Category. Most ambulance attendants have specific protocols for instituting intravenous therapy on trauma patients. They can also provide effective pain medication, where indicated, for patients with painful fractures, dislocations or soft tissue injuries. Some ambulance attendants are also trained in the use of special defibrillators for cardiac arrest victims. In some centres, advanced life support vehicles staffed with paramedics are available to provide advanced (rather than basic) cardiac life support. In summary, the ambulance service can provide the following:

1. Provide equipment not available to the First Aid Attendant.
2. Provide advanced pre-hospital care that First Aid Attendants are not licensed to do.
3. Provide transport to hospital. Even if an industrial ambulance or other transport vehicle is available, it may be beneficial to have the ambulance service rendezvous en route. The patient may benefit from the transfer to a better equipped vehicle with attendants who may be able to provide advanced pre-hospital care.

4. Provide patient transfers from the helipad or airport to hospital, if necessary. Precious minutes of the "golden hour" may be lost waiting for an ambulance to arrive at the airport if early contact was not made.

5. Ambulance dispatch can also help in mobilizing other agencies (e.g. police, fire, coast guard, rescue personnel) if their assistance is required. Ambulance dispatchers are also trained ambulance attendants. They are also able to provide advice regarding pre-hospital care to the First Aid Attendant.

The First Aid Attendant must think ahead and anticipate the patient's needs. By rapidly accessing the ambulance service where indicated, the patient's care is optimized. All emergency health care workers are part of a team, each with the same purpose — the optimal care of the sick and injured. Cooperation between First Aid Attendants and ambulance service personnel invariably results in faster and better care for the injured worker.

When contacting ambulance dispatch regarding assistance, the following information is essential. (See Table XVI-a.)

Contacting Ambulance Dispatch

It is always preferred that the Industrial First Aid Attendant who is with the patient contact ambulance dispatch directly rather than delegating this responsibility to assistants or office secretaries. In certain circumstances (e.g. critical patient, inaccessible phone), the Attendant may delegate the responsibility of contacting ambulance dispatch. However, it is essential that all information listed in Table XVI-a below be relayed to ambulance dispatch. Based on the information provided, ambulance dispatch will determine the type of ambulance response and the level of pre-hospital care required. Inaccurate or missing information can result in an inappropriate or delayed response which may adversely affect patient care.

TABLE XVI-a
Patient Information Required by
Ambulance Dispatch

1. Precise location of the patient
2. Age, sex of the patient
3. Mechanism of injury
4. Chief complaint(s)
5. Vital signs
6. Suspected diagnoses
7. Treatment rendered
8. Special equipment or manpower needed
9. Estimated time of arrival if an ETV or industrial ambulance is being used and a rendezvous is requested

AIR EVACUATION

Medical air evacuation has become increasingly common over the past few years. The Vietnam War experience showed a dramatic decrease in morbidity and mortality in trauma patients because of the rapid transport to hospital using helicopters. In some other provinces and countries, dedicated helicopters and medical personnel are specifically used as first responders for medical emergencies. Unfortunately, in British Columbia there are few dedicated air-evac helicopters with medical personnel immediately available to act as first responders. In remote areas, air evacuation is often a necessity because of the terrain and distance to hospital. The Industrial First Aid Regulations specifically state that it is the employer's responsibility to provide written procedures for transporting injured workers to medical aid. As with surface transports, this responsibility is often delegated to the First Aid Attendant. Medical air evacuation presents special problems for the First Aid Attendant.

Physiological Considerations of Air Evacuation

The medical effects resulting from the changes in altitude associated with an air evacuation can be profound. The following effects are important:
• Changes in barometric pressure;
• Variation in the partial pressure of oxygen with altitude;
• Effect of acceleration/deceleration and angle of climb/ descent.

Changes in Barometric Pressure

The air pressure decreases as the elevation above sea level increases. The laws of physics tell us that air-containing devices or organs will expand as the outside pressure decreases. On a medical air evacuation, the air inside an air splint (for example) will expand on takeoff and ascent to cruising altitude. This will result in further constriction around the patient's splinted extremity and may cut off the patient's circulation. Similarly, a partially filled glass IV bottle (or any other glass bottle) may explode as the air inside expands with ascent. For these reasons, air splints and glass containers are not recommended for aeromedical evacuations.

A patient with a pneumothorax may deteriorate significantly with ascent as a pneumothorax expands. Unless the aircraft is pressurized (unlikely), the only option is to maintain as low a flight altitude as weather conditions and terrain will permit.

The opposite effect occurs with a drop in altitude. During an air evacuation in our mountainous province, the Attendant is often faced with a variety of pressure changes as the pilot flies over a succession of mountain ranges.

The following table shows the expansion factor at different altitudes compared to sea level.

TABLE XVI-b

Altitude	Expansion Factor
Sea Level	1
5,000 Feet	1.2
8,000 Feet	1.33
10,000 Feet	1.5

Any gas-containing organ may be affected. The most common example of the effect of change in barometric pressure is pain in the ears or sinuses. This occurs most often in the individual with a cold or sinusitis.

Important injuries where pressure effects are potentially dangerous include:
- Open head injuries
- Facial fractures, especially involving the sinuses
- Open eye injuries
- Pneumothorax
- Decompression sickness
- Air emboli
- Gas gangrene

There are only two ways to overcome the detrimental effects of gas expansion:
- Maintain the flight altitude as close to sea level as possible (terrain and weather permitting).
- Use a pressurized aircraft.

Variation in the Partial Pressure of Oxygen with Altitude

The oxygen content of air decreases with altitude (the air is thin at high altitude). The level of oxygen in the circulating blood decreases dramatically with altitude, as shown in the following table.

TABLE XVI-c

Altitude (Feet)	Estimated Oxygen Content of Arterial Blood (%)
Sea Level	100
1,000 Feet	90
2,000 Feet	86
4,000 Feet	80
6,000 Feet	64
8,000 Feet	55

Ordinary commercial jets which cruise at altitudes of 30,000 feet or more are pressurized only to 8,000 feet! In normal subjects, the oxygen level in their blood is only 55% of normal. That is one of the reasons why patients with severe respiratory disease or pregnant patients near term are not allowed to fly without a doctor's letter.

In critically ill patients, the dramatic drop in the level of oxygen in the blood can be life threatening. The effect is more profound in patients with hemorrhage who also have a decreased blood volume.

The only remedies for the hypoxia under these circumstances are pressurization of the aircraft (helicopters are

TABLE XVI-d

Altitude Limit Above Sea Level	Cardiorespiratory Disease	Non-Cardiorespiratory Disease
2,000 feet	• chest pain with suspected heart attack • severe heart failure • severe respiratory failure	• decompression sickness • air emboli • penetrating eye injuries • severe facial injuries • open skull fracture
4,000 feet	• pneumothorax	• carbon monoxide poisoning • bowel obstruction
6,000 feet		• shock • coma • stroke • seizures
8,000 feet	• all other medical conditions necessitating aeromedical evacuation	

unpressurized) and the provision of supplementary oxygen. However, for certain conditions listed below, altitude limitations are still required. For all patients who require an aeromedical evacuation, a strict altitude limit of 8,000 feet is also mandatory.

Supplemental high-flow (10 Lpm) oxygen must be provided to the following air evacuation patients:
• All patients in the Rapid Transport Category
• Open eye injuries
• Facial fractures and/or a nosebleed with nasal obstruction
• Pneumothorax, chest injuries
• Bowel obstruction
• Decompression sickness
• Air emboli
• Patients with respiratory distress
• Chest pain with suspected heart attack
• Strokes, seizures
• Coma
• Spinal cord injuries

Effect of Acceleration/Deceleration and Angle of Climb/Descent

The G-forces experienced on takeoff and landing in fixed-wing aircraft can have detrimental effects on the air evacuation patient. The same forces that "drive you into the seat" on takeoff will cause redistribution of blood flow in the patient. For example, if the patient is lying down (supine or lateral) on takeoff, with the head forward, the forces will cause the redistribution of blood to the feet and away from the heart and the brain. This can have detrimental effects on patients with hemorrhagic shock who have decreased blood volume.

Similarly, if the angle of climb is quite steep on takeoff, the blood flow is redistributed to the feet. It is the same effect as if you stood the patient up.

The opposite effect occurs on descent and landing. These effects are minimal for helicopter evacuation because the flight cabin is usually maintained near horizontal and the G-forces are usually directed vertically rather than horizontally. However, for fixed-wing aircraft, the Attendant must take certain precautions to limit those effects.

Depending on the position of the head, the Attendant may have to elevate the legs or spine board to compensate for the effects of G-forces and the angle of climb. For example, if the patient is positioned feet forward, head back in the flight cabin, there is no adjustment required for takeoff and ascent. In that case, the blood is redistributed to the heart and brain (a good thing). However, on descent and landing, the legs or spine board should be elevated approximately six inches to compensate.

Medical Effects Related to the Flight Environment

There are other effects on a patient relating to the flight cabin in an aircraft:
1. Air sickness
2. Noise, turbulence, vibration
3. Electrical lighting
4. Humidity
5. Space limitations

1. Air sickness is relatively common during air evacuation. The following approaches are helpful in alleviating the problem.
   - All patients must be transported in the lateral or supine position. Administer oxygen if the patient is nauseous, dizzy or vomiting.
   - Have suction readily available and operational, if possible.
   - If no suction is available, the patient must be transported in the lateral position unless the patient can be quickly and easily rolled as required. Immobilized patients are best transported in the lateral position on a padded spine board.
   - Reassure the patient as much as possible.
2. Noise, turbulence and vibration make it difficult to hear and talk with the patient. Explain to the patient ahead of time that this may occur. For some patients, the noise and vibration is quite frightening and may make them agitated and anxious.

Splints, dressings or other equipment may loosen up or become undone. The Attendant must secure all splints, dressings and ties prior to takeoff. All first aid equipment must be secured, especially oxygen cylinders. The use of glass containers or objects is best avoided. Plastic, unbreakable containers are best.

3. Lighting is often poor and observing the patient may be difficult. Electrical supply may be variable and unreliable aboard an aircraft. The Attendant must bring along a flashlight and extra batteries. Only battery-powered devices are recommended. Cabin temperature may also be a problem, especially with ascent to altitude. The Attendant must take extra blankets to keep the patient warm.
4. The flight cabin atmosphere is very dry. The Attendant should add a bubble humidifier to the oxygen cylinder. It is best to administer humidified oxygen to the patient, if available.
5. Space limitations in the cabin make any medical procedures or first aid treatment difficult to perform. All necessary first aid procedures are best performed on the ground prior to takeoff. The Attendant must think ahead, anticipate problems and treat them on the ground.

In summary, altitude effects and flight environment considerations are of special clinical importance in aeromedical evacuation. The Attendant must consider these factors, especially in high-risk patients, when choosing between air evacuation and land transport. Furthermore, the Attendant must take extra precautions when evacuating the patient by air to prevent disastrous complications en route.

The current procedures for evacuation of injured workers may be outdated or deficient. The responsibility for review may be delegated to the First Aid Attendant. Policies and procedures for aeromedical evacuation at the work site must deal with the following items and concerns.
1. The need for an air evacuation
2. Aircraft selection
3. Pre-flight communication with flight crew
4. Pre-flight communication with ambulance dispatch and hospital
5. Checklist prior to aircraft arrival
6. Safety procedures around helicopters and fixed-wing aircraft
7. Pre-takeoff checklist
8. In-flight patient monitoring
9. Backup procedures in the event of equipment failure, unavailability of aircraft or poor weather conditions

Need for Medical Air Evacuation

Broad guidelines exist for determining the need for a medical air evacuation. Aeromedical evacuations do present some potential risks to the patient as discussed previously. There is also the small risk of crashing, which increases in poorer weather conditions. Finally, medical air evacuations are costly. Inappropriate use will, in the long run, create problems for both the employers and employees.

The following criteria are suggested for determining the need for medical air evacuation.

1. Land transport is impossible or unavailable.

    In certain remote areas, the only access may be by air. In other situations, the roads may be washed out or blocked, making land transport impossible.

2. Patient is in the Rapid Transport Category and total transport time by land to hospital significantly exceeds total transport time by air.

    Patients whose illnesses or injuries place them into the Rapid Transport Category must be transported to hospital as quickly as possible for definitive care. When calculating total transport time for air evacuation, the Attendant must factor in the time to find a helicopter or fixed-wing aircraft and its response time to the accident site. Although air travel is inherently faster than land transport, it may take significantly longer to organize an air evacuation and then await the aircraft's arrival. In those circumstances, land transport may be advised. Conversely, it may take an excessively long period of time for a land ambulance to arrive; in such circumstances, air transport may be advised. If the total time saved is 30 minutes or more, it is probably best to use air transport for patients in the Rapid Transport Category.

TABLE XVI-e

Summary of Emergency Conditions Requiring Rapid Transport to Hospital

Trauma

Mechanism of Injury:

1. Free fall greater than 20 feet
2. Severe deceleration in a motor vehicle accident
    *   High-speed accident and/or major vehicular damage
    *   Broken windshield, bent steering wheel or other significant damage to passenger compartment
    *   Victim thrown from the vehicle
    *   One or more vehicle occupants killed
    *   Victim involved in roll-over type accident
3. Pedestrian, motorcyclist or bicyclist struck at greater than 30 kph (20 mph)
4. Severe crush injuries

Anatomy of Injury:

1. Penetrating injury to the head, neck, chest, abdomen or groin
2. Two or more proximal long-bone fractures, i.e. femur, humerus
3. Flail chest
4. Extensive facial burns, inhalation injury or burns greater than 10% body surface area, especially if associated with any other trauma
5. Amputation of extremity other than toe or fingertip
6. Severe head injury defined as:
    *   Glasgow Coma Score less than or equal to 13
    *   Decreasing GCS by 2 or more
    *   Pupillary inequality greater than 1 mm and sluggish response to light
    *   Extremity weakness or paralysis, regardless of the GCS
    *   Depressed skull fracture
7. Spinal cord injury, paraplegia or quadriplegia

Primary Survey:

1. Partial or complete airway obstruction
2. Decreased level of consciousness (GCS less than or equal to 13)
3. Respiratory rate (less than 10 or greater than 30 per minute) or severe dyspnea
4. Absent radial pulses
5. Obvious circulatory shock

Other Conditions:

1. Chest injury with shortness of breath
2. Smoke or toxic gas inhalation, carbon monoxide poisoning
3. Decompression sickness
4. Air embolism
5. Penetrating eye injuries
6. Moderate or severe hypothermia
7. Near-drowning
8. Any limb-threatening injuries
9. Electrical injuries, especially with serious burns or loss of consciousness

Medical Emergencies

1. Cardiac arrest
2. Coma (GCS 8 or less)
3. Acute poisoning with any of the following:
   - Partially or completely obstructed airway
   - Respiratory rate less than 10 or greater than 30
   - Absent radial pulses
   - Altered mental status or decreased level of consciousness
   - If so directed by Poison Control Centre
4. Status epilepticus
5. Stroke
6. Heart failure
7. Shock
8. Severe shortness of breath
9. Chest pain with suspected heart attack
10. Suspected acute abdomen

For all other patients, land transport is recommended unless land access is impossible.

The decision to use air transport rests with the First Aid Attendant, taking into account all the risks and benefits. In some provinces and countries, the decision to use aeromedical evacuation is made by a dispatcher or a physician, based on the medical information provided by the First Aid Attendant.

The BC Ambulance Service operates an advanced air ambulance service for inter-hospital transport of patients. Specially trained paramedics, nurses or physicians are provided, depending on the patient's needs. Currently, only licenced physicians may request an air evacuation through the provincial dispatch office of the BC Ambulance Service. Nevertheless, the provincial dispatchers are available 24 hours a day and can provide advice and assistance to the Attendant who is trying to organize an air evacuation. In BC, the phone number is 1-800-742-8011.

Provincial dispatch is also responsible for coordinating ambulance transfers from the aircraft landing site to the hospital. The Attendant must think ahead, anticipating what will be required. Unless the landing pad is located at the hospital, a land ambulance will be required to transfer the patient to hospital. Provincial dispatch *must* be contacted in order to coordinate the transfer. When contacting provincial dispatch, the Attendant will be asked to provide pertinent medical information so that an appropriately trained and equipped crew will be dispatched to assist the Attendant on arrival.

Aircraft Selection

The aircraft selected for medical air evacuation must meet certain minimum criteria. The selection of an inappropriate aircraft will only delay the air evacuation, thereby losing precious time. The following minimum criteria must be met:

1. The aircraft must have a patient compartment large enough to accommodate the stretcher with the patient, the Attendant and all necessary equipment. There must be sufficient room for the Attendant to sit and/or kneel beside the patient and perform CPR. Do the seats have to be removed, or are they collapsible, in order to accommodate the stretcher?

2. Is the aircraft capable of carrying the extra weight over the terrain and distance required?

3. Does the aircraft, fully loaded, have sufficient range to make the trip with safety allowances?

4. Is there sufficient space in the patient compartment to rotate the patient to the lateral position, if necessary? Otherwise, the patient will have to be positioned in the lateral position prior to takeoff.

5. The door to the patient compartment must be sufficiently wide to accommodate a fully immobilized patient on a backboard or basket stretcher.

6. If night air evacuations are required, or where weather conditions are often poor, transport regulations may require two pilots, twin engine and IFR capabilities. These special situations must be discussed with the aircraft companies and possibly the federal transportation authorities. Alternative evacuation procedures may be required.

7. If fixed-wing aircraft are to be used, can the runway accommodate a fully loaded plane in all weather conditions?

8. Radio communications with hospital and/or ambulance dispatch are required.

9. The Attendant must be able to communicate directly with the pilot.

Pre-Flight Communication with the Flight Crew

The Attendant must contact the flight crew on a pre-arranged radio frequency and provide the following information:

1. Exact location and description of landing site (highway, field, dirt road, etc.). For fixed-wing aircraft, the length of the runway is also required (e.g. forestry grid coordinates are useful in logging operations).

2. An update on weather conditions, to include:
   - Cloud cover
   - Visibility (distance)
   - Fog, snow, rain
   - Wind velocity and direction, if known

3. Description of obstacles within half a mile on all sides of the landing area, including wires, towers, mountain peaks.

4. Type of signal to indicate landing area and important obstacles. Smoke bombs or flares are usually preferred because they also provide an estimate of ground wind velocity and direction.

5. An estimate of the time when darkness sets in at the landing site.

6. Determine the estimated time of arrival (ETA) for the aircraft at the accident site.

7. Ensure that the flight crew bring along any additional equipment that may be required (e.g. helicopter stretcher, extra oxygen cylinders, etc.).

Pre-Flight Communication with Provincial Dispatch and Hospital

The Attendant must communicate, if necessary, with provincial dispatch to organize the ambulance transfer from the final destination to the hospital. If not, precious time will be lost awaiting the ambulance when the patient arrives at the destination.

It is also extremely important that the Attendant inform the hospital (usually the emergency physician on duty) of the patient's transfer, including an estimated time of arrival. Proper hospital notification implies much more than simply leaving a message at the switchboard. It is best to discuss the case directly with the physician who will be attending the patient. Pertinent medical information and an estimated time of arrival must be provided so that the hospital will be adequately prepared. For example, physicians and nurses may have to be called in. By coordinating closely with the hospital, unnecessary treatment delays are avoided. Finally, the hospital personnel may be able to advise the Attendant with respect to stabilization, treatment and transport of the patient.

Checklist Prior to Aircraft Arrival

1. When possible, the landing site should be checked to remove all loose debris.

2. Where necessary, road blocks should be set up approximately one quarter mile on either side of the landing area.

3. Crowd control measures must be enforced. The Attendant must ensure that everyone is at least 100 to 200 feet away from the helicopter landing site, to avoid injury from flying debris caused by rotor downwash.

4. The Attendant must ensure that the landing site is well marked with signal flares or smoke bombs. They should be well clear of the actual landing site. All assistants must be briefed on the safety procedures for approaching the helicopter or fixed-wing aircraft and loading the patient.

Safety Procedures Around Helicopters and Fixed-Wing Aircraft

It is important that the following safety procedures be followed around aircraft.

1. A fixed-wing aircraft should not be approached until the pilot signals that it is safe to do so or the airplane has come to a full stop and the engines have been turned off.

2. For helicopters, the Attendant may have to direct the pilot's approach and landing. Stand at the side of the landing site, your back to the wind and arms outstretched forward, pointing to the landing site. The pilot may be unable to acknowledge instructions, even by radio.

3. After touchdown, await the pilot's instructions or signal to approach the helicopter.

4. Always approach or leave the machine from the front or side within the pilot's field of vision. Never approach or leave the helicopter from behind. On uneven terrain, it is always best to approach or leave the helicopter on the downslope side to avoid the main rotor.

5. Protect the patient from flying debris during landing.

6. The Attendant and assistants should crouch when approaching or leaving the helicopter to ensure adequate clearance from the main rotor.

7. Never carry anything above shoulder height when approaching or leaving the helicopter.

8. The patient should not be carried or lifted above the waist when being carried to or loaded into the helicopter.

9. Remove or fasten loose clothing (e.g. hats, jackets) so that they will not distract or interfere with personnel.

10. The Attendant and all assistants must wear eye protection (face shields or goggles) during takeoff and landing.

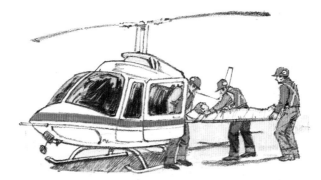

Always protect the patient from flying debris when the machine is landing

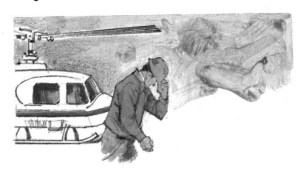

Crouch when approaching or leaving the machine for extra clearance from the main rotor

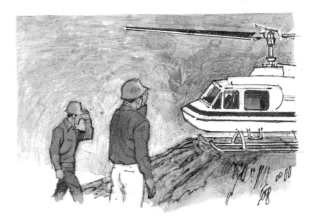

Approach or leave on the down slope side to avoid the main rotor

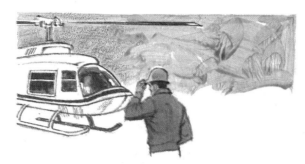

Approach or leave in the pilot's field or vision to avoid the tail rotor

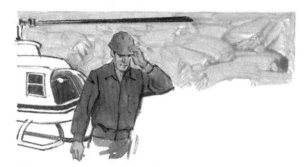

Hold onto hard hats when approaching or leaving the machine unless chin straps are used

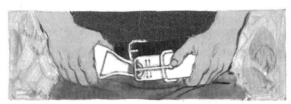

Fasten seat belts on entering the helicopter and leave them buckled until the pilot signals that it is safe to disembark

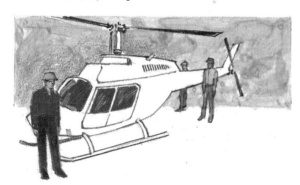

Do not touch the bubble or any of the moving parts, such as tail, rotor or linkage

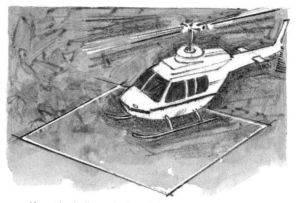

Keep the helispot (heli-pad) free from loose articles

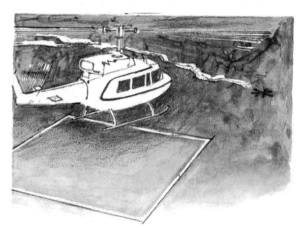

Keep signal fires well clear of the helispot

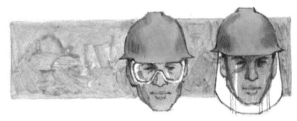

The Attendant and assistants should wear eye shields when the helicopter is landing and taking off.

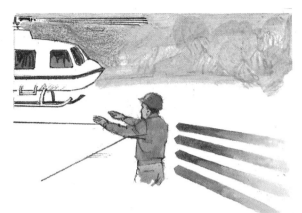

When directing the landing, stand with your back to the wind and arms outstretched toward the landing pad

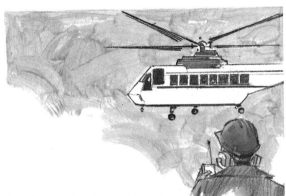

When directing the pilot by radio, the pilot will have both hands busy and cannot acknowledge instructions

Before the machine lands to pick up the patient, the Attendant should:
• Brief all assistants on safety procedures
• Keep all assistants and the patient out of the way at the side of the landing zone
• Have the assistants face away from the machine during landing and take-off
• Ensure each assistant knows what to do as soon as the pilot gives the signal to load the patient

Pre-Takeoff Checklist

This procedure is similar to the patient checklist prior to surface transport discussed previously.

1. Instruct the pilot not to take off until the pre-takeoff checklist has been completed by the Attendant.
2. Position and secure the patient appropriately.
3. Maximize patient comfort.
4. Check all splints, bandages and dressings.
5. Check and secure all equipment.
6. Ensure that there is an adequate supply of oxygen.
7. Remember to bring along the patient's medications, if possible. Bring along the patient's valuables.
8. Reassure the patient.
9. Repeat and record the patient's vital signs.
10. Confirm that the onboard radio is working. It is important that the Attendant is able to directly communicate with the pilot at all times.
11. Update provincial dispatch and the hospital with the patient's status and a revised estimated time of arrival, if possible.
12. Advise the pilot of any altitude limitations that may apply. For fixed-wing aircraft, the angle of climb may have to be reduced as well.

In-Flight Patient Monitoring

Guidelines for in-flight patient monitoring are identical to those outlined in the patient checklist during transport (see page 369).

Aeromedical evacuation can be truly life saving, provided that extra care is taken to avoid the pitfalls. The special physiological effects of air evacuation imply that the patient cannot be simply loaded into a plane or helicopter and taken away into the wild blue yonder. Because of all the intricacies involved in organizing and carrying out a proper air evacuation, it is essential that the First Aid Attendant organize evacuation drills with the aircraft company, flight crews and co-workers to evaluate and test the written policies and procedures in force at the work site. Only by pre-planning, reviewing and testing can the employer and the First Aid Attendant ensure that safe and efficient aeromedical evacuations are available for injured workers.

Appendix I
Emergency Childbirth

Be calm — don't be in a hurry to transport the patient.

Evaluate:

*   Is this her first child? If so, labour usually takes 12 to 15 hours; the period of labour with subsequent children is much shorter.
*   Listen to the mother and time the contractions.
*   If labour has just begun and there are no signs of immediate birth, transfer the mother to the nearest hospital. She should be placed on her left side, as this relieves pressure on the aorta and vena cava and will ensure that the baby has a good blood supply.

SIGNS OF IMMEDIATE BIRTH

*   The mother is having contractions every two minutes or less.
*   The mother says the baby is coming. BELIEVE HER.
*   The baby's head is visible at the vaginal opening (crowning).
*   The mother is straining and pushing down during contractions or feels she has to have a bowel movement.

DO NOT TRY TO DELAY THE DELIVERY BY ANY METHOD.

Signs that may indicate that labour is not progressing normally are:

*   Hemorrhaging (before, during or after the birth).
*   Weak contractions or contractions stop.
*   Prolapsed cord or malpresentation — breech (hips with legs up or feet first), face presentation or baby lies transversely in uterus.
*   Maternal distress, shock from loss of blood and dehydration from a long, difficult labour.
*   Fetal distress — If the baby is still in the uterus, it will pass meconium (feces) into the amniotic fluid if it is deprived of oxygen. The meconium will stain the amniotic fluid yellow, green or dark brown, depending on how much the baby passed.

Keep calm and reassure mother. Obtain medical help.

EMERGENCY CHILDBIRTH SUPPLIES

*   4 clean towels
*   2 folded sheets
*   1 receiving blanket for the baby
*   gauze squares
*   small rubber (ear) syringe
*   alcohol
*   sterilized scissors
*   sterilized ties or clamps (for umbilical cord)
*   diapers
*   safety pins
*   basin or pan (in case mother vomits)
*   blanket for mother
*   sanitary napkins
*   plastic bag or container for the afterbirth
*   flashlight, if the trip is at night

PROCEDURE TO ASSIST BIRTH

Wash hands. Get the supplies ready. Position mother on her back, knees raised, feet flat and thighs separated. Place clean towels or newspapers under her buttocks and a pillow under her head. If in a public place, provide for the patient's privacy. Talk to the mother about the procedures, to help put her at ease.

Stand by to assist the mother. Have her husband or friend stay at the mother's head to help reassure her and keep a constant check on her airway.

Be ready to support the baby and handle it very gently. Do not encourage pushing or bearing down as crowning progresses. Normally the baby will present face down. Have the mother take short breaths of air and blow out or pant, to slow delivery of the head and lessen the damage to the mother's perineum.

In the event that the water bag has not yet broken, carefully tear the bag open with a fingernail at the back of the baby's head. Peel it away from the baby's face.

Clean the baby's face, removing mucus and fluid from around the mouth and nose. Gently squeeze the baby's nose to get most of the mucus out. Using a bulb syringe, very carefully suction the baby's mouth and nose.

If the cord is around the baby's neck and is very loose, slip the cord over the head. If the cord is too tight and is choking the baby, use sterilized ties or clamps and tie the cord in two places, two inches apart, and cut between the ties; remove the cord from the baby's neck.

Do not try to pull the baby out. Gently support the baby and, on the next contraction, instruct the mother to bear down.

Be prepared to hold baby. CAUTION: it will be very slippery.

Clear mucus away from the baby's mouth and nose. Hold the feet slightly elevated with the head down to help drain away fluids from the airway. Keep the infant warm.

If the infant does not start breathing within 30 seconds, resuscitation procedures must be initiated.

Mother will rest between the next contractions. It usually takes up to 20 minutes to expel the placenta. Wrap the placenta in a towel and take it to the hospital for a doctor to examine.

Check uterus for firmness by palpating the abdomen just below the navel. If it is not firm and there is excessive bleeding, massage this area until it feels hard and firm.

It is not necessary to cut the umbilical cord unless medical care cannot be obtained for several hours. There is danger of infection through the open end of the cord if it is cut with unsterile equipment, so it is better to leave the cord uncut. However, it should be clamped or tied off while waiting for the placenta to be expelled. **Caution:** If the cord is not clamped or tied off, the placenta must be held above the baby in order to prevent baby from hemorrhaging from it.

Wait until pulsations stop (roughly five minutes). Use strips of sterile cloth if no clamps are available. Tie one strip at 10cm and another at 15cm from the baby's body. Cut through the umbilical cord between the ties with sterile scissors or a sterile razor blade. **Caution:** Make sure the ties are secure and there is no bleeding from the cut ends. Put on another tie close to the original tie if there is bleeding. Wrap the baby in a warm blanket and give to the mother to hold, as her body will keep the baby warm. Recheck for bleeding from the cord.

Clean the area around the vagina, place a sanitary napkin or clean cloth over the area. Some bleeding is normal. Cover the mother with a warm blanket and transport her to a hospital. Periodically monitor the firmness and size of the uterus.

INFANT RESUSCITATION

1. Establish unresponsiveness — gently shake the infant and call to him/her. If medical aid has not already been arranged, have someone call.
2. Establish breathlessness — maintain an open airway. Look, listen and feel for signs of breathing.
3. If the infant is not breathing, cover the mouth and nose with your mouth and administer two separate puffs, allowing deflation between breaths.
4. Establish pulselessness — while maintaining the head-tilt position, check circulation by assessing the brachial pulse.
5. If the pulse is absent, begin chest compressions. Position two fingers one finger's width below the nipple line. Vertical compressions are administered to a depth of 1.3-2.5 cm (½"-1") at the rate of 100/minute. The ratio is (5:1) five compressions to one ventilation.
6. Evaluate the infant's status after 10 cycles and re-evaluate the status every few minutes.

CHOKING INFANT/CHILD

In children, choking is commonly caused by the unexpected lodging of small objects (beads, marbles, etc.) or food (peanuts, candies, etc.) in the airway. Choking may also be caused by infection or allergies, which cause sudden swelling of the airway (e.g. croup).

A CHILD WHOSE AIRWAY IS PARTIALLY BLOCKED BECAUSE OF SWELLING (INFECTIOUS CAUSE) NEEDS PROMPT MEDICAL ATTENTION. Don't waste time attempting to relieve this type of obstruction: A child who has been ill with fever, a barking cough or croupy, noisy breathing, has a progressive airway obstruction and needs immediate transportation to the nearest medical facility.

A child who is choking on a small object (or seems to be choking) should be encouraged to persist with coughing and breathing efforts as long as his or her cough is effective. Relief of the obstruction should be attempted only if the cough is, or becomes, ineffective. ANY child who has difficulty breathing should be assisted.

A child who successfully clears his or her airway should be watched carefully. Referral to a physician is always mandatory.

PARTIAL AIRWAY OBSTRUCTION

With PARTIAL AIRWAY OBSTRUCTION, the victim may experience "good air exchange" or "poor air exchange".

What to Look For

— GOOD AIR EXCHANGE: The child can cough forcefully, breathe and cough again. There is often a wheezing sound between the coughs. Speech and/or crying are good signs that air exchange is still effective.

What to Do

— DO NOT INTERFERE with the child's attempts to clear his/her own airway. Encourage the child to keep up efforts to expel the foreign body with continued coughing. Stay with the victim at all times.

RELIEF OF COMPLETE AIRWAY OBSTRUCTION IN CHILDREN

The Heimlich Manoeuvre

If you observe a child who is unable to speak, breathe or cough, ask the child, "Are you choking?" Reassure the child that you are there to help. If it is obvious that the child has not succeeded in inhaling air, perform the Heimlich manoeuvre.

What to Look For

— POOR AIR EXCHANGE: The victim's cough is very weak and breathing is now increasingly difficult. If the child produces uneven and high-pitched, crowing noises as he attempts to breathe, there is partial obstruction with poor air exchange. The child's colour may turn bluish.

What to Do

— Treat this obstruction AS THOUGH IT WERE A COMPLETE AIRWAY OBSTRUCTION.

RELIEF OF COMPLETE AIRWAY OBSTRUCTION IN INFANTS

With COMPLETE AIRWAY OBSTRUCTION, the child cannot breathe, talk, cough or cry. The child may turn blue quite quickly from lack of oxygen. This child needs immediate assistance.

Back Blows

The infant is straddled over the rescuer's arm, with the head lower than the trunk (the head is supported by holding the baby's jaw). Supporting this arm on your thigh, deliver four back blows between the infant's shoulder blades, with the heel of your free hand.

Following the back blows, place your free hand along the infant's spine (the infant is now "sandwiched" in your arms) and turn the infant over onto your other thigh. The infant is now face-up. Supporting the infant's head (which is positioned lower than the trunk to utilize gravity), deliver four chest thrusts using TWO FINGERS ONLY. This manoeuvre is the same as in external cardiac compression.

This action is intended to dislodge the obstruction.

Tongue-Jaw Lift

After chest thrusts, open the infant's mouth gently. Grasp both the tongue and lower jaw between your thumb and forefinger, and lift upwards. This tongue-jaw lift will draw the tongue away from the back of the throat. IF YOU ARE ABLE TO SEE THE OFFENDING OBSTRUCTION, remove it carefully with your finger. Do not perform blind finger sweeps.

Continue these manoeuvres until the object is dislodged, the infant becomes unconscious or the infant reaches medical attention.

If the object you remove has been the cause of the obstruction, breathing may begin immediately. If breathing does not return naturally, provide rescue breathing. Watch carefully for the rise and fall of the chest. If the chest does not rise, reposition the head and try again. If rescue breathing is still unsuccessful, repeat your efforts to dislodge the airway obstruction.

Appendix II
Stress and the First Aid Attendant

STRESS FACTORS COMMON TO INDUSTRIAL FIRST AID ATTENDANTS

The role of the Industrial First Aid Attendant can be difficult both physically and emotionally. While the physical demands of the job can be met by maintaining good physical health, the emotional demands may be harder to cope with.

Although it is true that some stress is a useful and normal part of life, when stress becomes continuous or overwhelming, it is necessary to take steps to deal with it.

Following are stresses commonly experienced by Industrial First Aid Attendants:

1. Waiting for the call: Anxiety can be generated by just waiting for an emergency call, especially if the Attendant is not otherwise occupied. When the call does come, stress can increase as the Attendant moves into action.

2. On the way to the scene: The Attendant may be getting increasingly anxious/stressed while proceeding to the accident. He or she may feel scared, sick or shaky, wondering "What will I find?", "What if I can't handle it?"

3. Working alone: If the Attendant has no trained assistant or partner and is solely responsible for all emergency care and decision making, the responsibility may feel overwhelming.

4. Difficult environment: Bad weather, hazardous terrain and dangerous sites can add to the problems surrounding access, treatment, extrication and transport.

5. Difficulties and delays with transportation: In some locations, the Attendant may not be able to transport the patient immediately because of poor weather or inaccessible locations.

6. Shift work: Dual role and/or continuous shift changes may contribute to disturbed or altered sleep patterns, improper diet and lack of exercise, all of which may adversely affect the Attendant. Having the responsibility for a full-time job, as well as being the Attendant, may make life more difficult.

7. Supervisory hassles: Obviously, it is less stressful if the Attendant has good rapport with foremen and supervisors. The Attendant may, at times, feel caught between management, labour and the WCB.

8. Getting to know the workers: Often the Attendant will befriend the worker in an attempt to do a better job, but this may cause difficulties in treatment or if a major accident occurs. The Attendant may be placed in awkward situations, if workers try to take advantage of the situation. Also, in a major accident, treating "a friend" may make it harder.

9. Insufficient experience or practise: In the presence of major trauma or cardiac arrest, the Attendant's lack of experience or practise may affect their confidence.

10. Physical demands: Some sites and some accidents will require maximum physical effort and stamina from the Attendant.

11. Being separated from family and friends for long periods.

SUGGESTIONS FOR REDUCING STRESS FACTORS

1. Everyone feels anxious while waiting for an emergency call, so try to keep occupied if IFA is your only responsibility. Set aside time for study and practise as well as developing back-up plans for all possibilities. Mentally and/or physically "walk through" procedures you are uncertain about.

2. At the scene: If you freeze and cannot remember what to do — keep moving. Take some deep breaths, ensure no danger and check the airway. Once you start into action, you will function properly.

3. Keep physically fit: Nothing boosts confidence like being physically fit. It will also help reduce stress. Try to incorporate a regular exercise program into your day.

4. Skills update: If you are working alone, try to get together with another Attendant or an instructor to practise and update your skills. Be brutally honest with yourself in identifying your weak areas. Form an interest group of Attendants to meet periodically, correspond by mail or start a newsletter. Volunteer for activities such as riding third on a provincial ambulance. Confidence comes with experience and practise.

5. Learn from your experiences. Every first aid incident is a learning opportunity. Be realistic and have the courage to learn from your mistakes. Debrief yourself after each case to see if there is a better way to do

things. If there is a problem, review each case with another Attendant, your instructor or health care professional.

6. Share your worries. Sharing with people you trust does lighten the load and lessens anxiety.

7. Say "I don't know". Being able to say "I don't know" may take some practise but you will find this type of honesty will be rewarded. People who are confident and who keep current by continually learning are quite comfortable with saying it. Once you think you know it all, you stop learning. Besides, no one knows everything about their job.

8. Develop your sense of humour. A sense of humour at the appropriate time can reduce anxiety for you and those around you.

9. You are not alone. Remember all Attendants feel stressed at times and it is normal to feel *some* anxiety.

SOME RESOURCES

- WCB First Aid Section
- IFA Instructors
- Other Attendants
- Your personal physician
- Local community centres with fitness, nutrition and stress programs
- YMCA/YWCA
- Dial-a-Dietician
- Public Health and Community Health Services

Appendix III
Fatalities

In the presence of an obvious fatality, the Attendant may be the only person present who can bring order to an already emotionally charged scene. NOTE: IF THERE IS ANY DOUBT AS TO WHETHER THE PATIENT HAS BEEN KILLED, THE ATTENDANT DOES NOT HAVE THE AUTHORITY TO PRONOUNCE DEATH. Therefore, where doubt exists, the patient must be treated and transported to medical aid as if life-threatening conditions are present. Apply the appropriate treatments, as outlined in the manual, depending upon the patient's condition.

In cases of obvious death, it will be the responsibility of the Attendant to ensure that various people and agencies are notified. The Attendant must ensure that the employer, doctor, police and the local Workers' Compensation Board office are notified. The names of witnesses should be obtained and a record of the history of the accident should be made. The body of the worker MUST NOT be moved until the coroner gives permission to do so.

Where death has been certified by a medical doctor or coroner, proper care must be taken of the body. The coroner's office or local BC Ambulance Service ambulance crew, depending upon locale, may be responsible for transportation of the body. If it is necessary for the body to remain at the work site due to transportation difficulties, keep it in a cool isolated place. Dress any wounds and cover body openings with large ABD pads. Close the mouth and eyelids. DO NOT turn or incline the head to the side. Cover the body with a clean sheet or encase it in a body bag, if one is available.

In the presence of witnesses, collect and itemize (in quadruplicate) the personal belongings of the worker and have a witness sign the itemized list. Keep the personal belongings for the police.

Where practicable, the scene of any workplace accident involving a fatality should be left untouched, except for activity necessitated by rescue work or to prevent further failure of equipment or injuries. THE SCENE MUST NOT BE DISTURBED UNTIL THE ACCIDENT HAS BEEN INVESTIGATED BY AN OFFICER OF THE WCB OR UNTIL PERMISSION TO CLEAR THE SCENE HAS BEEN GRANTED BY AN OFFICER OF THE WCB.

Appendix IV
Measuring Body Temperature

MEASURING BODY TEMPERATURE BY THE ORAL METHOD

1. The Attendant should wash his or her hands. Explain the procedure of measuring the temperature to the patient.
2. Check the level of the mercury in the thermometer. If it is above 37°C, it will need to be shaken down.
3. To shake the mercury down, hold the thermometer securely at the top and between the thumb and index finger. Shake the thermometer down with a quick flip and twist of the wrist.
4. Place the thermometer in the patient's mouth, slightly to one side and under the tongue. Have the patient keep the lips closed to keep out cool air. Warn the patient not to bite down on the glass.
5. Leave the thermometer in the mouth for three to five minutes.
6. Remove the thermometer, record the reading and time and date.
7. Wash the thermometer, then return it to its sterilizing solution.

MEASURING BODY TEMPERATURE BY THE AXILLARY METHOD

The axillary method records the body temperature as about one degree lower (F°) than the oral temperature.
1. Follow the first three steps given for the oral method.
2. Place the thermometer high in the patient's axilla (armpit). The patient's arm must be tight against the lateral chest wall.
3. Leave the thermometer in place for 10 minutes.
4. Remove the thermometer and record the temperature, including the information that it was measured by the axillary method.
5. Wash the thermometer, then return it to its sterilizing solution.

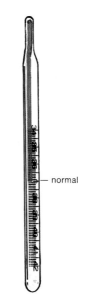

— normal

Standard Thermometer

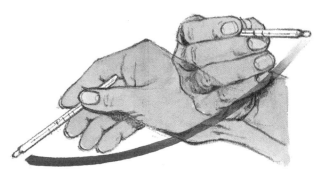

Shaking the mercury down

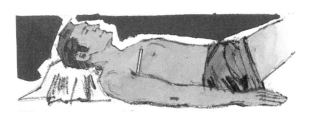

Axillary Method

Appendix V
WHMIS

WHMIS: WHAT DOES IT MEAN?

The Workplace Hazardous Materials Information System — WHMIS — is a major response to Canadian workers' rights to know more about safety and health hazards of materials used in the workplace.

WHMIS legislation became effective in October 1988. It provides employees, employers and suppliers nationwide with specific, vital information about hazardous materials (called "controlled products" in the legislation).

These are the key requirements of WHMIS:

1. controlled product labelling — to alert workers to the identity and dangers of products and to basic safety precautions;
2. material safety data sheets (MSDS) — technical bulletins that provide detailed hazard and precautionary information;
3. worker education and training programs;
4. protection of confidential business information.

THE LEGISLATION

Legislation to implement WHMIS has been enacted on both the federal and provincial/territorial levels. Federal requirements deal with the importation and sale of controlled products; provincial legislation covers the storage, handling and use of controlled products in the workplace. More specifically, the federal *Hazardous Products Act* and pursuant *Controlled Products Regulations* establish the criteria for including products in WHMIS; they also require suppliers to provide appropriate labels and material safety data sheets as a condition of sale and importation of those products.

Federal legislation balances a worker's right-to-know about hazardous products with industry's need to protect confidential business information (their proprietary formulas). A self-financing commission established by the *Hazardous Materials Information Review Act* oversees that aspect.

Provincial legislation, through amendments to occupational safety and health regulations, covers the responsibility of the employer to provide:

1. worker education on controlled products;
2. workplace labelling and identification;
3. a material safety data sheet (MSDS) where the employer produces a controlled product.

The equivalent requirements have been adopted for federally regulated workplaces, through amendments to the Canada Labour Code.

LABELLING

A set of universal labels has been adopted and is now in standard use across the country.

There are eight classes of materials, shown below with their corresponding symbols.

The labels are to be affixed to the supplier labels, which in turn are attached to the product container. The diagram below is an example of an acceptable format for a supplier label.

The following pages illustrate a typical MSDS and the nine sections providing important data about the different aspects of the product.

MATERIAL SAFETY DATA SHEET

PRODUCT
IDENTIFIER ♦

SECTION 6 — TOXICOLOGICAL PROPERTIES

ROUTE OF ENTRY

SKIN CONTACT ❑   SKIN ABSORPTION ❑   EYE CONTACT ❑   INHALATION ❑   INGESTION ❑

EFFECTS OF ACUTE EXPOSURE TO PRODUCT

EFFECTS OF CHRONIC EXPOSURE TO PRODUCT

EXPOSURE LIMITS	IRRITANCY OF PRODUCT	SENSITIZATION TO PRODUCT	CARCINOGENICITY
TERATOGENICITY	REPRODUCTIVE TOXICITY	MUTAGENICITY	SYNERGISTIC PRODUCTS

SECTION 7— PREVENTIVE MEASURES

PERSONAL PROTECTIVE EQUIPMENT

GLOVES (SPECIFY)	RESPIRATOR (SPECIFY)	EYE (SPECIFY)
FOOTWEAR (SPECIFY)	CLOTHING (SPECIFY)	OTHER (SPECIFY)

ENGINEERING CONTROLS (SPECIFY, E.G. VENTILATION, ENCLOSED PROCESS.)

LEAK AND SPILL PROCEDURE

WASTE DISPOSAL

HANDLING PROCEDURES AND EQUIPMENT

STORAGE REQUIREMENTS

SPECIAL SHIPPING INFORMATION

SECTION 8 — FIRST AID MEASURES

SPECIFIC MEASURES

SECTION 9 — PREPARATION DATE OF MSDS

PREPARED BY (GROUP, DEPARTMENT, ETC.)	PHONE NUMBER	DATE

Of special interest to the IFA Attendant are sections 6 through 8. **The First Aid Attendant should become familiar with the characteristics of all the products likely to be encountered in his/her own industry.**

It is recommended that copies of all relevant MSDSs be kept in one location where the IFA Attendant will have ready access to the information. The first aid room is an ideal location for such reference material.

WHMIS rules also require that appropriate MSDSs be available at the location in which the product is used, for the workers' reference.

As mentioned above, it is mandatory that the employer educate each worker on the risks and hazards associated with the use of all controlled products encountered in the performance of the worker's duties.

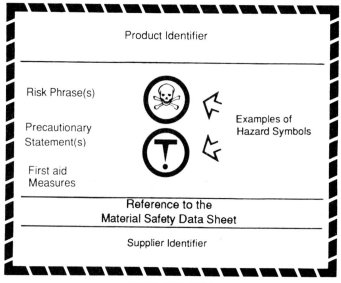

SUPPLIER LABEL

Class A: Compressed gas

Class B: Flammable and
combustible material

Class C: Oxidizing material

Class E: Corrosive material

LABELS

Division 1: Materials causing
immediate and serious toxic
effects

Division 2: Materials causing
other toxic effects

Division 3: Biohazardous
infectious material

Class F: Dangerously reactive
material

Class D: Poisonous and infectious materials

Appendix VI
Medical Terminology–Body Movement

Adducted — movement towards the midline of the body
Abducted — movement away from the midline of the body
Flexion — the act of bending
Extension — the act of straightening

Rotation — the process of turning around an axis (fixed point)
Inversion — the process of turning inward
Eversion — the process of turning outward

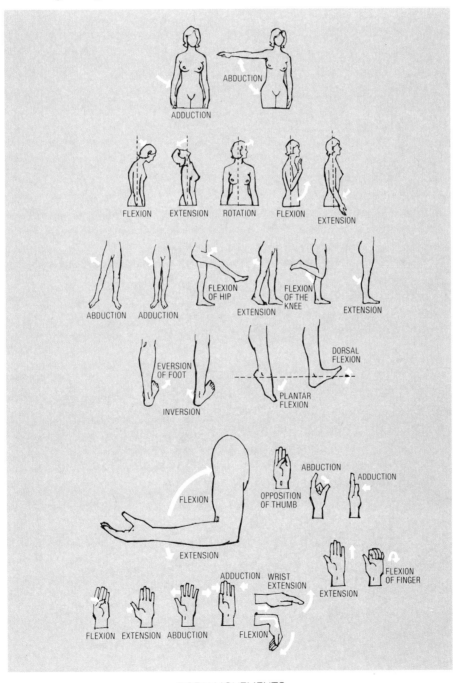

BODY MOVEMENTS

Glossary

USING THE GLOSSARY

To make it easier for the First Aid Attendant, the pronunciation as well as the meaning has been included on the more difficult words. Long and short vowels are marked as well as primary and secondary accents. Respellings have been done to indicate the proper phonetic sound.

DIACRITICS

These are marks over or under vowels to indicate pronunciation. Only two diacritics are used in this glossary: the *macron* (-) showing the long sound of vowels as the "a" in rāte and breve (˘) showing the short sound of vowels as the "e" in ĕver.

ACCENTS

These are marks used to indicate stress upon syllables. A single accent (′) is called a primary accent. A double accent (″) is called a secondary accent. The secondary accent indicates less stress upon a syllable than that given by a primary accent.

Example is: acetabulum (as″ĕ-tab′u-lum).

A

abdomen (ab-do′men): The large cavity below the diaphragm and above the pelvis.

abduction (ab-duk′shun): Movement of a limb away from the central axis of the body.

abrasion (ah-bra′zhun): The loss of a partial thickness of skin from rubbing or scraping on a hard or rough surface.

abruptio placentae (ah-brup′she-o placen′tae): Premature separation of a normally situated placenta.

abscess: A localized collection of pus in a cavity formed by disintegration of tissues.

acetabulum (as″ĕ-tab′u-lum): The large, cup-shaped depression on the external surface of the pelvic (innominate) bone, into which the head of the femur fits.

acetone (as′ĕ-ton): Colourless, volatile, liquid ketone used as a solvent of organic compounds.

acid (as′id): A substance which yields hydrogen ions in solution; has a pH less than 7.0.

acidosis (as″ĭ-do′sis): A state of increased acidity of body tissues and fluids.

acute (ah-kūt′): Having severe symptoms and a short course.

acute abdomen: A condition caused by an irritation or inflammation of the peritoneum.

Adam's Apple: The prominence of the thyroid cartilage of the larynx.

adduction (ad-duk′shun): Movement of a limb toward the central axis of the body.

adrenalin (ah-dren′ah-lin): A hormone which acts as a stimulant.

aerobic (a′er-ōb-ic): Requiring air or free oxygen to live.

air hunger: Distressed or laboured breathing; dyspnea.

air passage: Passage through which air enters and leaves the lungs.

airway: Passage through which air enters and leaves the lungs; a mechanical device used for maintaining unobstructed respiration.

alkali: A substance that yields hydroxyl ions in solution; a solution with pH greater than 7.0.

alveoli (al-ve′o-li): The air sacs of the lungs.

amniotic (am-nĭ-ot′ik) **fluid:** A liquid that surrounds the fetus in the uterus and protects it from injury.

amputation (ăm″pŭ-tā′shun): The removal of a limb or other part of the body.

amyl (ām′il) **nitrite:** A clear, yellowish liquid which, when inhaled as a vapour, will dilate coronary arteries; may be used in the treatment of cyanide poisoning.

anaerobic (ăn″ā-ĕr-ō′bik): Needing no oxygen to live.

anaphylactic (ăn-ă-fĭ-lăk′tĭk) **shock:** A condition, which may be rapidly fatal, resulting from severe allergic reaction.

anatomical (ăn″ă-tŏm′ik-al) **position:** When the body is standing erect, arms at the sides and palms forward.

anatomy (ăn-ăt-ō-mĭ): The study of body structure.

anesthetic (ăn″ĕs-thĕt′ĭk): A drug which causes loss of sensation in part or all of the body.

aneurysm (ăn′ū-rĭzm): Localized abnormal dilation of a blood vessel, due to congenital effect or weakness of the wall of the vessel.

angina (ăn-jĭ′nă) **pectoris** (pĕk″tōris): A distinctive type of pain which results from a deficiency of blood supply to the heart muscle.

anoxia (an-oks′ĭ-ă): Absence of oxygen.

anterior (an-te′rĭ-or): The front of the body surface.

antibiotic (ăn″-ti-bĭ-ŏt′ĭk): A chemical substance produced by a microorganism, which has the capacity to kill other microorganisms.

antidote (ăn″tĭ-dōt): An agent that counteracts a poison.

antiseptic (ăn″tĭ-sĕp′tĭk): A substance used to destroy bacteria.

anus (ā′nŭs): The opening of the rectum on the body surface.

aorta (ā-ōr′tă): The largest artery in the body; the main arterial trunk from which the systemic arterial system proceeds; arises from the left ventricle of the heart.

apnea (ăp-nē′ă): Cessation of breathing.

arc flash conjunctivitis (kon-junk″tĭ-vī′tus): Inflammation of the conjunctiva and/or the cornea, caused by excessive exposure to ultraviolet light, such as with welding.

arm: Upper limb distal to shoulder.

arrhythmia (ă-rith′mĭ-ă): Variation from the normal rhythm of the heart beat.

arteriole (ar-tē′rĭ-ōl): A minute arterial branch.

artery (ar′ter-ĭ): A muscular, thick-walled blood vessel that carries blood away from the heart.

articulate (ar-tik′u-lăt): A meeting place of two bones, forming a joint.

artificial ventilation: Any method used to force air in and out of the lungs of a person who is not breathing.

asphyxia (ăs-fĭk′sĭ-ă): Suffocation due to decreased oxygen and increased carbon dioxide in the blood.

aspirate: To draw in or out by suction.

aspiration (ăs-pĭ-rā′shŭn): The act of inhaling foreign material into the lungs.

asthma (ăz′mă): Disease of the lungs consisting of bronchial spasms.

asymmetry (ă-sĭm′ĕ-trĭ): Lack of correspondence of parts or organs on opposite sides of the body.

atherosclerosis (ath″er-o″skle-ro′sis): A form of hardening of the arteries.

atrium (ā′trĭ-um) (auricle, ō′rĭ-kl): Either of two receiving chambers of the heart from which blood passes to ventricles.

autonomic (ŏ-tō-nŏm′ĭk): Not subject to voluntary control.

autonomic nervous system: The section of the nervous system concerned with the function of the cardiac muscle, glands and smooth muscles. It is not subject to voluntary control.

autonomic reaction: An action carried out without conscious thought, such as breathing.

avulsion (ă-vŭl′shŭn): Tearing away of a body part or tissue.

axilla (ăks′ĭ-la): Armpit.

B

bacteria (băk-tĕr′ĭ-ă): Microscopic organism which may cause disease.

bag-valve mask: A portable unit consisting of a bag, a valve and a mask. Used to give artificial ventilation.

ball-and-socket: A type of joint with a wide range of movement, such as the shoulder and hip.

barotrauma (barŏ′-trawm′mah): Injury due to pressure.

basal (ba′sal) **fracture:** Fracture at the base of the skull.

bilateral (bĭ-lăt′ĕr-ăl): Pertaining to both sides.

bile: A greenish-yellow fluid secreted by the liver to aid in fat digestion.

bladder: A musculomembranous sac which collects and stores fluids.

bleb: A small blister or bubble in the skin.

blister: A collection of plasma or blood in or under the epidermis.

blood: The fluid circulating through the heart, arteries, capillaries and veins. It carries nutritive materials and oxygen to body cells and removes waste products and carbon dioxide.

blood pressure: The pressure of the blood in the body, usually given in millimeters.

blood volume: The total quantity of blood in the body, usually given in litres.

bone: The hard form of connective tissue that constitutes most of the skeleton.

botulism (bŏt′ū-lĭzm): An extremely severe type of food poisoning due to a neurotoxin produced in improperly canned or preserved foods.

bowel: See intestine.

brachial (brā′kĭ-ăl) **artery:** The main artery of the upper arm; a continuation of the axillary artery that branches into the radial and ulnar arteries at the elbow.

brain: The part of the central nervous system contained in the cranial vault.

brain stem: The stem-like portion of the brain connecting the cerebral hemispheres with the spinal cord.

bronchiole (brong′kĭ-ōl): A subdivision of the bronchi.

bronchospasm (brŏng′kŏ-spăzm): Spasmodic contraction of the smooth muscle coating of the bronchi, as occurs in asthma.

bronchus (brŏng′kŭs) (plural — bronchi, brŏng′kī): The primary division of the trachea, conveying air to the lungs. Bronchi transport air within the lungs.

bruise: A contusion; an injury due to hemorrhage into tissue from ruptured vessels. If it is superficial, discolouration of skin may result (see ecchymosis).

burn: Injury to tissue caused by contact with heat, flame, chemicals, electricity or radiation.

bursa: Small sacs containing fluid, found in the fascia under the skin, muscles or tendons. Situated in places where friction would otherwise develop.

bursitis (bŭr-si′tĭs): Inflammation of a bursa.

C

calcaneus (kal-kā′nē-us): The heel bone.

canthus (kăn′thŭs): The angular junction of the eyelids at either corner of the eyes, designated outer (lateral) and inner (medial).

capillary (kăp′ĭ-lăr′′ĭ): A minute vessel which joins arterioles and venules.

carbon dioxide (CO_2)**:** An odourless, colourless gas which is a normal by-product of body metabolism found in exhaled air.

carbon monoxide (CO)**:** A colourless, odourless, poisonous gas. When inhaled, it combines more readily with hemoglobin than oxygen, which causes central nervous system depression and asphyxiation.

cardiac: Pertaining to the heart.

cardiac arrest: Cessation of heart function.

cardiac compression: Artificial means of restoring circulation and the pumping action of the heart by external heart massage.

cardiac failure: See congestive heart failure.

cardiac muscle: The muscle of the heart.

cardiac tamponade (tăm′′pŏnăd′)**:** An accumulation of fluid in the pericardial sac, causing compression of the heart muscle.

cardial: Of the heart.

cardiogenic (kăr′′dĭ-ō-jĕn′ĭk) **shock:** A serious complication seen in myocardial infarction.

cardiopulmonary resuscitation (CPR): Artificial ventilation and external cardiac compression.

cardiovascular: Pertaining to the heart and blood vessels.

carotid artery: One of the main arteries of the neck supplying blood to the head.

carpal bones: The eight small bones of the wrist.

cartilage (kăr′tĭ-lĕj) (cartilaginous, kăr′′tĭ-lăj′ĭ-nŭs)**:** The gristle or white, elastic substance attached to articular bone surfaces and forming parts of the skeleton:

  cricoid (krī′koyd) — The lowest cartilage of the larynx.

  thyroid — The shield-shaped cartilage of the larynx.

caustic: A substance that burns or corrodes organic tissue.

cavity: A hollow or space.

cell: A mass of protoplasm containing a nucleus.

centigrade (Celsius): The temperature scale in which the freezing point of water is 0° and the boiling point at sea level is 100°.

central nervous system (CNS): The brain and spinal cord.

cerebellum (sĕr-ĕ-bĕl′um): Smaller posterior portion of the brain, mainly concerned with coordination of movement.

cerebral (sĕr′ĕ-brăl) **cortex:** That portion of the brain which governs thought, reasoning, memory, sensation and voluntary movement.

cerebral vascular accident (CVA): Commonly referred to as a stroke; the stoppage of circulation to a section of the brain.

cerebrospinal (sĕr′′ĕ-brō-spī′năl) **fluid (CSF):** The fluid which surrounds the brain and spinal cord and flows inside the central canal of the spinal cord and the four ventricles of the brain.

cerebrum (ser′e-brŭm): The main portion of the brain.

cervical spine: The first seven vertebrae of the spinal column.

chest: See thorax.

Cheyne-Stokes (Chān′Stōks): Respiration characterized by periods of apnea, interspersed with a crescendo respiration pattern.

chronic: Persisting for a long time.

chronic obstructive pulmonary disease (COPD): Illness that causes obstructive problems in the lower airways, such as chronic bronchitis, emphysema and, sometimes, asthma.

circulatory: Pertaining to the heart and blood vessels.

circulatory system: Consists of the heart, blood vessels and lymph vessels concerned with movement of blood and lymph.

clammy: Moist and cold.

clavicle: The collar bone; articulates with the sternum and scapula.

clot: A thrombus; a lump; a semi-solidified mass, as of blood or lymph.

coagulation (ko-ag′′u-la′shun): The process of changing from a liquid to a thickened or solid state; the formation of a clot.

coccyx (kŏk′siks) (coccygeal, kok-sij′ĭ-al): The tail bone; the lowest part of the spine, composed of four small, fused vertebrae.

collateral: Secondary or accessory, not direct or immediate; a small side branch, as of a blood vessel or nerve.

colon (kō′lon): The large intestine.

coma (kō′ma): Unconsciousness from which the patient cannot be aroused.

comatose: In a state of coma.

communicable disease: A disease which can be transmitted from one person to another.

concussion (kon-kush′un): A violent shaking or jarring; transient loss of normal brain function.

condyle (kon′dīl): The rounded prominence at the articular end of a bone.

congenital (kon-jen′ĭ-tal): Existing at or before birth.

congestive heart failure: Failure of adequate ventricular function, causing a back-up of blood or fluid into the lung.

coning: Brain stem compression due to increased intracranial pressure.

conjunctiva (kon′′junk-ti′vă): The delicate membrane that lines the eyelids and covers exposed surfaces of the eyeball.

conjunctivitis (kon′′junk′′ti-vī′tis): Inflammation of the conjunctiva.

conscious (kon′shus): Aware, knowing, alert mental faculties; awake.

consensual: Similar reaction by both pupils to a stimulus applied to only one.

constrict: Decrease in diameter; shrinking.

contaminated: Soiled with foreign matter.

contraction: In connection with muscles, implies shortening and/or tension.

contusion (kon-tu′zhun): A bruise; an injury that causes a hemorrhage into or beneath the skin but does not break the skin.

convulsion (kon-vul′shun): A violent, involuntary contraction or series of contractions of the voluntary muscles, a seizure or "fit".

cornea (kŏr′nē-ă): The transparent anterior part of the eye covering the iris and the pupil.

coronary (kor′o-nă-rī) **arteries:** The large arteries that branch from the ascending aorta and supply the heart muscle with oxygenated blood.

coronary artery disease: A disease which causes a progressive narrowing and eventual obstruction of the coronary arteries.

coronary occlusion (ŏ-klŭ-zhŭn): The blockage of a coronary artery.

coronary thrombosis (thrŏm-bō′sis): Blockage of a coronary artery by a clot.

costal arch (margin): The fused costal cartilages of ribs seven to ten; the arch forms the upper limit of the abdomen.

CPR: See cardiopulmonary resuscitation.

cramp: Painful involuntary contraction of muscle.

cranial (krā′ne-al): Referring to the skull.

cranial vault: The bony container for the brain.

crepitus (krĕp′ĭ-tŭs): The grating sound made by two fractured bone ends rubbing together; the bubbly sensation of air palpated in tissues.

cruciate (krŭ′shĭ-āt): Cross-shaped.

crush syndrome: Signs and symptoms of renal failure after crushing of a part, especially a large muscle mass.

cyanide (sī′ĭ-nīd′′): A highly poisonous substance used in extraction of gold and silver and also in the manufacture of synthetic rubber and textiles.

cyanosis (sī-ăn-ō′sis): A bluish discolouration of the skin and mucous membranes due to lack of oxygen.

D

decompression sickness: A formation of metabolically inert gas bubbles in the tissues and blood as a result of too rapid decrease in ambient pressure.

deformity: Distortion of any part or general disfigurement of the body.

dehydration (dē′′hī-drā′shŭn): Undue loss of water from the body or tissue.

delirium (dē-lir′ĭ-ŭm): A mental disturbance of relatively short duration, usually reflecting a toxic state. Marked by hallucinations, delusions, excitement, restlessness and incoherence.

dermis: The inner layer of the skin containing the skin appendages, hair follicles, sweat glands, nerves and blood vessels.

diabetes (dī′′ă-bē′tēz)**:** A disease of the pancreas characterized by deficient insulin secretion.

diabetic coma: Unconsciousness caused by uncontrolled diabetes.

diaphragm (dī′ă-fram)**:** The muscle which separates the thoracic cavity from the abdominal cavity.

diarrhea (dī-ă-rē′a)**:** Rapid movement of fecal matter through the intestine, resulting in poor absorption of water, nutritive elements and electrolytes. Produces abnormally watery stools.

diastole (dī-as′tō-lī)**:** The phase of the cardiac cycle in which the ventricles of the heart relax between contractions.

diastolic (dī-ăs-tol′ik) **blood pressure:** The measurement of blood pressure during diastole.

digestion: The act or process of converting food into chemical substances that can be absorbed into the blood and used by the body.

digit: A finger or toe.

dilate: To make or become larger or wider; expand, widen, enlarge.

disc: A circular or rounded flat plate, like the layer of cartilage between vertebrae.

disease: A definite morbid process, often with a characteristic set of symptoms.

dislocation: The displacement of the ends of two bones at their joint so that the joint surfaces are no longer in proper contact.

displacement: Movement to an abnormal location or position.

distal: Remote; farther from any point of reference; in the extremities, farthest from the point of junction with the trunk of the body.

distension: The state of being stretched out or enlarged.

duct: A passage with well-defined walls, especially a tubular structure for the passage of excretions or secretions.

duodenum (dū′′ō-dē′nŭm)**:** The first part of the small intestine.

dura mater: The outermost, toughest of the three meninges (membranes) of the brain and spinal cord.

dysfunction (dis-funk′-shun)**:** Disturbance or impairment.

dyspnea (disp-nē′ă)**:** Shortness of breath.

E

ecchymosis (ĕk-ĭ-mō′sĭs)**:** A discolouration of the skin resulting from subcutaneous and intracutaneous hemorrhage. Bluish at first, it changes later to a greenish-yellow because of chemical changes in the pooled blood.

eclampsia (ĕ-klamp′sĭ-ă)**:** One or more convulsions, not attributable to other cerebral conditions; a toxic condition of unknown etiology associated with some pregnancies.

ectopic (ĕk-tŏp′ĭk) **pregnancy:** Development of the fertilized ovum outside the uterus.

edema (ĕ-dē′mă)**:** A condition in which fluid escapes to the tissues from vascular or lymphatic spaces and causes local or generalized swelling.

embolism (ĕm′bō-lĭzm)**:** A blood clot or other plug, such as an air bubble or fat globule, obstructing local circulation.

emesis (ĕm′ĕ-sĭs)**:** The act of vomiting.

emetic: (ĕ-met′ic) An agent that causes vomiting.

emphysema (ĕm′′fĭ-sē′mă)**:** A chronic disease of the lung, characterized by extreme dilation of pulmonary air sacs and poor exchange of oxygen and carbon dioxide in the lungs.

endotoxic shock: A shock condition caused by endotoxin present in a bacterial cell.

enzyme: A protein capable of producing or accelerating some change in a given substance.

endotracheal (ĕn′′dō-tra′kē-al)**:** Within the trachea.

epicondyle (ĕp-ĭ-kŏn′dīl)**:** An eminence upon a bone above its condyle.

epidermis (ĕp′′ĭ-dĕr′mĭs)**:** The outermost layer of the skin.

epigastric (ĕp′′ĭ-găs′-trĭc)**:** The upper and middle region of the abdomen, located within the sternal angle.

epiglottis (ĕp′′ĭ-glŏt′ĭs)**:** The lid-like, cartilaginous structure overhanging the superior entrance to the larynx. It serves to prevent food from entering the larynx and trachea while a person is swallowing.

epilepsy: A chronic disorder characterized by intermittent attacks of brain dysfunction, usually associated with some alteration of consciousness. The attacks may be confined to impaired behaviour or may progress to a generalized convulsion.

esophagus (ē-sŏf'ă-gŭs): The tube extending from the pharynx to the stomach.

euphoria (ū-for'ĭ-ă): An exaggerated sense of well being.

eversion: The act of turning outward.

excretion (ĕks-krē'shŭn): The process of eliminating the residue of food and the waste products of metabolism.

expiration: The act of breathing out or expelling air from the lungs.

extension: Opposite to flexion; the act of straightening.

extradural (ĕks''tră-du'ral):Outside the dura mater.

F

Fahrenheit: The scale of temperature in which water freezes at 32° and boils at 212°, under standard conditions.

feces (fē'sēz): Waste matter discharged from the bowel, consisting of the undigested residue of food, intestinal mucosal cells, intestinal mucus, bacteria and waste material.

femoral artery: The principal artery of the leg.

femoral vein: The major vein of the leg.

femur (fē'mur): The longest and largest bone in the body, extending from the pelvis to the knee; the thigh bone.

fetus: Developing young in the uterus.

fever: An elevated body temperature.

fibula: The lateral and smaller of the two bones of the leg extending from just below the knee, forming the lateral wall of the ankle joint.

fissure (fish'ur): Any cleft or groove.

flail segment: That segment of the chest wall in a flail chest injury lying between the rib fractures and moving paradoxically with respiration.

flexion: The act of bending; the movement by which the two ends of any jointed part are drawn closer to one another (opposite to extension).

follicles (hair): A deep, narrow pit containing the root of the hair. The duct of the sebaceous gland opens into it.

foramen (fŏ-ră'mĕn) **magnum:** A large opening in the anterior, inferior part of the occipital bone between the cranial cavity and vertebral canal.

fossa (fŏs'să): A hollow or depressed area.

fracture: Any break in a bone:

closed — A fracture in which the broken bone does not break the skin.

comminuted — A fracture in which the bone has been splintered or crushed.

compound (open) — A fracture with an open wound over the fracture site.

compression — A fracture produced by compression.

depressed — A fracture of the skull in which a fragment is depressed.

greenstick — An incomplete fracture causing partial disruption, splintering or bending of a bone; it occurs in immature bones.

impacted — Broken bone ends firmly wedged together.

linear — A single fracture line in the bone of the skull caused by trauma.

simple (closed) — An uncomplicated fracture; one that does not cause disruption of the skin.

spiral — A fracture in which the fracture line twists around and through the bone.

transverse — A fracture extending from side to side, at right angles to the long axis of the bone.

frontal lobe: The anterior portion of the cerebrum of the brain; the site of emotional control.

frostbite: Injury to tissues caused by exposure to cold.

fused joint: A joint that forms a solid, immobile, bony structure.

G

gallbladder: A pear-shaped sac located on the undersurface of the liver; collects and stores bile.

ganglia (găng'glē-ăh) (plural of ganglion): A group of nerve cell bodies, located outside the central nervous system.

gangrene (gang'grĕn): Death of tissue, generally with loss of vascular supply. May be followed by bacterial invasion and putrefaction.

gastric juice: The digestive fluid secreted by the glands of the stomach; a thin, colourless liquid, containing mainly hydrochloric acid, pepsin and mucus.

gastroenteritis (gas''tro-en-ter-ĭ'tis): Inflammation of the stomach and intestine.

gastrointestinal: Pertaining to the stomach and intestine.

gelatinous (je-lat'ĭ-nus): Like jelly or softened gelatin.

genitalia (jen-ĭ-tal'ĭ-ă): The reproductive organs.

genitourinary (jen″ĭ-to-u′rĭ-ner″e) **system:** System including all the reproductive organs and the organs that manufacture and void urine.

germ: Pathogenic microorganisms, such as bacteria.

glenoid: Resembling a pit.

glottis: The vocal apparatus of the larynx, consisting of the vocal cords and the opening between them.

glucose: A simple sugar.

glycemia (glĭ-sē′mĭ-ă): Sugar in the blood.

glycogen: The form in which carbohydrates are stored in tissue.

greater trochanter: The greater of two bony processes below the neck of the femur; a broad, flat, lateral surface serving as a point of attachment for several muscles.

H

heart: The muscular pump of the cardiovascular system responsible for maintaining circulation of the blood.

heat exhaustion: Prostration due to an excessive loss of water and salt through sweating.

heat stroke: A condition that results from prolonged exposure to heat, causing a disturbance of the temperature-regulating mechanism of the body; also referred to as sunstroke.

hemarthrosis (hĕm-ăr-thrō′sĭs): Blood within a joint.

hematemesis (hĕm-ăt-ĕm′ē-sĭs): Vomiting of blood.

hematoma (hĕm-ă-tō′mă): A localized collection of blood in the tissues, as a result of injury or a broken blood vessel.

hemiplegia (hĕm-ĭ-plē′jĭ-ă): Paralysis of one side of the body.

hemoglobin (hĕm″ō-glō′bĭn): The oxygen-carrying pigment of the red blood cells.

hemopericardium (hĕ″mō-per″ĭ-kar′dē-ŭm): Blood in the pericardial sac.

hemoptysis (hē-mŏp′tĭ-sĭs): Coughing up blood as a result of bleeding from any part of the respiratory tract.

hemorrhage (hĕm′ē-rĭj): Escape of blood.

hemorrhagic (hĕm-ō-răj′ĭk) **shock:** Shock which results from a reduced blood volume.

hemostasis (hē-mŏs′tă-sĭs): Arrest of bleeding.

hemothorax (hē″mō-thō′raks): Bleeding into the pleural space or chest cavity.

hepatitis (hĕp″ă-tī′tĭs): Inflammation of the liver.

hinge joint: A joint that allows motion in only one place, such as the elbow and knee.

histamine (hĭs′tă-mĕn): A substance released from body cells which is partially responsible for allergic reactions.

hormones: A substance secreted by an endocrine gland that acts on other glands and organs of the body.

humerus: The bone of the upper arm which extends from the shoulder to the elbow.

hyper: Above, excessive.

hyperextension (hī″pĕr-ĕks-tĕn′shŭn): Extension of a limb or part beyond the normal limit.

hyperglycemia (hī″pĕr-glĭ-sē′mĭ-ă): Excess of glucose in the blood.

hypertension: High blood pressure.

hyperventilation: Excessive breathing.

hypo: Low.

hypoglycemia: An abnormally low concentration of glucose in the blood.

hypotension: Low blood pressure.

hypothermia: A decreased body temperature.

hypotonic (hī-po-tŏn′ĭk): A solution having less salt than normal body fluid.

hypovolemic (hī-po-vo-le′mĭc) **shock:** Shock resulting from an abnormally decreased amount of blood and fluids in the body.

hypoxemia (hī-pŏks-ē′mĭ-ă): Decreased oxygen in the blood.

hypoxia (hi-pŏks′ĭ-ă): Diminished availability of oxygen to the body tissues.

I

iliac (ĭl′ē-ăk) **crest:** The crest of the ilium, palpable just below the lower ribs.

ilium (ĭl′ĭ-ŭm): The lateral, flaring portion of the pelvic bone.

immobilize: To render incapable of movement.

impetigo (im-pĕ-ti′gō): A contagious skin infection.

incision: A cut or wound made by a sharp instrument.

infarct: Death.

infection: An invasion of the body by pathogenic microorganisms.

inferior: Situated below.

inflammation: A tissue response to injury or irritation of the cells.

ingest: To take food, drugs, etc. into the body by mouth.

inguinal (ing'gwĭ-nal)**:** Pertaining to the groin.

inguinal ligament: Fibrous band running from the anterior superior spine of the ilium to the spine of the pubis.

inhalation (inhaled)**:** The drawing in of air or other gases into the lungs; inspiration.

injection: The act of forcing a liquid through a needle or other tube through the skin into the body.

injury: A specific impairment of body structure or function caused by an outside agent or force. May be physical, chemical or psychological.

innominate (ĭ-nŏm'ĭ-nāt) **bone:** The bone forming one half of the pelvic girdle and arising from a fusion of the ilium, the ischium and the pubis.

inspiration: The act of drawing air into the lungs; inhalation.

insulin: A hormone secreted into the blood by the pancreatic islets that permits utilization of sugar by the body; also used for treatment of diabetes.

insulin shock: Severe hypoglycemia produced by excessive insulin.

intercostal: Between two ribs.

intertrochanteric (ĭn''tĕr-trŏ'kăn-tĕr-ĭk)**:** Between the greater or lesser trochanter.

intervertebral (ĭn-tĕr''-vĕr'tĕ-brăl)**:** Between two vertebrae.

intestine (small and large)**:**

small — The distal portion of the small bowel extending from the jejunum to the cecum.

large — The portion of the digestive tube extending from the ileocecal valve to the anus, comprising the cecum, colon and rectum; the large bowel.

intra-articular (ĭn''tră-ăr-tĭk'ŭ-lăr)**:** Within a joint.

intracranial: Within the cranium.

intravascular: Within a vessel or vessels.

inversion: A turning inward.

ipecac (ĭp'ĕ-kăk)**:** Substance that can cause vomiting.

iris: The coloured portion of the eye surrounding the pupil.

ischial (ĭs'kĭ-al) **tuberosity** (tu''bĕ-ros'ĭ-ti)**:** A protuberance on the inferior surface of the ischium lateral to the anus and bearing weight when a person is seated.

ischium (ĭs'kĭ-ŭm)**:** The posterior, distal portion of the hip bone.

J

joint: A point at which two or more bones articulate.

joint capsule: A fibrous sac with synovial lining which encases a joint.

jugular veins: Large veins that return blood from the head, neck and face to the superior vena cava.

K

kidneys: Two organs located in the retroperitoneal space that filter the blood and produce urine; they also regulate salt and water balance in the body.

L

laceration: A wound resulting from tearing or cutting of tissue.

lacrimal (lăk'rĭm-ăl)**:** Pertaining to tears.

lacrimal gland: Located at the upper, outer corner of the eye; secretes tears.

lactic acid: A metabolic product of the breakdown of glucose.

laryngectomy (lăr''ĭn-jĕk'tŏ-mĭ)**:** Partial or total removal of the larynx by surgery.

laryngospasm (lăr-ĭn'gŏ-spasm)**:** Reflex closure of the airway.

larynx (lăr'ĭnks)**:** The organ of voice production.

lateral: Pertaining to or situated at the side; away from the midline.

lens: The portion of the eye that focuses light rays on the retina.

lesion (lē'zhŭn)**:** Traumatic discontinuity of tissue or loss of function of a part.

lethargy (lĕth'ar-jĭ)**:** A condition of drowsiness or indifference.

ligament: A band of fibrous tissue connecting bones or cartilages, serving to support and strengthen joints.

liver: The large organ in the right upper quadrant of the abdomen that stores and filters blood, secretes bile, converts sugars into glycogen and performs many other metabolic activities.

lobe: A specific portion of an organ or gland.

lumbar spine: The five, individual vertebrae located between the thoracic vertebrae and the sacrum.

lungs: Two spongy organs of respiration contained in the thoracic cavity.

lymph: A colourless fluid formed in tissue spaces throughout the body; it is gathered into small vessels (lymphatics) which return it to central circulation.

lymph node (gland)**:** A rounded body of accumulations of lymph tissue found at intervals along the course of the lymphatic vessels.

lymphadenitis (lĭm-făd′′ĕn-ī′tĭs)**:** Inflammation of the lymph glands.

lymphangitis (lĭm′′fan-jī′tĭs)**:** Inflammation of the lymphatic vessel.

lymphocyte (lĭm′fō-sīt)**:** A type of white blood cell.

M

maceration (măs-ĕr-a′shun)**:** To soften by soaking.

malleolus (mă-le′o-lus)**:** The protuberance on each side of the ankle joint.

mandible: The bone of the lower jaw.

mastoid (mas′toyd) **process:** The projection of the mastoid portion of the temporal bone.

maxilla (mak-sĭl′ah)**:** The bone of the upper jaw.

medial: In or toward the midline or centre of the body.

mediastinum (mĕ′′dĭ-ăs-tī′nŭm)**:** The tissues and organs between the sternum and the thoracic vertebral column.

medulla (mĕ-dūl′lă) **oblongata** (ŏb′′lon-gă′tă)**:** That part of the brain stem continuous with the pons above the spinal cord below. Contains nerve cells that control vital functions such as respiration, circulation and the senses.

membrane: A thin layer of pliable tissue that covers a surface, lines a cavity or divides a space or organ.

meninges (mĕn-ĭn′jĕz)**:** The three layers of membranes that cover the brain and spinal cord — the dura mater, arachnoid and pia mater.

meningitis (mĕn-ĭn-jī′tĭs)**:** Inflammation of the meninges.

meniscus (mĕn-ĭs′kŭs)**:** Crescent-shaped fibrocartilage in the knee joint.

metabolism: All the physical and chemical changes that take place within an organism.

metacarpal bones: The five bones of the hand between the wrist (carpus) and the fingers (phalanges).

metatarsal bones: The five bones of the foot between the ankle (tarsus) and the toes (phalanges).

motor nerve: A nerve that causes a contraction in a skeletal muscle.

mucous membrane: The lining of certain body cavities.

mucus: A sticky semi-fluid secreted in mucous membranes.

muscle: A tissue which, by contraction, produces movement of an organ or part of the body:

    cardiac muscle — Specialized muscle which contracts rhythmically.

    skeletal muscle — Muscle attached to and moving the bones, generally under voluntary control.

    smooth muscle — Muscle comprising the walls of the internal organs, blood vessels, hair follicles and other appendages; generally it is not under voluntary control.

myo: Muscle.

myocardial (mī-ŏ-kar′dĭ-ăl) **infarction:** Damage or death of an area of the heart muscle (myocardium), resulting from a reduction in the blood supply.

myocardium: The middle and thickest layer of the heart wall; the cardiac muscle.

N

nausea (naw′sē-ă)**:** A feeling that vomiting may be imminent.

necrosis (nĕ-krō′sĭs)**:** Death of cells or localized tissue.

nerve: A collection of fibres in the cord-like structure, which conveys impulses between the central nervous system and some other region of the body.

nervous system: The brain, the spinal cord and the nerves.

neurogenic (nū-rŏ-jĕn′ĭk) **shock:** Shock produced by action of the nervous system, resulting in a generalized vasodilation.

neurological (nū-rŏ-lŏj′ĭk-ăl)**:** Relating to the diagnosis and treatment of disorders of the nervous system.

nitroglycerin (nī′′trŏ-glĭs′ĕr-ĭn)**:** A vasodilator used in the treatment of angina.

noradrenalin (nŏr′′ăh-drĕn′ăh-lĭn)**:** A hormone which causes generalized vasoconstriction to arteries.

O

occipital (ŏk-sĭp′ĭ-tăl) **lobe:** The most posterior portion of the cerebral hemisphere.

occiput (ŏk′sĭ-pŭt)**:** The back of the head.

occlusion (ŏ-kloo′zhun)**:** The act of closure or the state of being closed; an obstruction or a closing-off.

olecranon (ŏ-lĕk′răn-ŏn) **process:** The bony projection of the ulna at the elbow.

open wound: One in which the affected tissues are exposed.

orbit: The bony cavity containing the eyeball and its associated muscles, vessels and nerves.

organ: A collection of tissues that perform a special function.

orifice (or′ĭ-fĭs): The entrance or outlet of any body cavity.

oxygen: A colourless, odourless gas which supports combustion and is essential for life.

P

palate (păl′ăt): The roof of the mouth; the partition separating the nasal and oral cavities.

palpate (păl′pāt): To examine by feeling and pressing with the fingers and the palms of the hand.

palpitations (păl-pĭ-tā′shŭns): Awareness of a rapid, throbbing heart beat.

pancreas (păn′krē-ăs): A large, elongated gland situated transversely behind the stomach, between the spleen and the duodenum. It provides a major source of digestive enzymes and is the sole producer of the hormone insulin which regulates the metabolism of sugar.

paradoxical (păr′′ă-dŏk′sĭ-kăl) **movement:** The motion of the injured segment of a flail chest; opposite to the normal motion of the chest wall.

paralysis (pă-răl′ĭ-sĭs): The loss or impairment of motor function in a part due to lesion of the neural or muscular mechanism.

paranoia (păr′′ă-noy′ă): A mental disorder marked by delusions of persecution.

parietal (pă-rī′ĕ-tăl): Pertaining to the walls of a cavity.

patella (pă-tĕl′ă): The bone at the front of the knee; the kneecap.

pelvic cavity: The distal part of the abdominal cavity; contains the rectum, urinary bladder and internal sex organs.

pelvis: The bony ring connecting the trunk of the body to the lower extremities.

perfusion (pur-fū′zhŭn): The flow of blood which carries oxygen and nutrients to the cells and takes carbon dioxide,

acids and other wastes away.

pericardial (pĕr-ĭ-kar′dĭ-ăl) **cavity:** The potential space between the heart and the pericardium.

pericardial sac: The fibroserous membrane covering the heart.

perineum (pĕr′′ĭ-nē′ŭm): Area between the vaginal opening and the anus in females or scrotum and anus in males.

peripheral (pĕr-ĭf′ĕr-ăl) **nervous system:** The portion of the nervous system consisting of the nerves and ganglia outside the brain and spinal cord.

peristalsis (pĕr-ĭ-stăl′sĭs): A progressive wave-like movement that occurs involuntarily in hollow tubes of the body, most evident in the digestive tract. The simultaneous contraction and relaxation progresses slowly for a short distance as a wave that forces the contents of the tube along.

peritoneum (pĕr′′ĭ-tō-nē′ŭm): The serous membrane lying over the abdominal and pelvic organs; also lines the abdominal cavity.

peritonitis (pĕr′′ĭ-tō-nī′tĭs): Inflammation of the peritoneum.

phalanx (făl′ănks) (plural — phalanges): A bone of a finger or toe.

pharynx (făr′ĭnks): The cavity posterior to the nose and mouth and connecting with the esophagus and glottis; the throat.

photophobia (fō′′tō-fō′bĭ-ă): An abnormal visual intolerance to light.

phrenic (frĕn′ĭk) **nerve:** The motor nerve of the diaphragm.

physiology (fĭz′′ĭ-ŏl′ŏ-jĭ): The science of functions of living organisms and their parts.

pia mater (pī′ă mā′tĕr): The delicate, innermost meningeal membrane enveloping the brain and spinal cord.

placenta (plă-sĕn′tă) **previa** (prē′vĭă): A placenta located in the lower uterine segment. It partially or entirely covers the cervical opening, instead of lying in the proper position higher on the uterine wall.

plasma (plăz′mă): The liquid portion of whole blood.

platelet: (plăt′let) Part of the cellular portion of the blood; essential for blood coagulation.

pleura (ploo′ră): The serous membrane covering the lungs and lining the walls of the thoracic cavity.

pleural (ploo′răl) **space:** The potential space between the two layers of the pleura.

pneumonia (nū-mō′nĭ-ă): Inflammation of the lungs.

pneumothorax (nū-mō-thō′răks): The accumulation of air or gas in the pleural cavity, usually entering after a wound which penetrates the chest wall or lacerates the lung.

point tenderness: An area of tenderness limited to two or three centimetres in diameter. It can be identified through pain with gentle pressure. Point tenderness can be located in any area of the body.

pons (pŏnz): Part of the brain stem.

Pontocaine (Pŏn′tō-kān): A topical eye anesthetic.

popliteal (pŏp′′lĭt′ē-ăl) **artery:** The continuation of the femoral artery in the popliteal space.

posterior (pŏs-tē′rĭ-ŏr): Directed toward or situated at the back; opposite of anterior.

post-ictal (pōst-ĭk′tăl): A state immediately following a seizure.

pre-eclampsia (prē′′ē-klămp′sĭ-ă): A toxemia of late pregnancy characterized by hypertension, protein in the urine and edema, but without convulsions.

pressure point: Various locations on the body at which finger pressure may be applied to an artery for the control of hemorrhage.

process: A prominence or projection, as from a bone.

prolapse of cord: Protrusion of the umbilical cord ahead of the presenting part of the fetus in labour.

prone: The position of the body when lying face downward.

protuberance (prō-tū′bĕr-ăns): A projecting part.

proximal (prŏk′sĭm-ăl): Nearest to a point of reference, as to a centre or median line or to the point of attachment or origin.

psychogenic (sĭ-kō-jĕn′ĭk) **shock:** A fainting spell or state of shock, which has an emotional or psychological origin.

pubic (pū′bĭk) **symphysis** (sĭm′fĭ-sĭs): The site of fusion of the pubic bones at the anterior midline.

pulmonary (pŭl′mō-nĕ-rĭ): Pertaining to the lungs.

pulmonary artery: The large artery originating at the right ventricle of the heart, carrying blood to the lungs.

pulmonary embolism: An obstruction of the pulmonary artery or one of its branches by an embolus.

pulmonary vein: The large veins that originate in the lungs, carrying blood back to the heart.

pulse: The wave of increased pressure felt along the arteries as a result of ventricular contraction.

pupil: The opening at the centre of the iris of the eye.

pus: Tissue fluid containing the products of inflammation — white cells, bacteria and broken-down tissue.

R

radial artery: One of the major arteries of the forearm.

radius: The bone on the thumb side of the forearm.

rash: A temporary eruption on the skin.

rectum: The distal portion of the large intestine.

recumbent: Leaning back; reclining.

reduce (reduction): Restore to the normal place or relation of parts.

renal: Pertaining to the kidneys.

reproductive: Pertaining to the capacity of organisms to produce other organisms of the same kind.

respiration: The act of reviving a patient.

retina (rĕt′ĭ-nă): The lining of the back of the eye that receives visual images.

retrosternal (rĕ′′trō-ster′năl): Behind the sternum.

ribs: The long, flat, curved bones forming the wall of the thorax.

rigidity (rĭ-jĭd′ĭ-tĭ): Stiffness, inflexibility, immobility.

rotation (rō-tā′shŭn): Turning or rotating a body around its axis.

S

sacral (sā′krăl) **spine:** The five fused vertebrae which constitute the sacrum, a part of the pelvic girdle.

sacrum (sā′krŭm): Five fused vertebrae forming a triangular-shaped bone. It lies just below the lumbar vertebrae.

saline (sā′lēn′′): A solution containing salt.

saliva (să-lī′vă): The clear, alkaline secretion from the glands of the mouth.

scab: Coagulation of blood, pus, serum or a combination of these, forming a crust on the surface of an ulcer or wound.

scaphoid (skăf′oyd): One of the carpal bones.

scapula (skăp′ū-lă): The shoulder blade.

sciatic (sĭ-ăt′ĭk) **nerve:** A nerve extending from the base of the spine down the posterior aspect of the thigh, with branches throughout the lower leg and foot.

sclera (sklē′ră): The white, tough, outer coat of the eyeball.

sebaceous (sē-bā′shŭs) **gland:** A gland in the dermis, which secretes sebum.

sebum (sē'bŭm): An oily secretion of the sebaceous gland, which lubricates the skin.

seizure (sē'zhŭr): A sudden abnormal electrical discharge of brain cells.

semilunar (sĕm''ĭ-lū'năr) **cartilage:** One of the two intra-articular cartilages of the knee joint.

sensory nerve: A peripheral nerve that conducts impulses from a sense organ to the central nervous system.

septic shock: Shock resulting from severe bacterial infection.

septicemia (sĕp-tĭ-sē'mĭ-ă): Generalized blood poisoning.

septum (sĕp'tŭm): A partition; a dividing wall between two spaces or cavities.

serous (sĕr'ŭs) **membrane:** The membrane lining the walls of the body cavities and enclosing organs.

shock: A generalized depression of all body functions resulting from progressive failure of the cardiovascular system so that perfusion of tissues and organs is lost.

skeleton: The bones of the body.

skin: The outer covering of the body.

skull: The bones of the head.

spasm: Involuntary contraction of a muscle or a group of muscles.

spinal cord: That part of the central nervous system which extends from the foramen magnum to the upper end of the lumbar region:

> **canal** — A bony channel formed by the vertebral bodies and neural arches that contain and protect the spinal cord.

> **column** — All the vertebrae; the spine; the back bone.

spine: The vertebral column.

spinous (spī'nŭs): Pertaining to or like a spine.

spleen: An abdominal organ in the upper left-hand quadrant of the abdominal cavity.

sprain: Twisting or stretching of ligaments at the joint.

sputum (spū'tŭm): Matter ejected from the trachea, bronchi and lungs through the mouth.

sterile (stĕr'ĭl): Not fertile; free from living microorganisms.

sternomastoid (stur''nō-măs'toyd): Pertaining to the sternum and mastoid process.

sternum (stur'nŭm) (breast bone): The long, flat bone located in the midline of the anterior part of the thoracic cage.

stertorous (stĕr'tō-rŭs): The sound of noisy, partially obstructed breathing.

stomach: The hollow digestive organ that receives food material from the esophagus.

stove-in chest: See flail chest.

strain: An overstretching of a muscle.

stridor (strī'dŏr): A harsh, high-pitched respiratory sound.

stroke: A cerebrovascular accident.

subclavian (sŭb''klā'vē-ăn): Below the clavicle.

subclavian artery: The major artery located beneath the clavicle.

subcutaneous (sŭb''kū-tā'nē-ŭs): Beneath the skin.

subcutaneous emphysema: A condition where air escapes into the subcutaneous tissue, especially the chest wall, neck and face, causing a crackling sensation on palpation of the skin.

subdural (sŭb-dū'răl): Between the dura mater and arachnoid.

sublingual (sŭb-ling'gwăl): Beneath the tongue.

substernal (sŭb-ster'năl): Beneath the sternum.

subtrochanteric (sŭb''trō-kăn-tĕr'ĭk): Below the trochanter.

subungual (sŭb-ŭng'gwăl): Beneath a nail.

suffocate: To asphyxiate; to be unable to breathe.

superior: An organ or part that is located above another organ or part of the body.

supine: Lying flat, with the face upward.

supraclavicular (sū''pră-klă-vĭk'ū-lar): Above the clavicle.

supracondylar (sū''pră-kŏn'dĭ-lăr): Above a condyle.

suprasternal (sū''pră-stern'ăl): Above the sternum.

syncope (sĭn'kŭ-pē): Temporary loss of consciousness due to inadequate blood supply to the brain.

syndrome (sĭn'drōm): A group of signs and symptoms which characterize a condition or disease.

synovial (sĭn-ō'vĭ-ăl) **fluid:** Clear fluid secreted by the synovial membrane found in joint cavities, bursae and tendon sheaths.

synovial membrane: The inner lining of the articular capsule.

system: A set or series of interconnected or independent parts that act together in a common purpose or produce results impossible by action of one alone.

systemic: Pertaining to or affecting the body as a whole.

systole (sĭs′tŏ-lē) (systolic pressure): The contraction phase of the cardiac cycle.

systolic (sĭs′tŏl′ĭk) **blood pressure:** The higher blood pressure exerted by the blood on the arterial walls during ventricular contractions.

T

tachycardia (tăk′′ĭ-kar′dĭ-ă): Rapid heart beat.

tarsal bones: The seven bones that articulate between the lower leg and foot.

temporal (tĕm′por-ăl): Pertaining to the temple.

temporal artery: Located on either side of the face in front of the ear; supplying blood to the scalp.

temporal lobe: The lower lateral lobe of the cerebral hemisphere.

temporomandibular (tĕm′′pŏ-rŏ-măn-dĭb′ū-lar) **joint:** The articulation between the head of the mandible and the temporal region of the skull.

tendon: A fibrous cord which attaches a muscle to a bone.

tendon sheath: A tubular case or envelope surrounding a tendon.

tenosynovitis (tĕn′′ŏ-sĭn′′ŏ-vī′tĭs): Inflammation of a tendon sheath:

  infectious — Caused by microorganisms.

  mechanical — Caused by repetitive over-use.

tension pneumothorax: A condition that develops when air is continually forced into the chest cage outside the lung and is unable to escape; associated with compression of the lung and heart.

tetanus (tĕt′ă-nŭs): An infectious disease of the central nervous system caused by a bacterium which is found in soil, dust and the bowels of cows and horses.

thorax (thō′răks): The upper part of the trunk between the neck and the abdomen; the chest.

thrombosis (thrŏm-bō′sĭs): The formation or presence of a thrombus.

thrombus (thrŏm′bŭs): A solid mass formed in the heart or vessels from constituents in the blood.

tibia (tĭb′ĭ-ă): The shin bone.

tissue: A group or collection of similar cells which act together to perform a particular function.

tissue injury fluid: Plasma that accumulates in tissue spaces as a result of injury or irritation.

topical: Pertaining to a particular surface area.

tourniquet (toor′nĭ-kĕt): A bandage to be drawn tightly around a limb to stop circulation in the distal area.

toxemia (tŏks-ē′mĭ-ă): An abnormal condition associated with the presence of toxic substances in the blood.

toxic (toxin): Poisonous; pertaining to poison.

trachea (trā′kē-ă): The windpipe, the cartilaginous and membranous tube descending from the larynx and branching into the left and right main stem bronchus.

traction: The act of drawing or pulling.

transection (trăn-sĕk′shŭn): Division by cutting.

transfusion (trăns-fū′zhŭn): The introduction of whole blood or blood cellular components directly into the bloodstream.

trauma (traw′ma): An injury inflicted, usually suddenly, by some physical or psychological factor.

traumatic emphysema: Emphysema occurring as a result of trauma.

Trendelenburg (Trĕn-dĕl′ĕn-bŭrg): Position of the body with the head lower than the feet.

triage (trē-ahzh′): The sorting or selection of patients to determine the priority of care to be rendered to each.

trunk: The body, excluding the head and extremities.

U

ulcer (ŭl′sĕr): A lesion on the surface of the skin or a mucous membrane caused by the superficial loss of tissue, usually with inflammation.

ulna (ŭl′nă): The inner and larger bone of the forearm, on the side opposite the thumb.

ulnar artery: One of the two terminal branches of the brachial artery that extends medially down the arm to the palm.

ulnar nerve: Nerve controlling some of the flexor muscles of the forearm and most of the muscles of the hand.

umbilicus (ŭm-bĭ-lī′kŭs): The navel.

unconscious (ŭn-kŏn′shŭs): Insensible, incapable of responding to sensory stimuli or of having subjective experiences.

uremia (ū-rē′mĭ-ă): A toxic condition caused by retention of excessive by-products of protein metabolism in the blood.

ureter (ū′rē-ter): The fibromuscular tube which conveys urine from the kidney to the bladder.

urethra (ū-rē′thră): The membranous canal which conveys urine from the bladder to outside the body.

urinary (ū′rĭ-năr′′ĭ) **bladder:** The musculomembranous organ serving as a storage place for urine until it is discharged from the body.

urinary system: The organs concerned with the formation and passing of urine from the body.

urine: A fluid waste product, excreted by the kidneys, stored in the bladder and discharged through the urethra.

uterus (ū′tĕr-ŭs): The hollow muscular organ in the female that protects the fetus.

V

vagus (vā′gŭs) **nerve:** The tenth cranial nerve controlling motor and sensory functions of the chest and abdomen, as well as the head and neck.

varicose (văr′ĭ-kōs) **vein:** Enlarged or dilated tortuous veins.

vasoconstrictor (văs′′ō-kŏn-strĭk′tor): A substance that causes a narrowing of the diameter of the blood vessels.

vasodilator (văs′′ō-dĭ-lā′tor): A substance that causes a widening of the diameter of the blood vessels.

vein (văn): A blood vessel that carries blood towards the heart.

vena cava (vē′nă cā′vă) (superior, inferior): The largest veins of the body, which return blood to the right atrium of the heart.

venous (vē′nŭs): Pertaining to the veins.

ventilate: To move air in and out of the lungs.

ventricle (vĕn′trĭk-l): A thick-walled, muscular chamber of the heart that receives blood from the atrium and pumps it into the pulmonary or systemic circulation.

ventricular fibrillation (vĕn-trĭk′ū-lar fĭ′′brĭl-ā′shŭn): Rapid, ineffective contractions of the ventricular muscle.

venules (vĕn′ūls): Any of the small vessels that collect blood from the capillaries and join to form veins.

vertebrae (ver′tĕ-brā): The bones of the spinal column.

vertebral (ver′tĕ-brăl) **body:** The round, solid bone forming the front of each vertebra.

vertebral spine: The spinous process; the posterior projection of each vertebra.

vessels: Tubes or canals for conveying blood or lymph.

virus (vī′rŭs): A microscopic infectious agent.

vital signs: Measurement of body functions; include pulse, blood pressure, respiratory rate, temperature and level of consciousness.

vitreous (vĭt′rĭ-ŭs) **humor:** Transparent, gelatin-like substance, filling the inside of the eye.

vomitus (vŏm′ĭ-tŭs): Material ejected from the stomach by vomiting.

W

wrist drop: Caused by radial nerve injury characterized by the patient's inability to extend wrist or fingers.

X

xiphoid (zĭf′oyd) **process:** The cartilage at the lower end of the sternum.

Z

zygoma (zĭ′′gō′mă): Cheek bone.

Index